CANCER MEDICINE REVIEW

CANCER MEDICINE REVIEW

Richard M. Stone, MD

Assistant Professor of Medicine
Harvard Medical School
Dana-Farber Cancer Institute
Brigham and Women s Hospital
Boston, Massachusetts

Richard Essner, MD

Clinical Assistant Professor of Surgery
University of Southern California School of Medicine
Los Angeles, California
Assistant Director of Surgical Oncology
John Wayne Cancer Institute
Santa Monica, California

Arno J. Mundt, MD

Assistant Professor of Radiation and Cellular Oncology
University of Chicago Hospitals
Pritzker School of Medicine
Chicago, Illinois

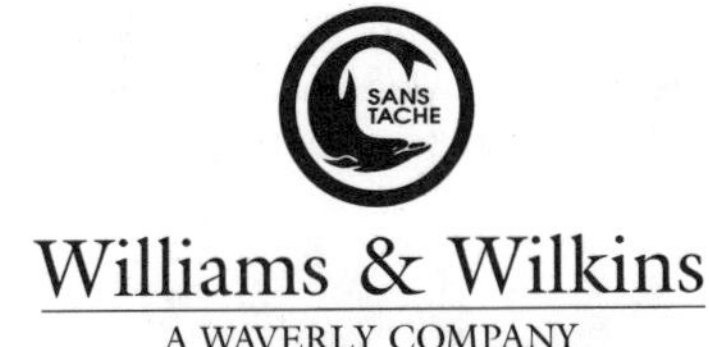

Williams & Wilkins

A WAVERLY COMPANY

BALTIMORE • PHILADELPHIA • LONDON • PARIS • BANGKOK
BUENOS AIRES • HONG KONG • MUNICH • SYDNEY • TOKYO • WROC

Editor: Jonathan W. Pine, Jr.
Managing Editor: Leah Ann Kiehne Hayes
Production Coordinator: Marette Magargle-Smith
Copy Editor: Arlene Sheir-Allen
Typesetter: Peirce Graphic Services, Inc.
Printer & Binder: Vicks Lithograph & Printing Co.
Binder: Vicks Lithograph & Printing Co.

Copyright © 1997 Williams & Wilkins

351 West Camden Street
Baltimore, Maryland 21201-2436 USA

Rose Tree Corporate Center
1400 North Providence Road
Building II, Suite 5025
Media, Pennsylvania 19063-2043 USA

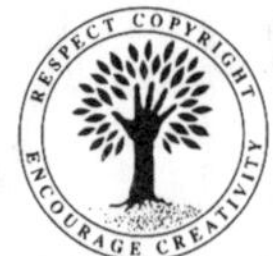

Accurate indications, adverse reactions and dosage schedules for drugs are provided in this book, but it is possible that they may change. The reader is urged to review the package information data of the manufacturers of the medications mentioned.

Printed in the United States of America

Library of Congress Cataloging-in-Publication Data

Cancer medicine review / editors, Richard M. Stone, Richard Essner,
  Arno J. Mundt.
      p.   cm.
   ISBN 0–683–30059–8
    1. Cancer—Examinations, questions, etc.   I. Stone, Richard M.
II. Essner, Richard.   III. Mundt, Arno J.
  [DNLM: 1. Neoplasms—examination questions.   QZ 18.2 C215 1997]
  RC262.C29115   1997
  616.99′4′0076—dc21
  DNLM/DLC
  for Library of Congress   96-48209
                                   CIP

The publishers have made every effort to trace the copyright holders for borrowed material. If they have inadvertently overlooked any, they will be pleased to make the necessary arrangements at the first opportunity.

To purchase additional copies of this book, call our customer service department at **(800) 638-0672** or fax orders to **(800) 447-8438.** For other book services, including chapter reprints and large quantity sales, ask for the Special Sales department.

Canadian customers should call **(800) 268-4178**, or fax **(905) 470-6780.** For all other calls originating outside of the United States, please call **(410) 528-4223** or fax us at **(410) 528-8550.**

Visit *Williams & Wilkins* on the *Internet:* http://www.wwilkins.com or contact our customer service department at **custserv@wwilkins.com**. Williams & Wilkins customer service representatives are available from 8:30 am to 6:00 pm, EST, Monday through Friday, for telephone access.

97 98 99 00 01
1 2 3 4 5 6 7 8 9 10

To Jane, Ben, Rebecca, Sarah, and Harry
—Richard M. Stone

To Sara
—Richard Essner

To my Father
—A.J. Mundt

PREFACE

We have attempted to provide a useful companion work for *Cancer Medicine*. This textbook is the most up-to-date and complete reference book that is available on the biology, diagnosis, epidemiology, and treatment of cancer. Because of its vast scope, readers may wish to test their proficiency in one or more of the areas covered in this seminal work. We hope that *Cancer Medicine Review* will provide such an opportunity.

The organization of *Cancer Medicine Review,* with questions that are grouped by general themes, will allow the reader to devote energies to those specific areas he or she needs to review. Moreover, the style of four or five possible responses—with only one being the correct response—is analogous to the type of questions on the American Board of Internal Medicine Examination in Oncology as well as the In-service Examination in Surgical Oncology. Therefore, *Cancer Medicine Review* should aid the student in board examination preparation.

The authors of *Cancer Medicine Review* are indebted to the editors of the *Cancer Medicine* textbook for their support and guidance. We would especially like to acknowledge the Herculean efforts of Dr. James Holland. It was his vision and enthusiasm that was responsible for the conception and successful completion of this review book. Dr. Holland's efforts to elicit major contributions by most of the chapter authors were indispensable. We would also like to express our gratitude to those individuals who, despite having apparently completed their work for *Cancer Medicine,* were called upon to deliver excellent questions for the editors' review. One of the very strengths of *Cancer Medicine Review* is that many of the questions were written by the chapter authors themselves, individuals with world-renowned expertise in the field, who are well aware of the key issues in their own field. The question-writing contributors should be praised for their interest in enhancing the educational value of *Cancer Medicine.*

The authors also gratefully acknowledge the dedication of Leah Hayes, our managing editor at Williams & Wilkins. Without the stalwart secretarial support at the Dana-Farber Institute provided by Fannie Fong, Valerie Barges, and Cindy Civetti, the successful completion of *Cancer Medicine Review* would have been impossible.

We appreciate any comments and suggestions from our readers as we look forward to future editions of *Cancer Medicine Review.*

CONTRIBUTORS

David H. Abramson, MD
Clinical Professor of Ophthalmology
New York Hospital–Cornell Medical
Center
New York, New York

Erik Barquist, MD
Fellow in Trauma and Critical Care
Division of General Surgery
University of Miami School of Medicine
Miami, Florida

Stephen Barrett, MD
Consumer Advocate
Member, Board of Directors
National Council Against Health
Fraud, Inc.
Allentown, Pennsylvania

Lawrence W. Bassett, MD
Iris Center Professor of Breast Imaging
Department of Radiological Sciences
University of California, Los Angeles,
School of Medicine
Los Angeles, California

Robert C. Bast, Jr., MD
Internist and Professor of Medicine
Harry Carothers Wiess Chair for
Cancer Research
Head, Division of Medicine
The University of Texas M.D.
Anderson Cancer Center
Houston, Texas

Poonam V. Batra, MD, FCCP, FACR
Professor of Radiological Sciences
University of California, Los Angeles,
School of Medicine
Los Angeles, California

Jonathan S. Berek, MD, FACOG, FACS
Professor and Vice-Chair
Chief of Gynecology and Gynecologic
Oncology
Johnson Comprehensive Cancer
Center
University of California, Los Angeles,
School of Medicine
Los Angeles, California

Ross S. Berkowitz, MD
William H. Baker Professor of
Gynecology
Harvard Medical School
Director of Gynecologic Oncology
Co-Director, New England
Trophoblastic Disease Center
Brigham and Women's Hospital
Boston, Massachusetts

Smita Bhatia, MD
Staff Physician
City of Hope National Medical Center
Duarte, California

A. Philippe Chahinian, MD
Professor of Medicine
Division of Neoplastic Diseases
Mount Sinai School of Medicine
New York, New York

Gary L. Clayman, DDS, MD
Associate Professor of Head and
Neck Surgery
The University of Texas M.D.
Anderson Cancer Center
Houston, Texas

Steven K. Clinton, MD, PhD
Clinical Associate of Medicine
Dana-Farber Cancer Institute
Harvard Medical School
Boston, Massachusetts

Jeffrey I. Cohen, MD
Senior Investigator
Laboratory of Clinical Investigation
National Institutes of Health
Bethesda, Maryland

O. Michael Colvin, MD
Director, Duke Comprehensive
Cancer Center
Duke University Medical Center
Durham, North Carolina

Ana Maria Comaru-Schally, MD, MS
Professor of Clinical Medicine
Tulane University School of
Medicine
New Orleans, Louisiana

Arnold M. Conforti, MD
Senior Fellow in Surgical Oncology
John Wayne Cancer Institute
Santa Monica, California

James L. Connolly, MD
Associate Professor of Pathology
Harvard Medical School
Director of Anatomic Pathology
Division
Department of Pathology
Beth Israel Hospital
Boston, Massachusetts

Christopher P. Crum, MD
Associate Professor of Pathology
Harvard Medical School
Director, Division of Women's
Perinatal Pathology
Brigham and Women's Hospital
Boston, Massachusetts

Lisa M. DeAngelis, MD
Associate Professor of Neurology
Cornell University Medical College
Chief, Neurology Service
Memorial Sloan-Kettering Cancer
Center
New York, New York

George D. Demetri, MD
Assistant Professor of Medicine
Harvard Medical School
Dana-Farber Cancer Institute
Boston, Massachusetts

Ira J. Dunkel, MD
Clinical Assistant
Department of Pediatrics
Memorial Sloan-Kettering Cancer
Center
New York, New York

Ann M. Dvorak, MD
Professor of Pathology
Harvard Medical School
Senior Pathologist
Beth Israel Hospital
Boston, Massachusetts

Harold F. Dvorak, MD
Mallinckrodt Professor of Pathology
Harvard Medical School
Chief, Department of Pathology
Beth Israel Hospital
Boston, Massachusetts

Ezekiel J. Emanuel, MD, PhD
Assistant Professor of Medicine
Division of Cancer Epidemiology and
Control
Dana-Farber Cancer Institute
Boston, Massachusetts

Richard Essner, MD
Clinical Assistant Professor of Surgery
University of Southern California
School of Medicine
Los Angeles, California
Assistant Director of Surgical
Oncology
John Wayne Cancer Institute
Santa Monica, California

Michael S. Ewer, MD, MPH
Internist, Associate Professor of
Medicine
Medical Specialties/Cardiology
The University of Texas M.D.
Anderson Cancer Center
Houston, Texas

Eric R. Fearon, MD, PhD
Maisel Professor of Oncology
Associate Professor of Internal
Medicine, Human Genetics and
Pathology
University of Michigan Medical Center
Ann Arbor, Michigan

Arnold S. Freedman, MD
Associate Professor of Medicine
Harvard Medical School
Dana-Farber Cancer Institute
Boston, Massachusetts

Emil Frei III, MD
Director and Physician-in-Chief,
Emeritus
Dana-Farber Cancer Institute
Richard and Susan Smith
Distinguished Professor of Medicine
Harvard Medical School
Boston, Massachusetts

William J. Fulkerson, Jr., MD
Associate Professor of Medicine
Duke University Medical Center
Durham, North Carolina

George T. Gallagher, DMD, DMSc
Associate Professor of Oral Pathology
Department of Oral Medicine and
Diagnostic Sciences
Harvard School of Dental Medicine
Boston, Massachusetts

Edward G. Grant, MD
*Vice Chairman of Radiological
Sciences
University of California, Los Angeles,
School of Medicine
Chairman, Department of Radiology
Veterans Administration Medical
Center, West Los Angeles
Los Angeles, California*

Gerald M. Haase, MD
*Clinical Professor of Surgery
Department of Pediatric Surgery
The Children's Hospital
Denver, Colorado*

John D. Hainsworth, MD
*Associate Director
Sarah Cannon Cancer Center
Centennial Medical Center
Nashville, Tennessee*

Yusuf A. Hannun, MD
*Associate Professor of Medicine
Duke University Medical Center
Durham, North Carolina*

Harold A. Harvey, MD
*Professor of Medicine
Hershey Medical Center
Pennsylvania State University
Hershey, Pennsylvania*

James F. Holland, MD
*Distinguished Professor of Neoplastic
Diseases
Director Emeritus, Derald H.
Ruttenberg Cancer Center
Mount Sinai Medical Center
New York, New York*

Stephen B. Howell, MD
*Professor of Medicine
University of California, San Diego
La Jolla, California*

T. Scott Jennings, MD
*Director, Division of Gynecologic
Oncology
Medical University of South Carolina
Charleston, South Carolina*

Elwood V. Jensen, MD
*Professor, Institute for Hormone and
Fertility Research
University of Hamburg
Hamburg, Germany*

Roy B. Jones, PhD, MD
*Director, Bone Marrow Transplant
Program
Department of Medicine
University of Colorado Health
Sciences Center
Denver, Colorado*

Ralph C. Jones, LtCdr, MC, USN
*Clinical Assistant Professor of
Surgery
Uniformed Services University of the
Health Sciences
Bethesda, Maryland
Senior Research Fellow
Department of Surgical Oncology
John Wayne Cancer Institute at St.
John's Hospital
Santa Monica, California*

A. Robert Kagan, MD
*Chief, Radiation Oncology
Kaiser Permanente
Los Angeles, California*

Philip W. Kantoff, MD
*Director, Genitourinary Oncology
Department of Medicine
Dana-Farber Cancer Institute
Boston, Massachusetts*

Steven M. Keller, MD
*Associate Professor of Surgery
Albert Einstein College of
Medicine
Bronx, New York*

Samuel Kenan, MD
*Professor of Orthopedics
New York University School of
Medicine
Director of Orthopedic Oncology
Service
Orthopedic Institute
New York, New York*

B.J. Kennedy, MD
*Regents' Professor of Medicine,
Emeritus
Masonic Professor of Oncology,
Emeritus
Division of Medical Oncology
University of Minnesota Medical
School
Minneapolis, Minnesota*

Catherine E. Klein, MD
Associate Professor of Medicine
Divisions of Hematology and Medical Oncology
University of Colorado Health Sciences Center
Denver Veterans Affairs Medical Center
Denver, Colorado

Elise C. Kohn, MD
Chief, Signal Transduction and Prevention Unit
Laboratory of Pathology
National Cancer Institute
National Institutes of Health
Bethesda, Maryland

Mark G. Kris, MD
Associate Professor of Medicine
Cornell University Medical College
Chief, Thoracic Oncology Service
Department of Medicine
Memorial Sloan-Kettering Cancer Center
New York, New York

Donald W. Kufe, MD
Professor of Medicine
Harvard Medical School
Deputy Director
Dana-Farber Cancer Center
Chief, Division of Cancer Pharmacology
Boston, Massachusetts

Joanne Kurtzberg, MD
Professor of Pediatrics
Duke University Medical Center
Durham, North Carolina

Steven A. Lieberman, MD
Assistant Professor of Internal Medicine
University of Texas Medical Branch
Galveston, Texas

Beryl McCormick, MD
Associate Radiation Oncologist
Department of Radiation Oncology
Memorial Sloan-Kettering Cancer Center
New York, New York

Catherine M. McLachlin, MD, FRCPC
Assistant Professor of Pathology
University of Western Ontario
Pathologist
Victoria Hospital
London, Ontario
Canada

Ari Melnick, MD
Fellow in Neoplastic Diseases
Mount Sinai Medical Center
New York, New York

John C. Morris, MD
Assistant Professor of Medicine
Division of Neoplastic Diseases
Mount Sinai Medical Center
New York, New York
Visiting Scientist
Clinical Gene Therapy Branch
National Center for Human Genome Research
Bethesda, Maryland

Charles S. Morrow, MD, PhD
Assistant Professor of Biochemistry
Associate Professor of Pediatrics
Bowman Gray School of Medicine
Winston-Salem, North Carolina

Donald L. Morton, MD
Medical Director and Surgeon-in-Chief
John Wayne Cancer Institute at St. John's Hospital
Santa Monica, California
Professor and Chief, Emeritus, Surgery/Oncology
University of California, Los Angeles, School of Medicine
Los Angeles, California

Arno J. Mundt, MD
Assistant Professor of Radiation and Cellular Oncology
University of Chicago Hospitals
Pritzker School of Medicine
Chicago, Illinois

Scott Murphy, MD
Professor of Medicine
Thomas Jefferson University
Chief Medical Officer
American Red Cross Blood Services
Penn-Jersey Region
Philadelphia, Pennsylvania

Craig R. Nichols, MD
Associate Professor of Medicine
Indiana University School of Medicine
Indianapolis, Indiana

William D. Odell, MD, PhD, MACP
Professor and Chairman
Department of Internal Medicine
University of Utah Medical Center
Salt Lake City, Utah

Takao Ohnuma, MD, PhD
Professor of Neoplastic Diseases
Mount Sinai School of Medicine
Attending Physician
The Mount Sinai Hospital
New York, New York

Roger J. Packer, MD
Chairman, Department of Neurology
Children's National Medical Center
Professor of Neurology and
Pediatrics
George Washington University
Washington, D.C.

William Plunkett, PhD
Hubert L. and Olive Stringer Professor
of Medical Oncology
Professor of Medicine (Pharmacology)
Division of Clinical Investigation
The University of Texas M.D.
Anderson Cancer Center
Houston, Texas

Jerome B. Posner, MD
Chairman
Department of Neurology
Memorial Sloan-Kettering Cancer
Center
New York, New York

Kristjan T. Ragnarsson, MD
Dr. Lucy G. Moses Professor and
Chairman
Department of Rehabilitation
Medicine
Mount Sinai Medical Center
New York, New York

Kenneth V.I. Rolston, MD, FACP
Professor of Medicine
Chief, Section of Infectious
Diseases
Department of Medical
Specialties
The University of Texas M.D.
Anderson Cancer Center
Houston, Texas

Andrew V. Schally, PhD, DSci, MDhc
Professor of Medicine
Head, Section of Experimental
Medicine
Tulane University Medical School
Chief, Endocrine, Polypeptide and
Cancer Institute
Veterans Affairs Medical Center
New Orleans, Louisiana

Stuart J. Schnitt, MD
Associate Professor of Pathology
Harvard Medical School
Associate Director of Surgical
Pathology
Department of Pathology
Beth Israel Hospital
Boston, Massachusetts

Leanne L. Seeger, MD
Associate Professor of Radiological
Sciences
Chief, Musculoskeletal Radiology
University of California, Los Angeles,
Center for Health Sciences
Los Angeles, California

Michail Shafir, MD
Associate Clinical Professor of
Surgery and Neoplastic Diseases
Mount Sinai School of Medicine
New York, New York

Brenda Shank, MD, PhD
Chairman and Professor of Radiation
Oncology
Mount Sinai School of Medicine
Director and Attending Physician
Radiation Oncology
Mount Sinai Hospital
New York, New York

Gerald Shklar, DDS, MS
Head, Department of Oral Medicine
and Oral Pathology
Harvard Medical School
Boston, Massachusetts

Robert Silber, MD
Professor of Medicine, Emeritus
New York University Medical
Center
New York, New York
Clinical Professor of Medicine
Duke University Medical Center
Durham, North Carolina

Richard T. Silver, MD
Clinical Professor of Medicine
Cornell University Medical
College
Director, Section of Clinical Oncology
Chemotherapy Research
Attending Physician
New York Hospital–Cornell Medical
Center
New York, New York

Stephen T. Sonis, DMD, DMSc
Professor of Oral Medicine
Chief, Division of Oral Medicine, Oral and Maxillofacial Surgery and Dentistry
Brigham and Women's Hospital
Boston, Massachusetts

Richard Statman, MD
Senior Clinical Fellow
John Wayne Cancer Institute
Santa Monica, California

Richard J. Steckel, MD
Chair, Department of Radiological Sciences
University of California, Los Angeles, School of Medicine
Los Angeles, California

Richard M. Stone, MD
Assistant Professor of Medicine
Harvard Medical School
Dana-Farber Cancer Institute
Brigham and Women's Hospital
Boston, Massachusetts

Victor F. Tapson, MD
Assistant Professor of Medicine
Duke University Medical Center
Durham, North Carolina

Ayalew Tefferi, MD
Assistant Professor of Medicine
Mayo Clinic and Mayo Foundation
Rochester, Minnesota

Michael E. Trigg, MD
Professor of Pediatrics
Director, Pediatric Bone Marrow Transplantation
University of Iowa Hospital and Clinics
Iowa City, Iowa

Donald L. Trump, MD
Professor of Medicine and Surgery
University of Pittsburgh
Deputy Director for Clinical Investigations
Pittsburgh Cancer Institute
Pittsburgh, Pennsylvania

Nazim S. Turhal, MD
Fellow in Neoplastic Diseases
Mount Sinai Medical Center
New York, New York

Bert Vogelstein, MD
Professor of Oncology
Johns Hopkins School of Medicine
Investigator
Howard Hughes Medical Institute
Baltimore, Maryland

Ralph R. Weichselbaum, MD
Harold H. Hines, Jr., Professor and Chairman
Department of Radiation and Cellular Oncology
University of Chicago Hospital
Director, Chicago Tumor Institute
University of Chicago
Chicago, Illinois

Ainsley Weston, PhD
Associate Professor of Community Medicine
Mount Sinai Medical Center
New York, New York

Antoinette J. Wozniak, MD
Assistant Professor of Medicine
Division of Hematology-Oncology
Wayne State University
Detroit, Michigan

CONTENTS

CHAPTER 1

Cancer Biology and Epidemiology

DIRECTIONS: Each question below contains five suggested responses. Select the best response to each question.

QUESTIONS

Question 1.1. **Which of the following characteristics of cell proliferation distinguish normal from neoplastic cells?**

a) Only normal cells fail to grow exponentially over time.
b) Neoplastic cells display shorter cell cycle time compared with their normal counterparts.
c) Neoplastic cells display an increased growth fraction or a higher percentage of cells in the cell cycle at a given time.
d) Neoplastic cells spend less time in the S-phase (DNA synthesis phase) compared with their normal counterparts.
e) Mitosis requires less time in neoplastic cells compared with normal cells.

Question 1.2. **Which of the following changes in the retinoblastoma gene product is oncogenic?**

a) Overproduction of retinoblastoma protein
b) Activating mutation that prevents normal regulation of the retinoblastoma protein's effect on stimulating proliferation
c) Mutation that prevents phosphorylation of retinoblastoma protein
d) Mutation that allows overphosphorylation of retinoblastoma protein
e) Overabundance of messenger RNA coding for the retinoblastoma gene product

Question 1.3. **Overexpression of the *bcl-2* gene is thought to lead to cancer because:**

a) Normal cell death is prevented.
b) Cells are more likely to enter the cell cycle.
c) Cell cycle time is shortened.
d) Cells become more sensitive to external growth factors.
e) Growth promoting signals are enhanced.

Question 1.4. **Restriction fragment length polymorphisms (RFLPs) have contributed to our understanding of the pathophysiology of neoplastic transformation because:**

a) They are typically found only in proto-oncogenes.

b)   They are involved in DNA binding.

c)   They define the promoter regions of critical genes.

d)   Their presence close to important genes for a given cancer allows linkage analysis.

e)   They tend to be more abundant in cancer cells compared with non-neoplastic cells.

Question 1.5. **You are called by a gastroenterologist who has identified a patient who has thousands of adenomatous polyps in the colon and rectum. The patient reported a history of several other family members (a brother, an aunt, and a grandparent) who were told that they had colonic polyps of this type. The patient is likely to have which of the following genetic abnormalities?**

a)   Deletion in the short arm of chromosome 17

b)   A microsatellite chromosome

c)   Deletion or mutation in the retinoblastoma gene on chromosome 13

d)   Deletion of a portion of the long arm of chromosome 5

e)   Loss of chromosome 11

Question 1.6. **A 45-year-old patient with adenocarcinoma of the colon is seen for evaluation. He has three siblings, one of whom died of metastatic colon cancer at age 49. His mother had a colon cancer resection at age 56. Two of his mother's brothers also died of colon cancer. His maternal grandmother died of ovarian cancer. Which of the following genetic abnormalities is most likely to have played a role in the development of colon cancer in this patient?**

a)   Inactivation of a gene important in preventing progression through the cell cycle

b)   Mutation in a gene responsible for DNA repair

c)   Activation of a gene responsible for promoting proliferation

d)   Alteration of a gene coding for a DNA–binding transcription factor

e)   Overexpression of a growth promoting gene

Question 1.7. **Which of the following is the least well-documented hormonally related risk factor for the development of breast cancer?**

a)   Early age at menarche

b)   Late age at menopause

c)   Nulliparity

d)   Late age at first full-term pregnancy

e)   Weight

Question 1.8. **Which of the following is a documented risk factor for the development of endometrial carcinoma?**

a)   Oral contraceptive pill use (combined estrogen and progesterone)

b)   Multiple pregnancies

c)   Progesterone withdrawal therapy

d)   Estrogen replacement therapy

e)   Use of an intrauterine device

Question 1.9. **All of the following statements regarding skin cancer are true EXCEPT:**

a)   Nonmelanoma skin cancer accounts for approximately 30% of all cancers diagnosed yearly.

b)   A direct causal role exists between sunlight exposure and the induction of skin cancer.
c)   The incidence of basal and squamous cell carcinomas of the skin is directly correlated with cumulative sun exposure.
d)   Melanoma is found predominantly on non–sun-exposed areas and is not associated with sunlight exposure.
e)   The incidence of all types of skin cancer is increasing.

Question 1.10.   All of the following genetic sunlight-sensitive disorders are autosomal recessive disorders EXCEPT:

a)   Xeroderma pigmentosa
b)   Cockayne's syndrome
c)   Trichothiodystrophy
d)   Basal cell nevus syndrome
e)   All of these disorders are autosomal recessive.

Question 1.11.   Which of the following statements regarding xeroderma pigmentosa (XP) is false?

a)   XP is an autosomal recessive disease.
b)   Median age of onset of symptoms is 1 to 2 years of age.
c)   The frequency of cancers in XP patients is approximately 2000 times that seen in the general population.
d)   XP is associated with an increased risk of squamous and basal cell carcinomas of the skin but not an increased risk of melanoma.
e)   All are true.

Question 1.12.   Which of the following statements concerning retrovirally mediated oncogenesis is true?

a)   Retroviruses require an oncogene sequence for replication.
b)   The addition of a retroviral sequence to a cellular proto-oncogene allows the creation of a transforming protein.
c)   Retrovirally mediated oncogenes cause the formation of polyclonal tumors.
d)   The duration between infection and transformation is several months or more.
e)   Only adult eukaryotic cells can be induced to transform.

Question 1.13.   In which of the following ways will retroviral vectors be most likely useful in the treatment of cancer?

a)   To reverse the malignant phenotype by replacement of a tumor suppressor gene
b)   To reverse the malignant phenotype by inhibition of proto-oncogene function
c)   To reverse the malignant phenotype by replacement of a missing or defective gene
d)   To kill malignant cells by delivering a gene to destroy such cells
e)   To cause lytic viral infection that is specific for cancer cells

Question 1.14.   In which of the following neoplasms is the pathophysiologic role of Epstein-Barr virus best established?

a)   Nonkeratinizing nasopharyngeal carcinoma
b)   Hodgkin's disease

c) Kaposi's sarcoma
d) Burkitt's lymphoma
e) Leiomyosarcoma

Question 1.15. **Which of the following tumors is most closely associated with schistosomal infection?**

a) Cholangiocellular carcinoma
b) Breast cancer
c) Non-Hodgkin's lymphoma
d) Hepatocellular carcinoma
e) Bladder carcinoma

Question 1.16. **Which of the following statements concerning the association of viral infection with the development of hepatocellular carcinoma is correct?**

a) Chronic hepatitis C virus infection usually leads to hepatocellular carcinoma without intervening cirrhosis of the liver.
b) The integration of hepatitis B virus DNA is obligatory.
c) Inactivation of the retinoblastoma gene product by hepatitis B virus is required.
d) Hepatitis B virus infection leads to cirrhosis, which is required for the development of hepatocellular carcinoma.
e) Even in an endemic area, most patients with hepatocellular carcinoma do not have evidence of a prior infection with hepatitis B virus.

Question 1.17. **A 54-year-old woman is found to have suspicious calcifications as revealed by her annual routine mammogram. No palpable lesion is identified on physical examination. A fine needle aspiration under the guidance of mammography is hypocellular and reveals unremarkable ductal cells and apocrine metaplastic cells. At this point, the physician should:**

a) Continue to recommend annual routine mammography
b) Recommend more frequent mammography, such as every 6 months
c) Recommend a blind surgical biopsy
d) Recommend a surgical biopsy after needle localization of the suspicious calcification guided with mammography
e) Recommend a mastectomy

Question 1.18. **All of the following are advantages of magnetic resonance imaging (MRI) for patients who have tumors of the central nervous system compared with computed tomography EXCEPT:**

a) Contrast between normal tissues and tumor is better.
b) MRI does not involve the use of ionizing radiation.
c) MR images can be generated in any plane (not just the axial plane).
d) MRI is capable of detecting calcifications within tumors.
e) All of the above are advantages.

Question 1.19. **A 60-year-old man has a solitary left midcervical lymph node from which biopsy reveals metastatic cancer. Which of the following statements regarding the work-up and treatment of this patient is false?**

a) The most likely primary site is located in the head and neck region.
b) Compared with a patient who has an enlarged supraclavicular lymph node, an unlikely primary site is the lungs.

c)   If no primary site is found, treatment should be directed to the involved neck.
d)   The standard approach in this patient is a combination of chemotherapy and radiotherapy.
e)   An endoscopic examination of the upper aerodigestive tract is mandated.

Question 1.20.   Which of the following statements regarding radiologic imaging is true?

a)   In the case of mass occupying lesions, MRI can generally provide a precise diagnosis.
b)   Intravenous contrast should always be used in evaluating musculoskeletal tumors with MRI.
c)   MRI is superior to computed tomography (CT) in evaluating the intramedullary extent of a tumor.
d)   In most instances, either MRI or CT can be used for tumor staging; both examinations are not necessary.
e)   In the patient who has a known primary tumor, new onset of bone pain, and negative or equivocal radiographs, CT should be the next imaging modality undertaken.

Question 1.21.   A 55-year-old woman felt a hard mass in the upper outer quadrant of her right breast. Needle aspiration failed to obtain fluid. Which ONE of the following is NOT a reason to perform a mammogram before biopsy of the suspicious solid mass?

a)   To better define the nature of the mass
b)   If cancer is present, to determine if there is an extensive intraductal component
c)   To detect unexpected cancer in the same or other breast
d)   To rule out multifocal carcinoma
e)   To defer a biopsy if the mammogram is negative

Question 1.22.   A 50-year-old woman had a screening mammogram that revealed a cluster of indeterminate calcifications in the left upper-inner quadrant. A decision was made to perform a core needle biopsy of this lesion. Regarding imaging-guided core needle biopsy of the abnormality, which one of the following statements is NOT true?

a)   Core biopsy should be guided by stereotactic mammography.
b)   Atypical duct hyperplasia is a benign diagnosis that would need no further work-up.
c)   Core biopsy can usually determine whether a carcinoma is invasive or noninvasive.
d)   Five core specimens will usually provide enough tissue to make the diagnosis.
e)   Definitive results will require concordance of pathologic, mammographic, and clinical findings.

Question 1.23.   A 40-year-old woman had a mammogram that showed some calcifications. The conclusion of the report stated: "Final Assessment: Probably benign findings." Regarding the "Final Assessment" on standardized mammography reports, which ONE of the following statements is true?

a)   It indicates the composition of the breast tissue based on proportion of fatty and fibroglandular tissue.

b)   It indicates the likelihood of malignancy on a scale of 1 to 5, including a specific management recommendation.
c)   It provides an overall risk factor assessment, taking into account family history, age, and other risk factors.
d)   It applies only to diagnostic mammography, never screening mammography.
e)   It was not intended to be included on written mammography reports.

Question 1.24.   Which of the following statements is true regarding positron emission tomography (PET) imaging with glucose-2-fluoro-2-deoxy-D-glucose (FDG)?

a)   PET FDG is useful in the diagnosis of primary brain tumors and the detection of tumor recurrence following therapy.
b)   Tissue inflammation results in increased FDG uptake.
c)   PET FDG can be used in the detection of primary breast cancers as well as the detection of axillary nodal metastases.
d)   PET is currently used as a clinical tool in cancer medicine.
e)   All of the above are true.

Question 1.25.   Iodine 131 (I 131) is not useful in the treatment of patients who have which type of thyroid carcinoma?

a)   Papillary
b)   Follicular
c)   Medullary
d)   Mixed papillary-follicular
e)   I 131 is useful in all types of thyroid carcinoma

Question 1.26.   Chemoprevention trials in breast cancer have shown that:

a)   Contralateral breast cancer occurs at a rate of 0.8% yearly, and a slightly increased rate of ovarian cancer exists with fenretinide treatment.
b)   Tamoxifen chemoprevention trials currently show the same risk of contralateral secondary tumors in patients who are treated with a placebo.
c)   Women entering the tamoxifen chemoprevention trial must demonstrate a fourfold increase in risk before starting the study.
d)   Fenretinide and tamoxifen have been shown in laboratory studies to be more effective alone than in combination to suppress mammary carcinogenesis.
e)   Fenretinide can cause ocular toxicity.

Question 1.27.   A 62-year-old man has lost 30 pounds during the course of 1 year. He is 6 feet tall and now weighs 155 pounds. On physical examination, a 3-cm, hard, nontender mass is found in the left supraclavicular fossa. No other physical or laboratory abnormalities are found, except for a serum alkaline phosphatase that is moderately elevated. A needle biopsy of the mass reveals poorly differentiated adenocarcinoma of unknown origin. On further questioning, the patient recalls a decrease in caliber of his stools over the past 6 months, and he has been experiencing intermittent "constipation" during the same period. Otherwise, he has not been symptomatic. What follow-up diagnostic studies would you recommend to determine the appropriate management regimen for this patient?

a)   Posteroanterior and lateral chest radiographs (followed by a chest CT, if the chest radiographs are negative or equivocal)

b)   Sigmoidoscopy (to be followed by a barium enema)
c)   Abdominal CT scan
d)   All of the aforementioned
e)   None of the aforementioned

Question 1.28.   Regarding the use of tamoxifen as a chemopreventive agent, its mechanism of action is most accurately described as:

a)   Tamoxifen has a strong estrogen-inducing effect on human mammary tissue.
b)   Tamoxifen has neither anti-estrogen or estrogen agonist effects on breast tissue.
c)   Tamoxifen has no role in the treatment of estrogen receptor–negative carcinomas.
d)   Tamoxifen suppresses insulin-like growth factor 1 in breast cancer.
e)   Tamoxifen does not induce synthesis of transforming growth factor-beta.

Question 1.29.   The action of retinoids as chemoprevention agents is most likely based on:

a)   Action through the steroid receptor family
b)   Control of normal differentiation and proliferation of a number of cells, except those of mesenchymal origin
c)   Control of carcinogenesis
d)   Control of cell growth
e)   Interference with the anti-estrogenic effects of tamoxifen

Question 1.30.   A 42-year-old woman is found to have atypical squamous cells of undetermined significance (ASCUS) on her annual routine Pap smear. At this point, her physician should:

a)   Continue to recommend an annual routine Pap smear
b)   Recommend more frequent Pap smears, such as every 4 to 6 months
c)   Recommend colposcopy
d)   Recommend cone biopsy
e)   Recommend simple hysterectomy

Question 1.31.   A 37-year-old man is seen with diffuse adenopathy without signs of infection. A lymph node biopsy is performed. The lymph node should be:

a)   Placed in the standard fixative, 10% formaldehyde, and sent to the pathology department
b)   Frozen in liquid nitrogen
c)   Saved for electron microscopy
d)   Kept fresh until the pathologist can examine
e)   Smeared on slides for cytologic evaluation

Question 1.32.   A biopsy of a liver mass reveals an undifferentiated malignant tumor. Immunocytochemistry is performed and reveals the tumor to be keratin positive. On the basis of this finding, the pathologist concludes:

a)   The tumor is metastatic squamous cell carcinoma.
b)   The tumor is a carcinoma.
c)   The tumor is not a lymphoma.
d)   The tumor is not a sarcoma.
e)   Additional studies need to be performed.

Question 1.33. **A 35-year-old woman has a non-palpable rounded density with microcalcifications that are visible on mammogram. A mammographically directed biopsy reveals "fibrocystic changes." The clinician should:**

a) Reassure the patient that all is well and advise her to have another mammogram at age 40
b) Inform the patient that "fibrocystic changes" are pre-malignant and advise bilateral mastectomy
c) Advise the patient to return in 1 year for follow-up physical examination and mammography
d) Conclude that the mammographic and pathologic findings do not correlate well and institute immediate follow-up to determine whether the mammographically discovered lesion was indeed removed
e) Conclude that the rounded density was a cyst

Question 1.34. **A 15-year-old female is seen with pain and fullness around the distal femur. The most appropriate initial imaging modality is:**

a) MRI
b) CT
c) Radionuclide bone scan
d) Plain radiographs
e) Ultrasound

Question 1.35. **A major advance in the use of monoclonal antibodies (MoAB) in the diagnosis and treatment of cancer is the development of technetium 99m–labeled MoAB fragments. The advantages of labeled MoAB fragments compared with whole MoAB molecules include all of the following EXCEPT:**

a) A decreased human anti-mouse antibody (HAMA) response
b) Increased rate of clearing from the circulation
c) Higher ratio of tumor to background
d) Less likelihood of hepatotoxicity
e) All of the aforementioned

Question 1.36. **Which of the following radionuclides is currently used in the treatment of symptomatic bone metastases?**

a) Rhenium 186
b) Samarium 153
c) Strontium 89
d) Iodine 123
e) Phosporus 32

Question 1.37. **Which of the following cancers is NOT among the top five misdiagnosed conditions in the United States, according to the Physician Insurers Association of America?**

a) Breast cancer
b) Prostate cancer
c) Lung cancer
d) All of the aforementioned
e) None of the aforementioned

Question 1.38. **Sonography has a wide array of uses throughout the body. All of the following could potentially be examined with ultrasound EXCEPT:**

a)   Hepatic metastases
b)   Pulmonary abscess
c)   Dilatation of the common bile duct
d)   Deep venous thrombosis of the legs
e)   Pancreatic cancer

Question 1.39. **Scrotal sonography can be used for the evaluation of all of the following EXCEPT:**

a)   Identification of a varicocele
b)   Differentiation between hydrocele and spermatocele
c)   Differentiation of intratesticular mass from extratesticular mass
d)   Identification of residual lymphoma
e)   Differentiation between embryonal carcinoma and seminoma

Question 1.40. **Color Doppler sonography is a useful technique in all of the following EXCEPT:**

a)   Upper extremity venous thrombosis
b)   Carotid artery involvement by cervical tumor/adenopathy
c)   Differentiation of malignant from benign breast masses
d)   Iliac vein thrombosis

Question 1.41. **Endovaginal and transrectal pelvic sonography are excellent techniques to:**

a)   Stage ovarian carcinomas
b)   Screen the general population for ovarian cancer
c)   Differentiate benign from malignant prostatic masses
d)   Identify small submucosal leiomyomas

Question 1.42. **All of the following are characteristics of tumor initiators EXCEPT:**

a)   Causes an irreversible genetic change
b)   Necessary event for malignant conversion
c)   Typically modifies molecular structure of DNA
d)   Causes selective clonal expansion of at-risk cells
e)   Consistent with chemical carcinogenesis

Question 1.43. **Each of the following represents a major mechanism for DNA repair EXCEPT:**

a)   RNA-based repair
b)   Direct DNA repair
c)   DNA-nucleotide excision repair
d)   Base excision repair
e)   DNA mismatch repair

Question 1.44. **Which of the following statements concerning aflatoxins is correct?**

a)   They are metabolites of *Helicobacter pylori.*
b)   They typically contaminate fruits.
c)   They require activation by the hepatic cytochrome system.
d)   The carcinogenic metabolite binds to pyrimidine bases.
e)   They are leukemogenic.

Question 1.45. **The pathologic examination of the ipsilateral axillary lymph node of a patient with the diagnosis of ductal carcinoma in situ is positive for metastatic cells. On re-review of the breast lesion pathology slides, which of the following would you expect to find?**

a)   No increase in microvessel formation in the primary tumor
b)   An absence of infiltrating tumor cells in the biopsy
c)   A different histologic subtype in the breast from that found in the axillary lymph nodes
d)   A break in the integrity of the duct basement membrane
e)   Atrophy of the lobules

Question 1.46. **Many new markers of the aggressiveness of malignancy have been uncovered recently. All of the following have been associated with clinical cancer progression EXCEPT:**

a)   Loss of E-cadherin expression on colon cancer specimens
b)   Increased expression of *nm23* in breast cancer specimens
c)   Proliferation of microvessels on staining of the tissue with antibody to von Willebrand's factor
d)   Production of scatter factor/HGF by the tumor
e)   Elevated plasma concentrations of and immunostaining of tumors for MMP-2 Type IV collagenase

Question 1.47. **Invasion is the hallmark of malignancy; however, it may also be found in physiologic states. Which of the following conditions are not associated with an invasive phenotype?**

a)   Bone remodeling
b)   Angiogenesis
c)   Inflammatory exudate
d)   Wound healing
e)   Serous transudation

Question 1.48. **A 55-year-old man is seen with a rapidly deteriorating clinical course and is found to have hepatocellular carcinoma as revealed by CT scan and liver biopsy. Serum hepatitis B surface antigen (HBsAg) test results are reactive. His 52-year-old asymptomatic wife is tested and is also found to have serum positive for HBsAg. Her levels of serum transaminases, bilirubin, and albumin are within normal range. Her abdominal ultrasound reveals no hepatic lesions or cirrhotic changes. What would you recommend to the patient's wife?**

a)   Alpha-interferon 10 million units three times a week for 12 weeks
b)   Alpha-interferon 3 million units three times a week for 6 months

c)   Hepatitis B vaccine
d)   No treatment
e)   Hepatitis immunoglobulin

Question 1.49.   **A 60-year-old woman was found to have a platelet count of 92,000/μL as revealed by a routine blood test. Bone marrow biopsy showed an increase in megakaryocytes and normal myeloid and erythroid maturation. Liver spleen scan and abdominal ultrasound showed splenomegaly. No hepatic masses were seen. Viral hepatitis serology studies showed reactive anti-hepatitis C viral antibody, reactive anti-HBs, and nonreactive HbsAg. Blood tests showed albumin, 3.5 g/dL; aspartate aminotransferase (AST), 85 U/L; alanine aminotransferase (ALT), 110 U/L; and bilirubin 1.2 mg/dL. What would you recommend for this patient?**

a)   Alpha-interferon 3 million units three times a week for 6 months
b)   Hepatitis B vaccine
c)   No treatment
d)   Liver biopsy
e)   Abdominal CT scan

Question 1.50.   **A 62-year-old man with known reactive serum anti-HCV and a previous history of heavy alcohol abuse that was discontinued 2 years previously is seen with worsening hepatic encephalopathy, refractory ascites, and hepatorenal failure. The patient has had recurrent variceal hemorrhage from portal hypertension for the past 2 years. Abdominal MRI showed a 2-cm mass in the right hepatic lobe. Serum alpha-fetoprotein level is elevated to 400 ng/mL. Treatment with oral lactulose fails to improve the encephalopathy. How would you approach this patient?**

a)   Biopsy of liver mass
b)   Refer for hepatic arterial chemoembolization
c)   Alpha-interferon 3 million units three times a week
d)   Refer for orthotopic liver transplantation
e)   Supportive care only

Question 1.51.   **A 42-year-old woman has recently completed lumpectomy, radiotherapy, and adjuvant chemotherapy for adenocarcinoma of the right breast. She returns for routine follow-up and reports that she has started consuming a Far Eastern herbal extract and requests your advice concerning diet and nutritional approaches that may prevent the development of a second breast cancer in herself and reduce the risk of breast cancer in her two teenage daughters. You suggest the following:**

a)   Consume a multivitamin and mineral supplement, with additional vitamin E, beta carotene, and selenium.
b)   Follow a vegetarian diet and consume only those foods labeled as "natural" or "organic."
c)   Consume a diet with total fat reduced to less than 10% of energy.
d)   Refer to the dietary guidelines for cancer prevention recently updated by the American Cancer Society and offer a consult with a dietitian.
e)   All of the aforementioned.

Question 1.52. **The claim that high doses of vitamin C are effective in treating cancer is based on studies published by Drs. Linus Pauling and Ewan Cameron during the late 1970s. Which one of the following statements are TRUE?**

a)   The data were not collected properly.
b)   The studies were improperly designed.
c)   The dose of vitamin C was too low to produce optimal results.
d)   The data were sufficiently promising that further studies should be done.
e)   None of the aforementioned are true.

Question 1.53. **If a patient expresses interest in a particular questionable method, which option would be most sensible?**

a)   Advise the patient to ask the provider for the names of persons who have used the treatment, so the patient can obtain firsthand reports on whether the treatment works.
b)   Ask the patient to obtain written information from the provider so that the two of you can review it together.
c)   State that if the treatment is used, you will discharge the patient from your care.
d)   Advise that as long as the patient obtains standard treatment, there is no harm in obtaining "alternative" treatments as well.
e)   Advise the patient to contact the American Holistic Medical Association for further information.

Question 1.54. **The "START" or restriction point in the cell cycle precedes mitosis and commits the cell irreversibly to cell division. Which one of the following is correct?**

a)   The START point refers to a point in G0 (resting phase of the cycle), which when passed, commits the cell to division.
b)   It refers to initiating synthesis of genes during the S phase of the cell cycle.
c)   It refers to a point late in G1 in a cell cycle that commits the cell to DNA synthesis (to the S phase).
d)   It refers to a point late in G1 which, if passed, commits the cell to division.
e)   In normal cells, alkylating agents rarely cause cycle arrest in G2.

Question 1.55. **All of the following statements regarding proto-oncogenes are correct EXCEPT:**

a)   Proto-oncogenes are generally normal growth regulatory genes.
b)   Diffuse large-cell lymphoma grows rapidly because of excessive *c-myc* gene product.
c)   Excessive production of *c-myc* gene product results when a strong promoter is translocated to the *c-myc* gene.
d)   Point mutations of the *ras* gene lead to a continuous "on" switch in signal transduction upstream from transcriptional activation, which leads to cell proliferation.
e)   *C-myc* gene amplification has been noted in small-cell lung carcinoma and neuroblastoma.

Question 1.56. **Knudsen's two-hit hyopthesis is consistent with all of the following EXCEPT:**

a) The fusion of normal with neoplastic cells results in hybrid cells that are neoplastic.
b) The familial loss of one allele of a tumor suppressor gene does not result in cancer.
c) The retinoblastoma gene is deleted or mutant in patients who have retinoblastoma.
d) The sibling of a 5-year-old with retinoblastoma and no family history is likely to have two normal Rb alleles in his fibroblasts.
e) A 5-year-old with retinoblastoma and a brother with retinoblastoma might have two Rb allele deletions in his tumor and one in his normal fibroblasts.

Question 1.57. **All of the following statements regarding control of cellular proliferation are correct EXCEPT:**

a) Loss of heterozygosity (LOH) refers to loss of one of the two alleles in the tumor genome as compared with normal tissue from the same patient.
b) LOH is rare in normal cells but common and nonrandom in tumor cells.
c) LOH, along with cytogenetic studies of human tumors, has led to, and presumptively will continue to identify areas on the genome where tumor suppressive genes exist.
d) Loss of a retinoblastoma gene occurs in more than 70% of patients who have small-cell lung carcinoma.
e) Retinoblastoma protein must be dephosphorylated to allow the cell to enter S phase.

Question 1.58. **All of the following statements regarding molecular control of the cell cycle are correct EXCEPT:**

a) Cyclin dependent kinases (CDKs), along with cyclins, which are the regulatory subunits of CDKs, are primarily responsible for the transit of cells through the various stages of the cell cycle.
b) The CDK/cyclin–driven cell cycle progression is under the control of inhibitors, that is, under negative control.
c) The retinoblastoma gene product transcriptionally activates genes that inhibit *cdk* function.
d) The Rb gene is the gatekeeper for the restriction point. When Rb becomes phosphorylated, the gate opens, and the cell proceeds through its cycle.
e) Certain oncogenic viral protein products, for example, human papillomavirus type E7, may complex with and inactivate RB protein and thus have an effect comparable to deletion of a tumor suppressor gene.

Question 1.59. **The slow growth rate of micrometastasis in the adjuvant breast cancer setting might be explained by all of the following EXCEPT:**

a) All of the tumor cells are "resting," that is, in the G0 phase, which means that they are not in active cycle.
b) The cell cycle time in the micrometastasis is long.
c) A balanced rate of tumor cell proliferation and programmed cell death exists.

d)   There is genetic programming for tumor angiogenesis factor production.
e)   Lower oxygenation occurs within the tumor.

Question 1.60.   All of the following statements regarding lymphoid cells are correct EXCEPT:

a)   B cells originate in the marrow, and T cells originate in the thymus.
b)   T cells cannot be distinguished from B cells by routine stains.
c)   Each clone of B cells interacts with a specific antigen and T-cell products to produce antibodies.
d)   Both T and B cells can produce a highly diverse array of surface receptors.
e)   Both T and B cells respond to alloantigens.

Question 1.61.   All of the following statements regarding the immune system are correct EXCEPT:

a)   Almost all cytokines, such as interferon gamma, interleukins, and tumor necrosis factor are produced by T cells and macrophages.
b)   Epitopes are the simplest forms of an antigenic determinant to which antibodies bind.
c)   Epitopes may consist of protein, glycoprotein, carbohydrate, and lipid moieties.
d)   Binding of antibody to epitope depends on precise complementarity between the epitope and antibody binding site.
e)   After repeated antigen exposure, subsequently produced antibodies display decreasing affinity for the epitope.

Question 1.62.   Antibody diversity is generated by all of the following EXCEPT:

a)   Somatic recombination of immunoglobulin gene segments
b)   Germ line mutations
c)   Somatic mutation within complementarity determining regions (hypermutable regions)
d)   Variable region of H chain gene in which there are recombinations of segments from a library of more than a hundred variable, six joining, and thirty diversity segments
e)   High-affinity, antibody-producing cells that are selected through signals received following binding of surface Ig by the appropriate antigen

Question 1.63.   Different monoclonal antibodies prepared against human leukocytes and tumor cells have led to all of the following conclusions EXCEPT:

a)   There are defined "clusters of differentiation" known as CD groups.
b)   Tumor cells almost never express CD determinants for multiple cell lineages.
c)   T cells help B cells produce immunoglobulin.
d)   The specific Ig produced is influenced by the array of cytokines present.
e)   IL-2, IL-4, and IL-5 drive IgM production.

Question 1.64.   All of the following statements regarding lymphocyte trafficking are correct EXCEPT:

a)   Mature T cells traffic through the peripheral circulation, and return through venous and post-capillary venules to the skin and lymph nodes.
b)   T cells can recognize antigenic peptides that are either on the surface of antigen-presenting cells or free in the circulation.

c)   Binding of the T-cell receptor to an antigen generates a primary signal that traverses the membrane, which activates protein tyrosine kinases on the cytoplasmic side of the receptor.
d)   After antibody-antigen binding, a signal is then transduced through a series of protein phosphorylations, including activation of protein kinase C and the release of intracellular calcium.
e)   Complete lymphocyte activation requires one or more co-stimulatory signals.

Question 1.65.   All of the following statements regarding T cells are correct EXCEPT:

a)   Mature T cells express either CD4 helper or CD8 cytotoxic suppressor antigens, but not both.
b)   Mature T cells constitute approximately 20% of normal blood lymphocyte, 35% of lymph node cells, and 50% of splenic lymphocytes.
c)   An immunologically functioning T-cell clone results from encountering an appropriately presented and relevant antigen in the presence of co-stimulatory factors and cytokines.
d)   Long-lived memory T cells represent persistence of the clone after clearance of the foreign antigen.
e)   CD4 positive cells can be subdivided based on their ability to produce different specific cytokines such as TNF-alpha, GM-CSF, and IL-3.

Question 1.66.   All of the following are characteristics of natural killer cells EXCEPT:

a)   CD56 (NKH1) and IL-2 receptor expression
b)   Intracytoplasmic granules
c)   A binding site or surface receptor for the Fc region of IgG
d)   The inability to exercise antibody-dependent, cell-meditated cytotoxicity (ADCC)
e)   The ability to destroy tumor cells in the absence of specific IgG antibody

Question 1.67.   Mircoorganisms have been closely linked to the etiology of all the following neoplasms EXCEPT:

a)   Acute T-cell leukemia/lymphoma
b)   Colon cancer
c)   Nasopharyngeal carcinoma
d)   Cervical carcinoma
e)   Hepatoma

Question 1.68.   All of the following statements regarding major histocompatibility complex (MHC) antigens are correct EXCEPT:

a)   Class I antigens (HLA-A, B, and C) are cell surface proteins expressed by almost all normal cells.
b)   Class I antigens are associated with a β_2-microglobulin molecule, which is released in the blood and correlates with tumor burden for many neoplasms.
c)   Class II antigens are expressed primarily on lymphoreticular and endothelial cells. They may be induced in epithelial cells by inflammation or gamma interferon.
d)   MHC class I gene products are inappropriately expressed in many neoplasms. Such expression is associated with the ability of malignant cells to evade the immune system and produce metastases.

e)   Cells whose MHC class I gene product expression is down-regulated are more resistant to cytotoxic T lymphocytes and natural killer cells.

Question 1.69.   **All of the following statements regarding oncofetal antigens are correct EXCEPT:**

a)   They are expressed during fetal development, but not in normal adult tissues.
b)   They may be expressed in neoplasia, but not in benign diseases such as chronic hepatitis and ulcerative colitis.
c)   Human chorionic gonadotropin (hCG) is the most sensitive oncofetal protein for monitoring microscopic tumor deposits.
d)   Alpha fetoprotein (AFP) is the best marker for the diagnosis and monitoring of hepatoma.
e)   CA 125 levels are commonly elevated in colon cancer.

Question 1.70.   **All of the following statements regarding oncofetal antigens are correct EXCEPT:**

a)   If the hCG level returns to normal after chemotherapy for gestational choriocarcinoma and remains low for 4 months, there is a 50% likelihood that the patient is cured.
b)   Detectable levels of interleukin-10 predict a poor prognosis in patients with non-Hodgkin's lymphoma.
c)   Serum levels of β_2-microglobulin allow for evaluation of response in myeloma.
d)   Serum levels of IL-2 receptor correlate with disease activity in adult T-cell leukemia.
e)   Serum levels of the ICAM-1 intercellular adhesion molecule correlate with disease activity in certain childhood solid tumors.

Question 1.71.   **A solitary pulmonary nodule is highly likely to be benign when:**

a)   It is greater than 3 cm in size.
b)   It remains stable in size for 2 or more years.
c)   Eccentric calcification is present.
d)   Irregular spiculated margins are present.
e)   It is associated with endocrine-related symptoms.

Question 1.72.   **The role of CT in the preoperative staging of lung cancer is:**

a)   To detect cancer in enlarged intrathoracic nodes
b)   To differentiate inflammatory versus neoplastic enlargement of lymph nodes
c)   To detect microscopic metastasis in normal-size nodes
d)   To detect hilar or mediastinal invasion or lymphadenopathy
e)   To accurately detect chest wall invasion by peripheral lung cancer in the absence of rib destruction or mass lesion

Question 1.73.   **You have been caring for a 59-year-old woman who has breast cancer metastatic to the lungs and bones. After she failed hormonal treatments, you treated her with doxorubicin, and when her tumor progressed, you switched the patient to navelbine. During the last two cycles of navelbine, her CEA level has begun to rise, and the nodules as revealed by chest radiograph have begun increasing in size. Simultaneously, the patient's shortness of breath has progressed, and her performance status has been decreasing so that she now spends approximately 50% of the day in bed or on the couch.**

The day before a scheduled office visit, she is brought to the emergency room by her husband and daughter. The patient is tachypneic, with a blood gas that shows PO$_2$ of 60 mm Hg and an oxygen saturation of 88% (on 50% inspired oxygen). The chest radiograph shows further enlargement of her tumor nodules, with right lower lobe opacity. Despite the hypoxia and anxiety it is causing, the patient is awake, alert, and oriented to person and place.

You begin to inform the patient of her situation. She asks a few questions. You outline your plan and raise the possibility of intubation and mechanical ventilation. The patient immediately rejects the idea, saying that she does not want to be "hooked up to machines." Her daughter interrupts, stating that she would not want her mom to die and that the decision for a ventilator can be put off. Her mother retorts that she is clear and her mind is made up; she again states that she does not want to be "hooked up to machines," whether the decision is made now or later and even if it means she might die.

The patient is admitted to the hospital. She is treated with oxygen and antibiotics for presumed post-obstructive pneumonia. That night, the patient experiences respiratory arrest. At the urging of the daughter and husband who are present, the house staff intubates the patient. You arrive after the patient has been transferred to the intensive care unit on a ventilator. You talk with the daughter and husband who insist that the patient continue to be treated and remain on the ventilator. They reiterate their contention that she remain on the ventilator and express the hope that the treatments for pneumonia will work and she will improve enough to get off the ventilator. What is the ethically correct course of action?

a) Because the patient is incompetent, the family should decide how she should be treated. Therefore, you follow the wishes of the daughter and husband to keep the patient on the ventilator and continue treatments for post-obstructive pneumonia.

b) Because this is a complex ethical and legal problem, you call the hospital attorney, with the plan to go to court to obtain an order to stop the ventilator.

c) Because the patient clearly expressed her wishes regarding the mechanical ventilator to you, you gently tell the family that you must stop the ventilator to honor the patient's wishes.

d) Because this is a common problem, you talk to the chief of oncology who tells you that turning off the ventilator is the correct thing to do, but that you should nevertheless continue it because dead patients cannot sue, but surviving families can.

e) Because this is a complex ethical and legal problem, you decide to call the ethics committee to determine the right answer.

Question 1.74.   A patient's tumor is found to be resistant to several chemotherapeutic agents. What is the most likely molecular explanation for this phenomenon?

a) Mutation in *p53*
b) Increased expression of *Bcl-2*
c) Absent expression of p-glycoprotein
d) Mutated *ras*
e) Expression of nm 23

Question 1.75.   **Tumor promoters are agents that enhance (promote) the development of tumors in animal models following initiation of DNA damage by a carcinogen. Many of these tumor promoters are now known to act on components of signal transduction. These effects include:**

a)   Activation of protein kinases
b)   Activation of protein phosphatases
c)   Reduction of cellular levels of calcium
d)   Direct activation of transcription factors
e)   Amplification of cell surface receptors

Question 1.76.   **As a diagnostic modality for directing the treatment of patients with metastatic cancer and an unknown primary site, radiologic imaging is:**

a)   The most important diagnostic modality available for planning therapy and for estimating prognosis
b)   Frequently contributory to a decision on management, in conjunction with the laboratory and physical findings
c)   Primarily useful to rule out an unknown primary that might be amenable to treatment for palliation
d)   Never useful in directing the management of patients with widespread metastatic disease
e)   Primarily useful to protect the physician against subsequent medical-legal challenges

Question 1.77.   **A 63-year-old man who is seen with bilaterally enlarged lymph nodes in the upper neck but with no other symptoms or findings undergoes a needle biopsy that yields an "undifferentiated" carcinoma. A subsequent diagnostic work-up using radiologic imaging studies to determine the primary site:**

a)   Is not likely to produce useful results, regardless of which radiologic imaging technique is employed
b)   Should be directed primarily to determine the total extent of metastatic disease
c)   Could be used most productively to examine the upper aerodigestive tract with a cross-sectional imaging method like MRI, following a careful endoscopic examination
d)   Should concentrate on ruling out the most prevalent metastasizing primary cancer by means of a CT of the chest
e)   Should concentrate on ruling out a primary in the abdomen, preferably through barium studies and/or a CT examination

ANSWERS

Answer 1.1.   **The answer is (c).**

All tumor cells are believed to multiply exponentially in the initial period following the transformation event. A "flattening out" of the growth rate over time occurs due to an increase in cell loss, nutritional depletion of tumor cells, or lengthening of cell cycle time. However, the percentage of cells not in the cell cycle (ie, in the G0 phase) is higher in normal cells than in cancer cells. In other words, tumor cells are more likely to enter G1 phase and less likely to exit the cell cycle, which leads to an increased growth fraction in cancer cells. Conversely, cancer cells do not grow faster (have shorter cell cycle times) or require less time to complete DNA synthesis or undergo mitosis. Another assessment of the growth fraction is the labeling index, which is a measure of the number of cells synthesizing DNA at any given time; this index typically employs thymidine incorporation to label such S-phase cells by autoradiography.

For Detailed Discussion: (1) Chapter 1, "Cell Proliferation and Differentiation."

Answer 1.2.   The answer is (d).

Tumor cells are less likely, compared with their normal counterparts, to remain at the G1-S cell cycle boundary (ie, be on "hold" before DNA synthesis). In nontumorigenic cells, the retinoblastoma protein is produced throughout the cell cycle; however, phosphorylation by enzymes such as G1 cyclin kinase complexes inactivates this protein, thereby releasing cells from G1 arrest. p53 protein phosphorylation also aids in allowing release from the pre–DNA synthesis phase. As such, both retinoblastoma and p53 protein are tumor suppressor proteins whose normal function provides an important control against overproliferation. Inactivation of the normal suppressor function of these proteins (as might occur by an inability to become dephosphorylated) or by deletion or truncation could result in loss of normal regulation mitigating against proceeding through the cell cycle, which would thereby lead to neoplastic transformation.

For Detailed Discussion: (1) Chapter 1, "Cell Proliferation and Differentiation."

Answer 1.3.   The answer is (a).

In addition to inactivation of tumor suppressor genes and activating mutations in growth-promoting proto-oncogenes, potentially oncogenic genes also include those that code for proteins that prevent or interfere with the normal process of programmed cell death. The *bcl-2* gene product may interact with mitochondrial or other intercellular membranes, thereby preventing an oxygen-dependent apoptotic signal. For example, the translocation between chromosome 14 and 18, characteristic of many follicular lymphomas, allows overexpression and thereby places the *bcl-2* gene under the control of the immunoglobulin heavy chain gene promoter.

For Detailed Discussions: (1) Chapter 1, "Cell Proliferation and Differentiation." (2) Thompson et al. Apoptosis in the pathogenesis treatment of disease. Science 1995; 267:1456.

Answer 1.4.   The answer is (d).

Restriction fragment length polymorphisms are areas of DNA, generally in noncoding regions, that vary among individuals in the population. These variants may be detectable by Southern blot due to a nucleotide change creating or destroying the recognition site for a restriction endonuclease enzyme or creating variable fragments of altered length due to a variable number of tandem repeat (or *alu*) sequences between restriction sites. RFLPs are stably inherited. If an RFLP is in close proximity to a gene important in the development of human cancer, then the finding of a given RFLP associated with a cancer "maps" the gene for that disease. Furthermore, the loss of genetic material from a tumor (specifically, the loss of an RFLP in the noncancer cells in this individual) defines a loss of heterozygosity and may be a hallmark of a tumor suppressor gene.

For Detailed Discussion: (1) Chapter 2, "Molecular Biology." (2) Miki et al. A strong candidate for the breast and ovarian cancer gene: BRCA-1. Science 1994;266:66.

Answer 1.5.   **The answer is (d).**

Familial adenomatous polyposis, an autosomal dominant disorder, is characterized by thousands of benign adenomatous polyps in the colon and rectum in affected individuals. There is essentially a 100% incidence of malignant degeneration in patients who do not undergo colectomies. Linkage studies have determined that the gene responsible for this disease resides on the long arm of chromosome 5q21 and is termed the "adenomatous polyposis coli (APC) gene." This gene encodes a ubiquitously expressed protein that may be involved in linking the cytoskeleton to E-cadherin, an adhesion molecule on the cell surface. As such, this protein may signal a "brake" on proliferation in the event of certain cell-cell interactions. More than two thirds of patients who have familial adenomatous polyposis can be shown to have a germ-line mutation of the APC gene. Patients inheriting a defective APC gene would only require one abnormality in the other allele for colonic cells to undergo a neoplastic transformation, which implies that APC is a typical tumor suppressor gene. Moreover, virtually all colorectal cancers harbor somatically mutated APC alleles.

For Detailed Discussion: (1) Chapter 6, "Tumor Suppressor and DNA Repair Gene Defects in Human Cancer." (2) Polakis P. Mutations in the APC gene and their implications for protein structure and function. Curr Opin Genet Develop 1995;5:66.

Answer 1.6.   **The answer is (b).**

The diagnosis of hereditary nonpolyposis colon cancer (HNPCC) requires a kindred that contains at least three affected relatives, two of whom are first degree with at least two generations being affected; also, at least one of the affected individuals must be under the age of 50. Female members of such kindreds also have a high risk of endometrial and ovarian cancer. Cancers in patients from these kindreds display expansions or contractions of simple short repeated sequences of DNA known as microsatellites. Microsatellite instability in such cancers is similar to that observed in simpler organisms, such as yeast that may display "mismatch repair" gene defects. Defects in this system fail to allow correction of errors made during DNA replication. The biochemical similarity between colon cancers in patients who have HNPCC and mismatch repair defects in yeast led to the cloning of human homologues of the genes *hMSH2* (mapping to chromosome 2p16) and *hMLH1* (located at chromosome 3p21). These two genes account for germ line mutations in 50% and 33% of HNPCC kindreds, respectively. HNPCC patients inherit one inactivated DNA repair gene from the affected parent and acquire a defect in the other during tumorigenesis. When both the alleles are inactivated, mutations may accumulate in rapid succession, thereby accelerating the transition from benign to malignant neoplasia. Approximately 15% of apparently sporadic colorectal cancers can be shown to demonstrate similar alterations in mismatch repair activity.

For Detailed Discussion: (1) Chapter 6, "Tumor Suppressor and DNA Repair Gene Defects in Human Cancer." (2) Modrich P. Mismatch repair, genetic stability, and cancer. Science 1994;266:1959.

Answer 1.7. **The answer is (c).**

There is considerable epidemiologic evidence that suggests that estrogen is the primary stimulant for breast cell proliferation; exposure to progesterone may also play a role in enhancing mitotic activity of breast tissue. In simple terms, the influence of these hormones translates into: the more ovulatory cycles, the greater the risk of breast cancer. Case-control studies have demonstrated an approximately 20% decrease in risk for each year in which there is a delay in menarche. Extreme physical activity during adolescence, which tends to delay the onset of ovulation, appears to reduce the risk of breast cancer. Moreover, women whose natural menopause occurs before the age of 45 have approximately half the breast cancer risk of those whose menopause occurs after the age of 55. Although early age for the first birth is protective, women who have a very late first full-term pregnancy actually are at a higher risk of breast cancer than are women who never have had children. Although pregnancy produces a long-term reduction in risk, gestation does appear to carry a short-term increase in the incidence of breast cancer, perhaps due to the high levels of bioavailable estradiol associated with early pregnancy. The relative risk of breast cancer decreases in populations that consume low per capita quantities of fat. Nutrition can modify age at menarche as well as body weight, which appears to be a risk factor based on increased peripheral synthesis of sex steroids.

For Detailed Discussion: (1) Chapter 14, "Hormones and the Etiology of Cancer." (2) Henderson BE, et al. Do regular ovulatory cycles increase breast cancer risk? Cancer 1985;56:1206.

Answer 1.8. **The answer is (d).**

The frequency of mitotic activity in cells that line the endometrium correlates with the risk of endometrial cancer. Because such activity is primarily controlled by unopposed estrogens, estrogen replacement therapy without co-administration of progestational agents (which are primarily anti-estrogenic and decrease endometrial proliferation) is a risk factor. Multiple pregnancies, which also expose the uterus to progestational compounds as well as estrogens, decrease risk. Obesity, like estrogen replacement therapy, increases the circulating concentration of estrogen, thereby increasing the risk of uterine cancer. Women who take unopposed estrogens for 5 or more years have an approximately three- to fivefold increase in risk compared with women who have never used such therapy. It is interesting that the aggressiveness of an individual cancer in those who use estrogen is lower than among nonusers, presumably due to the increased screening performed on individuals using this drug. Tamoxifen, considered to be an estrogen antagonist, acts as an estrogen with regard to uterine tissue. As such, tamoxifen use is associated with a slightly increased risk of endometrial cancer.

For Detailed Discussion: (1) Chapter 14, "Hormones and the Etiology of Cancer."

Answer 1.9. **The answer is (d).**

Nonmelanoma skin cancers are by far the most common cancers diagnosed in the United States each year. Overall, they account for approximately 30 to 40% of all cancers. The incidence is increasing sharply and may be considered a quiet 20th century epidemic. There is ample epidemiologic and laboratory evidence that provides a direct causal role of sunlight exposure in the induction of skin cancer. Both basal cell and squamous cell carcinomas are found primarily on sun-exposed skin areas, and their incidence is correlated with cumulative sun exposure. Although melanoma shows a weaker dependence on total sunlight exposure, it is also associated with exposure to sunlight.

For Detailed Discussion: (1) Chapter 16, "Ultraviolet Radiation Carcinogenesis." (2) Fitzpatrick TB, et al. Sunlight and skin cancer. N Engl J Med 1985;313:818.

Answer 1.10. **The correct answer is (d).**

All of the listed disorders represent increased sensitivity to ultraviolet B and C wavelengths due to recessive mutations except basal cell nevus syndrome (BCNS). BCNS is an autosomal dominant disorder with high (>97%) penetrance. The principal manifestations of BCNS are multiple tumors (50 to 100), primarily occurring on sun-exposed skin, that usually appear at puberty and during the second and third decades of life.

For Detailed Discussion: (1) Chapter 16, "Ultraviolet Radiation Carcinogenesis."

Answer 1.11. **The correct answer is (d).**

Xeroderma pigmentosa (XP) is a rare autosomal recessive disorder occurring at a frequency of approximately 1:250,000 live births in the United States. Affected patients (homozygotes) have sun sensitivity that results in progressive degenerative changes of sun-exposed surfaces that often lead to neoplasia. The median age of onset of symptoms is age 12, with skin rapidly taking on the appearance of that seen in individuals who have years of sun exposure. The frequency of skin cancer (squamous and basal cell and melanoma) is increased approximately 2000 times compared with that seen in the general population under 20 years of age.

For Detailed Discussion: (1) Chapter 16, "Ultraviolet Radiation Carcinogenesis."

Answer 1.12. **The correct answer is (c).**

Oncogene-transducing retroviruses are generally replication-incompetent because most or all of their structural genes (eg, *gag, pol, env*) are replaced by an oncogene. An oncogene is related to, but not identical to, a proto-oncogene that encodes a protein important in normal cellular proliferation. The proto-oncogenes that are transduced are not merely appended onto a retroviral sequence, but rather are potentially extensive changes occurring within the proto-oncogene sequence itself as a requirement for the generation of transforming activity. Tumors produced by a retroviral infection via transduction of an oncogenic gene into the host genome generally occur acutely (within 2 weeks) and yield a high efficiency of transformation, thereby causing the formation of polyclonal tumors. Most oncogene-transducing retroviruses are replication incompetent and may yield tumors when cells of young or old animals are infected. In some cases, normal development of the immune system can cause the regression of such virally mediated tumors. Because of the inability of an onco-genic retrovirus to replicate due to the lack of normal functional genes, co-infection with a "helper virus" is required. This helper virus is a replication-incompetent virus that contains the information required for packaging the defective transforming retro-viral genome to allow infection of the host cell. Another type of transforming retro-virus, which is replication competent and contains an entire set of structural genes, is much less efficient in inducing in vitro tumor formation compared with oncogene-transducing viruses. In this case, the provirus must be inserted in a location close to a proto-oncogene, and, due to the rarity of the transforming event, a monoclonal tu-mor may be formed.

For Detailed Discussion: (1) Chapter 20, "RNA Tumor Viruses."

Answer 1.13.   **The correct answer is (d).**

Retroviral vectors can be used to deliver a gene of interest to a target cell. A retroviral-based vector may infect multiple cells simultaneously and deliver a single copy of genetic information into a target cell. Moreover, the host range of such viruses could be targeted to a particular cell type by specifically altering the type of envelope proteins used by the virion.

Any specific genomic RNA can be added to the genome of a retroviral vector, as long as the genomic RNA contains the appropriate packaging signals. However, the generation of helper or wild-type viruses that in and of themselves could be oncogenic, is a theoretical problem that must be minimized before the clinical ap-plication of the strategy. Also, insertional mutagenesis by the vector could be onco-genic if a viral enhancer element is inserted proximal to genes involved in prolifera-tion. Because retroviral vectors may carry only one or few genes, they hold great promise for genetic deficiency diseases such as adenosine deaminase deficiency or Lesch-Nyhan syndrome; however, neoplastic transformation in human cells re-quires multiple genetic alterations; therefore, replacement of an inherently inactive tumor-suppressor gene may not reverse the neoplastic phenotype. The most impor-tant current application of retrovirology to cancer therapy is the use of vectors that directly carry an anticancer gene product that can be specifically delivered to can-cer cells. For example, a retroviral vector carrying the tumor necrosis factor gene has infected tumor infiltrating lymphocytes, which may then travel to the specific tumor from which they were derived and elicit antineoplastic activity due to very high lev-els of tumor necrosis factor produced by the transduced cells.

For Detailed Discussion: (1) Chapter 20, "RNA Tumor Viruses."

Answer 1.14.   **The correct answer is (a).**

The malignancies associated with Epstein-Barr virus (DNA viruses that have the ca-pacity to establish both latent and lytic infection) fall into two categories: those that occur shortly after a viral infection and those that occur long after infection. Tumors occurring early after EBV infection are generally caused by latent virus integration into the genome of B lymphocytes, which can lead to lymphoproliferation, especially in the setting of a defective immune system. On the other hand, Burkitt's lymphoma and nasopharyngeal carcinoma become manifest long after primary EBV infection; viral gene expression may not be central to the growth of a neoplasm in these cases. An important type of EBV-related disease are lymphoproliferative disorders that occur in patients who are immunosuppressed due to bone marrow or solid organ transplantation; these disorders are usually classified as lymphomas, frequently of the immunoblastic variety. Tissue studies of patients who have African Burkitt's lymphoma, a high-grade malignant lymphoma that typically occurs in the face or abdomen in children, offer serologic evidence that this condition is strongly associated with EBV infection. However, only approximately 20% of Burkitt's lymphoma cases in the United States are associated with the EBV virus, compared with 90% in Africa. The precise etiologic association between EBV and endemic Burkitt's lymphoma is not known, but it may involve the expansion of B lymphocyte proliferation due to EBV infection. Such enhanced proliferation may favor the chance occurrence of a chromosomal translocation that places the *c-myc* proto-oncogene under the control of immunoglobulin gene-related transcriptional enhancers. Nasopharyngeal carcinoma, which typically causes a metastatic lymph node in the jugular chain, bloody nasal discharge, nasal speech, or unilateral otitis media (secondary to compression of the eustachian tube), displays a nonkeratinizing squamous cell histology and is universally associated with high levels of antibodies to EBV antigens in the serum of affected patients. The relationship of Hodgkin's disease and leiomyosarcomas in AIDS patients to EBV infection is less clear. A herpesvirus distinct from EBV has been detected in tissues from patients who have classic Kaposi's sarcoma.

For Detailed Discussion: (1) Chapter 21, "Herpesviruses."

Answer 1.15. **The correct answer is (e).**

The association between schistosomal infection and neoplasia of the bladder, particularly squamous cell carcinoma, is overwhelming. Long-standing and severe infections are predisposing factors. *Schistosoma haematobium* is the schistosomal species most closely linked to the development of bladder carcinoma. Squamous cell carcinoma of the bladder is markedly over-represented only in areas where infection with *S. haematobium* is endemic. The precise etiologic reason why infection with this parasite leads to bladder carcinoma is not clear; bladder inflammation that may generate potentially carcinogenic metabolites has been one proposed factor. Schistosomal infection has more tenuous links to breast cancer and hepatocellular carcinoma (only if cirrhosis is concomitant) and rarely, to non-Hodgkin's lymphoma. The liver fluke *Opisthorchis viverrini,* which is endemic in Thailand, is associated with a high incidence of cholangiocarcinoma.

For Detailed Discussion: (1) Chapter 24, "Parasites."

Answer 1.16. **The correct answer is (b).**

Chronic hepatitis B virus infection is a definitive risk factor for the development of hepatocellular carcinoma. Essentially all of these cancers in endemic areas occur in patients whose blood studies show serologic markers of previous hepatitis B virus infection. Although hepatitis B virus–infected individuals who also have cirrhosis are at higher risk, cirrhosis is absent in approximately one quarter of patients who have hepatocellular carcinoma in endemic areas. Although exposure to other agents, such as aflatoxin, cigarettes, oral contraceptives, or alcohol may be contributing factors, the insertion of hepatitis B virus DNA sequences into the hepatic cell genome appears to be required for the development of hepatocellular carcinoma. The oncogenic mechanism of the hepatitis B virus is not clear, although production of proliferation-inducing cytokines; transactivation activity of hepatitis B virus gene products (ie, protein); oncogene activation; and tumor suppressor gene inactivation (particularly the long arm of chromosome 11p; the retinoblastoma gene on chromosome 13q is also disturbed in a few cases) may be involved. Hepatitis C virus is also associated with the development of hepatocellular carcinoma. Except in rare cases, the inflammation associated with cirrhosis due to hepatitis C infection is required to induce carcinogenesis, presumably on the basis of continuous cell regeneration because of the chronic inflammation.

For Detailed Discussion: (1) Chapter 23, "Hepatitis Viruses."

Answer 1.17.   **The answer is (d).**

Mammography, physical examination, and fine needle aspiration of either palpable lesions or suspicious lesions that are revealed by mammogram are supplementary to one another for the early detection of breast cancer. The finding of a suspicious lesion on any one of the three tests is an indication for immediate surgical biopsy. If no palpable lesion is identified, the biopsy should be guided by mammographic findings. Many of the nonpalpable suspicious lesions indicated on mammogram are carcinoma in situ, which can be difficult to sample even with surgical biopsy, let alone fine needle aspiration. A benign result indicated on fine needle aspiration under this circumstance should not be interpreted as indicating that the suspicious lesion indicated on mammogram is benign.

For Detailed Discussion: (1) Chapter 31, "Principles of Cancer Pathology."

Answer 1.18.   **The correct answer is (d).**

Because of the limited physical access to the patient, MRI is not well suited for the scanning of very ill patients, particularly those who are on life support systems. MR imaging allows superior contrast between normal tissue and tumor (T2-weighted images) than is possible with CT. The multiplanar capability of MRI is also an important advantage of this technique. Unlike CT images that are restricted to the axial plane, MRI is capable of imaging in any plane. Unlike CT, MRI is not capable of detecting areas of calcification within tumors.

For Detailed Discussion: (1) Chapter 32, "Introduction to Principles of Imaging."

Answer 1.19.   **The answer is (d).**

The cervical lymph nodes represent the most common metastatic site for squamous cell carcinoma of unknown primary origin. In patients who have midcervical lymph nodes, the primary tumor is typically within the head and neck region. In contrast, patients who have a supraclavicular lymph node are more likely to have a primary lung tumor. When no primary site is identified, treatment should be given locally to the involved neck. Neck dissection alone is reserved for only a select group of patients who have small lymph nodes in the submandibular and submental regions.

The majority of patients are treated with a combination of surgical resection and postoperative radiotherapy. Most radiation oncologists recommend treatment to the nasopharynx, oropharynx, and hypopharynx. The role of chemotherapy currently remains investigational.

For Detailed Discussion: (1) Chapter 33, "Imaging Cancer of Unknown Primary Site."

Answer 1.20.   The answer is (d).

Findings indicated on MRI in patients who have bone marrow abnormalities are often nonspecific. Malignant and benign bone tumors, infection, and trauma may all appear similar. Correlation with the patient's clinical history is extremely important. In general, radiographs provide the most useful clinical information when dealing with bony lesions. Intravenous contrast enhancement is rarely needed for MR imaging and generally does not add clinically useful information to the diagnosis. MRI and CT can both provide information regarding the intramedullary extent of tumor, and either can be used to locally stage musculoskeletal neoplasms. In the patient who has a known primary tumor and new onset of bone pain, plain radiographs should be obtained. If there is a strong clinical suspicion of metastatic disease, MRI should be undertaken.

For Detailed Discussion: (1) Chapter 37, "Cross-Sectional Imaging of Musculoskeletal Neoplasms."

Answer 1.21.   The answer is (e).

A mammogram may show the nature of the mass to be definitely benign—for example, a typically calcified degenerating fibroadenoma. Thus, a biopsy could potentially be avoided. The prebiopsy mammogram could also identify an extensive intraductal component of a carcinoma. Because the intraductal component is nonpalpable and should be removed to decrease the possibility of recurrence of tumor, this would be very useful. Also, a prebiopsy mammogram could reveal an unexpected focus of carcinoma, possibly multifocal cancer or contralateral carcinoma. A biopsy should not be deferred because the mammogram is negative.

For Detailed Discussion: (1) Chapter 38, "Imaging the Breast."

Answer 1.22.   The correct answer is (b).

Calcifications are not expected to show up on ultrasonography, and stereotaxis is needed to assure that the needle core samples are directed to the correct site. Although not 100% accurate, core needle biopsy can usually determine whether a carcinoma is intraductal or invasive, which is one of the advantages of core needle biopsy over fine needle aspiration cytology. Although five core specimens are usually adequate for the evaluation of a mass, more samples are usually taken for mammographically detected—usually 10 specimens are taken. Atypical duct hyperplasia is difficult to differentiate from ductal carcinoma in situ by core needle biopsy, because it may coexist with ductal carcinoma in situ. An excisional biopsy is recommended whenever a core biopsy results in this pathologic diagnosis. Some clinical reports have indicated that approximately half of these patients will have ductal carcinoma in situ at re-excision.

For Detailed Discussion: (1) Chapter 38, "Imaging the Breast."

Answer 1.23. **The correct answer is (b).**

Although the composition of the breast tissue should be indicated in the standardized mammography report, this is not the same as the Final Assessment. The Final Assessment of the Breast Imaging Report indicates the likelihood of malignancy on a scale of 1 to 5, based on the mammographic findings. Each of the Final Assessment categories has a "negative" (1) or "benign findings" (2) final assessment that indicates a recommendation for routine screening. A "probably benign finding" (3) indicates that the likelihood of malignancy is low (probably less than 2%). Therefore, a biopsy would be unreasonable in most cases, and a short-term follow-up mammogram, usually within 6 months, is normally done to establish stability of the finding. A "suspicious abnormality" (4) designation indicates that the likelihood of malignancy is great enough that biopsy should be considered. For lesions that are "highly suggestive of malignancy" (5), the probability of malignancy is so great that the surgeon may decide on either a one-stage or two-stage procedure.

In the one-stage procedure, the patient is informed of the results and treatment options. At surgery, a frozen sectioning is performed to confirm the diagnosis before proceeding to definitive treatment. In the two-stage procedure, a biopsy is performed first for tissue diagnosis, and this can be a needle biopsy. Then, should the diagnosis be confirmed, a surgery is scheduled for definitive treatment. Screening mammograms usually have a Final Assessment of "Negative" or "Benign Findings." Often, an abnormality found on screening mammography needs further work-up before a Final Assessment can be made. Then, the conclusion of the report will recommend "additional work-up." However, sometimes the findings of screening examinations are definitive enough to make a Final Assessment. The Final Assessment should appear on all diagnostic examinations. Risk assessment is not part of the standardized reporting system. Because the final assessment is intended to eliminate equivocation as to the interpretation and the recommendations of the interpreting physician, it should be on the written report.

For Detailed Discussion: (1) Chapter 38, "Imaging the Breast."

Answer 1.24. **The correct answer is (e).**

PET is now used as an investigative and a clinical tool in cancer medicine. PET imaging with FDG (PET-FDG) is useful in both imaging and the quantification of glucose metabolism in patients who have malignant tumors. One of the first sites in which PET-FDG has been applied is in the central nervous system. PET-FDG scans are capable of not only diagnosing a primary tumor but also of detecting recurrent disease following therapy. Another promising site in which PET-FDG scans have been studied is the breast. PET-FDG imaging appears capable of detecting primary breast tumors, involvement of axillary nodes, and systemic metastases.

For Detailed Discussion: (1) Chapter 40, "Radionuclide Imaging in Cancer Medicine."

Answer 1.25. **The correct answer is (c).**

Iodine 131 has been effectively used in the treatment of differentiated thyroid carcinoma. Treatment with ^{131}I delivers a high concentration of radiation (doses approach 50,000 cGy) selectively to the tumor. ^{131}I is currently the treatment of choice for residual functioning tissue within the thyroid bed following total thyroidectomy of recurrent localized disease, as well as of systemic metastases. ^{131}I therapy is effective only in tumors that metabolize iodine. Although papillary and follicular carcinomas of the thyroid metabolize iodine, medullary carcinomas do not. The standard approach to patients who have medullary thyroid carcinoma is total thyroidectomy and functional neck dissection.

For Detailed Discussion: (1) Chapter 40, "Radionuclide Imaging in Cancer Medicine."

Answer 1.26. **The correct answer is (e).**

Fenretinide, a retinoid derivative, is administered with a monthly 3-day drug holiday to prevent ocular toxicity. Contralateral breast cancers occur at a rate of 0.8% per year in patients who receive fenretinide. This drug may suppress the rate of ovarian cancer. Tamoxifen has been shown to have superior results over a placebo in preventing breast cancer. Women entering the tamoxifen chemoprevention trial must demonstrate a twofold increase in developing breast cancer.

For Detailed Discussion: (1) Chapter 29, "Chemoprevention of Cancer."

Answer 1.27. **The correct answer is (b).**

The answer rests on a value judgement (how far to go diagnostically, to achieve—at best—a limited benefit). With the symptoms and findings mentioned, the patient almost certainly has a primary carcinoma of the colon with widespread metastases, including a "Virchow's node". He probably has liver involvement as well. Therefore, the only clinical management issue is how best to palliate him after conversion of his designation from an "unknown primary" to a "known primary" tumor (ie, demonstration of a carcinoma of the colon). Palliation could be aided by performing sigmoidoscopy and perhaps a barium enema. A limited colonic resection and/or ostomy procedure might then be considered to avoid the development of a complete bowel obstruction. Chemotherapy would be the only possibility for systemic palliation. Alternatively, the patient's prognosis could be established through clinical observation alone, and the response to palliative chemotherapy could be gauged simply by following the supraclavicular lesion. In summary, establishing that the patient did have a colonic primary tumor might be worthwhile to reduce the likelihood, through limited surgery, of the complication of a bowel obstruction. Any further diagnostic studies would be elective and probably unnecessary.

For Detailed Discussion: (1) Chapter 33, "Imaging Cancer of Unknown Primary Site."

Answer 1.28. **The answer is (d).**

Tamoxifen has been shown to have both estrogen agonist and antagonist properties. In human breast cancer, tamoxifen has predominately an antiestrogen effect, and is generally used in patients whose tumors are known to be estrogen-receptor–positive. Tamoxifen induces the synthesis of transforming growth factor-beta (TGF-B) and induces insulin-like growth factor 1, which is a mutagen for breast cancer. These properties of tamoxifen may explain its efficacy, albeit limited, in estrogen receptor–negative tumors.

For Detailed Discussion: (1) Chapter 29, "Chemoprevention of Cancer."

Answer 1.29.   **The correct answer is (a).**

The intracellular receptors for retinoids and thyroid hormone both belong to the steroid receptor family. These receptors are involved in the selective regulation of transcription of specific genes that control cell growth and differentiation. Retinoids are also responsible for maintaining normal differentiation and proliferation of mesenchymal cells as well as arresting the process of carcinogenesis. Retinoids are necessary for stem cells to mature and differentiate. Retinoids and tamoxifen have a synergistic effect in chemoprevention.

For Detailed Discussion: (1) Chapter 29, "Chemoprevention of Cancer."

Answer 1.30.   **The correct answer is (b).**

Several management options exist for patients whose smears are interpreted as ASCUS, depending on the clinical circumstances and whether the diagnosis of ASCUS is further qualified. These options include the following:

1. Follow-up by repeat Pap smears every 4 to 6 months for 2 years is acceptable, particularly when the diagnosis is not qualified further or a reactive process is favored. When the patient has three consecutive negative smears, the patient can be monitored according to routine screening protocols. If a second ASCUS report occurs in the 2-year period, the patient should be considered for colposcopy.
2. If specific infections are identified, repeat the Pap smear after appropriate treatment. However, treatment is not indicated in the absence of a specific diagnosis of infection.
3. If the patient is postmenopausal and not receiving hormone replacement therapy, repeat the Pap smear after a course of topical estrogen therapy. If ASCUS persists, colposcopy should be considered.
4. If the patient is at high risk (previous high-grade lesion, poor compliance for follow-up, and so on), colposcopy could be considered.
5. If the diagnosis of ASCUS is qualified by a statement indicating that a neoplastic process is favored, the patient should be managed as if she had a diagnosis of low-grade squamous intraepithelial lesion.

For Detailed Discussion: (1) Chapter 31, "Principles of Cancer Pathology."

Answer 1.31.   **The answer is (d).**

Different types of specimens require different work-ups. In this case, the clinical suspicion is that of lymphoma. In order to properly diagnose and subcategorize a lymphoma, special studies need to be performed that require both fresh frozen tissue and unusual fixatives. Ideally, the pathologist should be notified before the biopsy is performed in order to carefully plan the course of action, with the clinician performing the procedure in order not to compromise the valuable tissue sample.

For Detailed Discussion: (1) Chapter 31, "Principles of Cancer Pathology."

Answer 1.32.   The answer is (e).

Most antigens are not totally specific. Although keratin staining is usually seen in carcinomas rather than other malignant tumors, it has been reported in lymphomas, melanomas, sarcomas, and so on. As a general principle, a select panel of antibodies rather than a single marker is useful in pinpointing the site of origin of a metastatic lesion. In this case, if keratin is positive while leukocyte common antigen and melanoma-associated antigen are negative, the most likely diagnosis is metastatic carcinoma.

For Detailed Discussion: (1) Chapter 31, "Principles of Cancer Pathology."

Answer 1.33.   The answer is (d).

One of the most important principles to remember is that a negative biopsy does not rule out the possibility of carcinoma unless one is sure of the adequacy of sampling. If a specific lesion is removed and appropriately sectioned, that is a definitive diagnosis. In this case, the findings are nonspecific, and the mammographic appearance does not correlate well with the pathologic findings. The first comparison would be the preoperative mammogram and a specimen mammogram (if one was obtained). If no specimen mammogram was obtained, a repeat mammogram should be performed as soon as compression could be tolerated by the patient. If the calcified nodule has been removed, the patient should be reassured; routine follow-up would be appropriate. If not, additional surgery is warranted.

For Detailed Discussion: (1) Chapter 31, "Principles of Cancer Pathology."

Answer 1.34.   The answer is (d).

Evaluation of the patient with musculoskeletal pain and/or swelling should almost always begin with radiographs. If an aggressive or malignant-appearing bone lesion is identified, cross-sectional imaging should be undertaken to evaluate the full extent of the lesion. If the bony lesion is calcified or shows matrix mineralization on plain radiographs, CT may be the most useful modality. In the case of a purely lytic lesion, MRI is often the modality of choice. Radionuclide bone scans are useful to evaluate for bony metastatic disease. Ultrasound plays no role in the evaluation of a bone tumor.

For Detailed Discussion: (1) Chapter 37, "Cross-Sectional Imaging of Musculoskeletal Neoplasms."

Answer 1.35.   The answer is (e).

Radiolabeled MoAB can be directed against a variety of tumor antigens associated with specific tumor types; use of MoAb labeled with different radionuclides is currently under investigation. The use of MoAB fragments instead of whole immunoglobulin G molecules has a number of advantages. Tc 99m–labeled fragments are less immunogenic, which results in a decreased HAMA response. These fragments are also cleared from the circulation more quickly. Labeled fragments have a higher tumor-to-background ratio, which can be reached earlier following injection, thus facilitating tumor detection.

For Detailed Discussion: (1) Chapter 40, "Radionuclide Imaging in Cancer Medicine."

Answer 1.36. **The correct answer is (c).**

Radionuclides can be used both for tumor imaging and therapy in patients who have a variety of malignancies. The most commonly used radionuclides for imaging include gallium 67 and thallium 201. Bone-seeking radionuclides represent a promising approach in the treatment of patients who have symptomatic bony metastases from a wide variety of primary tumors. Strontium 89 is currently the only radionuclide approved in the United States for the treatment of bony metastases. Other bone-seeking radionuclides currently under investigation for the treatment of bony metastases are samarium 156 and rhenium 186. Iodine 123 is not a bone-seeking radionuclide. Instead, 1 123 is a non–beta-emitting isotope of iodine used in the diagnostic evaluation of patients who have thyroid carcinoma.

For Detailed Discussion: (1) Chapter 40, "Radionuclide Imaging in Cancer Medicine."

Answer 1.37. **The correct answer is (b).**

The Physician Insurers Association of America is an organization that is comprised of professional liability insurers owned or managed by physicians. Their statistics have demonstrated that the top five misdiagnosed conditions in the United States are: (1) breast cancer, (2) lung cancer, (3) appendicitis, (4) acute myocardial infarction, and (5) ectopic pregnancy. Cancers in the top-20 list of conditions that result in the largest payouts by malpractice insurers were cancers of the breast, lung, colon, rectum, and anus.

For Detailed Discussion: (1) Chapter 92, "Legal Aspects of Cancer."

Answer 1.38. **The answer is (b).**

Real-time and Doppler sonography are able to visualize most soft-tissue structures and blood vessels. The physics of ultrasound, however, renders penetration of materials that are acoustically dissimilar impossible. For that reason, structures that lie beneath bone or behind air may be impossible to see. As such, pulmonary abscesses and other lesions within the lung are usually impossible to visualize because of overlying air.

For Detailed Discussion: (1) Chapter 39, "Ultrasound in Cancer Medicine."

Answer 1.39. **The answer is (e).**

Ultrasound is an excellent method of determining whether or not lesions are solid or fluid-filled; differentiation can usually be made between those that require surgery (intratesticular masses) versus those that do not (extratesticular masses). Additionally, the various extratesticular lesions such as hydrocele, varicocele, or spermatocele are usually readily differentiated sonographically. Sonography, however, is unable to differentiate between the various types of intratesticular malignancies, because their features tend to be identical.

For Detailed Discussion: (1) Chapter 39, "Ultrasound in Cancer Medicine."

Answer 1.40.   **The answer is (c).**

Work continues toward finding specific Doppler signals that would allow differentiation of benign versus malignant masses in many organs. Unfortunately thus far, this technique has been unsuccessful in the breast because of frequent overlap in the vascular signals and color Doppler patterns when comparing benign lesions to malignant lesions.

For Detailed Discussion: (1) Chapter 39, "Ultrasound in Cancer Medicine."

Answer 1.41.   **The answer is (d).**

Endovaginal sonography affords excellent images of the internal characteristics of both the uterus and ovaries. Therefore, small masses such as submucosal leiomyomas are readily identified as discrete hypoechoic lesions by virtue of producing a mass effect on the endometrial canal. On the other hand, CT has proved more effective in staging tumors than ultrasound, because it can depict pelvic sidewall disease and nodal adenopathy. Regarding the differentiation of benign from malignant nodules in the prostate, little can be done with any imaging technique, and biopsy is generally required. Finally, although endovaginal sonography is capable of identifying small ovarian masses, the low prevalence of this disease in the general population would not render any screening modality cost effective.

For Detailed Discussion: (1) Chapter 39, "Ultrasound in Cancer Medicine."

Answer 1.42.   **The answer is (d).**

Tumor initiation is a necessary, but not sufficient, step in the change from benign growth to malignant conversion and ultimately to tumor progression. The initiating event is a primary and irreversible change or mutation in a cell that *may* eventually yield a tumor. Such an initiating event is typically a mutation in a proto-oncogene or a deactivation of a tumor suppressor gene; such an event is best typified by a chemical carcinogen that covalently modifies the structure of DNA, often by formation of an adduct between the chemical carcinogen and a nucleotide. Tumor promotion is a selective clonal expansion of initiated cells that produces a large population of cells at risk for further genetic changes and ultimately malignant conversion. Tumor promoters are usually not mutagenic and not carcinogenic alone, but may reduce the latency for tumors after exposure to an initiator, or may lower the dose of initiator required to incite the entire process.

For Detailed Discussion: (1) Chapter 13, "Chemical Carcinogenesis."

Answer 1.43.   **The answer is (a).**

Suicide enzymes involved in DNA repair include alkyl-transferases, which are capable of removing an alkyl group from an alkylated base to a cysteine residue without requiring DNA strand scission. An endonuclease may remove a distorted piece of DNA, thereby leaving the intact stand as a template to be "patched" by 5′ to 3′ polymerization with subsequent ligation-free ends. This so-called DNA-nucleotide excision repair mechanism is defective in the cancer predisposition syndrome, xeroderma pigmentosum. A covalently modified segment of DNA may be removed by a base excision repair catalyzed by a glycosylase enzyme. This is useful for repair of small alkyl groups that are adducted to DNA base. If non-alkylated bases are opposite from non-complementary Watson-Crick bases, then DNA mismatch repair is required to correct this problem. Large pieces of DNA are often removed to correct such mismatched pairings. A GATC recognition sequence is usually required for this process.

For Detailed Discussion: (1) Chapter 13, "Chemical Carcinogenesis."

Answer 1.44.   The answer is (c).

Aflatoxins (there are at least four subtypes) are *Aspergillus* spp metabolites that may contaminate cereals, grains, and nuts. They require activation by enzymes in the cytochrome P-450 reductase system. The aflatoxin-8,9-oxide is reactive and binds covalently to the N7 position on deoxyguanosine (this is a purine base, and the chemical does not bind with pyrimidine bases).

For Detailed Discussion: (1) Chapter 13, "Chemical Carcinogenesis."

Answer 1.45.   The answer is (d).

The hallmark of invasion is the loss of integrity of the barrier to invasion, in this case, the epithelial basement membrane. A key component of invasion is the ability to locally degrade the basement membrane to provide a point of departure for invasive cells. The initial diagnosis was that of in situ carcinoma, one that cannot be supported by the finding of metastatic cells in the axillary lymph nodes. Careful review and further sectioning of the primary lesion might uncover loss of basement membrane integrity. With lymph node metastasis, one would expect to find other hallmarks of invasive cancer in the primary lesion, such as microvessel formation and infiltrating tumor cell (of the same histologic subtype found in the node). Atrophy is unrelated to the diagnosis of cancer.

For Detailed Discussion: Chapter 9, "Invasion and Metastasis."

Answer 1.46.   The answer is (b).

Loss of E-cadherin, an epithelial adhesion factor, has been demonstrated in progressive metastatic colon cancer. Scatter factor/HGF is a factor that induces migration of tumor cells and endothelial cells. Transfection of scatter factor/HGF into non-metastatic cells makes them metastatic, whereas introduction of E-cadherin can abrogate metastatic potential. Neovascularization has been shown to be a predictive marker for poor prognosis in breast cancer, ovarian cancer, and prostate cancer, as well as other cancers. Increased MMP-2 production, whether documented by immunostaining of tumors or measured in plasma, portends invasive disease and a poor prognosis. In contrast, *nm23* is a gene that in most cancers studies is lost in metastatic disease and transfection of which is associated with loss of the metastatic phenotype but not the malignant phenotype. Therefore, increased expression of *nm23* would be a marker not of clinical cancer progression but of a better phenotype and reduced metastatic potential.

For Detailed Discussion: (1) Chapter 9, "Invasion and Metastatis."

Answer 1.47. **The answer is (e).**

The critical components of invasion are cell-cell and/or the cell-extracellular matrix/basement membrane adhesion, local proteolytic degradation of the extracellular matrix, and migration. All of these events require translocation of cells and local environmental remodeling. In bone modeling, osteoblasts and osteoclasts migrate within the bone, locally degrading and relaying bone matrix and anchoring themselves to the matrix. Wound healing and neovascularization require fibroblasts and endothelial cells, respectively, to interact with the local environment to fill in the wound with fresh matrix and cells or, in the case of angiogenesis, to form capillary sprouts that then open to form new capillaries. Adhesion, proteolysis, and migration are actively at work in those settings. In the development of inflammatory exudates, inflammatory cells must sense the stimulus, adhere to vascular cells and basement membranes, and translocate across a proteolyzed rent in the basement membrane to migrate into the site of infection. Thus, invasion, although the hallmark of malignancy when it is unregulated, can be found physiologically in many normal processes of the body. Not listed is embryonic development and placental implantation and development, other events that require regulation invasion. Serous transudation occurs without inflammatory cells, and invasion does not occur.

For Detailed Discussion: (1) Chapter 9, "Invasion and Metastasis."

Answer 1.48. **The answer is (d).**

Alpha-interferon at 5 million units daily or 10 million units three times a week has been shown in randomized trials to be more effective in HBsAg seroconversion than no therapy. Factors predictive of favorable response to alpha-interferon include high serum transaminase levels, low serum HBV DNA levels, and active hepatic necro-inflammation. Patients who have normal ALT levels and high serum HBV DNA rarely respond to alpha-interferon. Lower doses of alpha-interferon (3 million units three times a week), which are effective for chronic HCV infection, are not satisfactory for an HBV infection. The use of hepatitis B vaccine in seropositive patients is controversial, and is not generally given despite anecdotal reports of seroconversion in some patients. Hepatitis immunoglobulin is effective in preventing HBV infection when administered to seronegative patients following exposure to HBV, such as needlestick puncture and postdelivery from an infected mother.

For Detailed Discussion: (1) Chapter 23, "Hepatitis Viruses."

Answer 1.49. **The answer is (d).**

Alpha-interferon 3 million units three times a week for 6 months is the only treatment effective for chronic HCV infection. Forty-one percent of treated patients had normalization of serum ALT, and 70% of responders had an improvement in necro-inflammation of the liver as revealed by biopsy. Favorable predictors of response include the absence of advanced inflammation or cirrhosis as revealed by liver histology and low levels of HCV RNA. Patients should therefore undergo liver biopsy to assess the degree of necro-inflammation of the liver to determine the probability of response to alpha-interferon. Hepatitis B vaccine is ineffective for chronic HCV infection.

For Detailed Discussion: (1) Chapter 23, "Hepatitis Viruses."

Answer 1.50.   **The answer is (d).**

Patients who have advanced cirrhosis and chronic HCV infection rarely respond to alpha-interferon. Patients who undergo orthotopic liver transplantation and are found to have a small hepatocellular carcinoma (less than 5 cm) have an excellent prognosis, with survival similar to that of patients who undergo transplantation and do not have hepatocellular carcinoma. Because this patient has demonstrated alcohol abstinence for 2 years, he is a good candidate for orthotopic liver transplantation. Liver biopsy and hepatic arterial chemoembolization are high-risk procedures in patients who have end-stage liver disease, and, given the excellent survival of patients with a small hepatocellular carcinoma following transplantation, these procedures are not indicated for this patient.

For Detailed Discussion: (1) Chapter 23, "Hepatitis Viruses."

Answer 1.51.   **The answer is (d).**

Breast cancer is one of the malignancies that is associated with an affluent life-style. It has been postulated that dietary factors play a central role in the increased risk noted in women of North America and much of Europe. Although this patient is at risk of a second primary tumor, and the risk of breast cancer in her first-degree family members is slightly increased, they are also at risk for many other diseases common in our affluent society. The dietary recommendations for this woman and her family should include the knowledge derived from studies of nutrition and cardiovascular disease, hypertension, diabetes, osteoporosis, and other illnesses. There are no studies indicating that supplement use will prevent breast cancer. Products that are of no documented benefit include vitamin and mineral supplements from reputable pharmaceutical companies or the diverse array of poorly characterized and unregulated products sold by many stores or practitioners of "alternative" medicine. A vegetarian diet can be a healthy approach to eating, but it is not necessary in order to achieve the current guidelines for cancer prevention that have been provided by various organizations. Foods labeled "natural" and "organic" have no proven benefit, and understanding of these terms is complicated by the fact that the laws and regulations concerning their use are vague and rarely enforced. The precise role of dietary fat in breast cancer and determining what the ideal intake of dietary fat is remain controversial. Recommending less than 10% fat calories in the diet is considered excessive by most experts and would require major changes in the types of food chosen, and perhaps this dietary goal would put the individual at risk for inadequate intake of various vitamins and minerals. The updated guidelines provided by the American Cancer Society, National Cancer Institute, and United States Department of Agriculture provide a very reasonable starting point for dietary changes to prevent malignancies and other chronic diseases characteristic of our society. Few oncologists have the knowledge or time to provide practical instruction concerning the dietary recommendations. The best resource for assisting in patient education in diet and nutrition is a registered dietitian.

For Detailed Discussion: (1) Chapter 28, "Nutrition in the Etiology and Prevention of Cancer."

Answer 1.52.   **The answer is (b).**

No data other than the claim by Nobel laureate Pauling support the activity of vitamin C in human cancer. Study design for such a major claim requires random allocation of patients of identical stage to a treatment regimen with and without vitamin C. Anecdotal descriptions do not suffice.

For Detailed Discussion: (1) Chapter 96, "Questionable Cancer Therapies."

Answer 1.53.   **The answer is (b).**

Hearsay is unreliable. Desperate patients may seek help out of lack of confidence that the treatment prescribed will work, and they should not be ostracized nor lionized for their aspiration. Review of written material may uncover facts that help the patient understand the physician's opinion, and may avoid dangerous confounding drug interactions.

For Detailed Discussion: (1) Chapter 96, "Questionable Cancer Therapies."

Answer 1.54.   **The answer is (d).**

The restriction point or start site in the cell cycle was originally discovered when normal cells, at low serum concentrations, accumulated at a point during late G1 phase. The addition of serum to the culture allowed the cells to proceed through the cycle. Once past the restriction point, the cells were committed to DNA synthesis and usually cell division. The restriction point is not a component of the G0 or S phases of the cell cycle.

For Detailed Discussion: (1) Chapter 1, "Cell Proliferation and Differentiation."

Answer 1.55.   **The answer is (b).**

Proto-oncogenes are normal growth regulatory genes that may cause neoplasia when altered as a result of mutations, deletions, translocations, amplifications, or other factors. Juxtaposition of the immunoglobulin gene—which has a strong promoter during B-cell development—with the *c-myc* gene leads to a hybrid gene whose product causes excessive cell proliferation, that is, cancer. This applies particularly to Burkitt's lymphoma with characteristic t(8;14), but not to large-cell, non-Hodgkin's lymphoma. Gene amplification of *c-myc,* which may be evidenced cytogenetically (by double minutes and homogeneously staining regions) as well as by molecular biology probes, commonly occurs in neuroblastoma and in small-cell lung carcinoma, but not in gastric or esophageal cancer.

For Detailed Discussion: (1) Chapter 5, "Oncogenes."

Answer 1.56. **The answer is (a).**

The first laboratory evidence for a substance in normal cells that suppressed neoplasia was the observation that hybrids of normal and neoplastic cells were phenotypically normal. Knudsen's studies of retinoblastoma (Rb) strongly suggested that there was a familial and a nonfamilial type of retinoblastoma. The familial type was seen at a younger age, was multifocal, and was associated with a family history suggesting recessive genetic traits. He then developed the two-hit hypothesis. For the familial type, one hit (mutant or deleted allele) was present in the germ line. A subsequent acquired hit (mutation) in the opposite allele would equate to loss of tumor suppressor activity, and therefore cancer. For the acquired type of retinoblastoma, two mutational hits in the *Rb* genes would be required for overt neoplasia, a much less likely event than the one environmental hit required in the familial type.

For Detailed Discussion: (1) Chapter 6, "Tumor Suppressor and DNA Repair Gene Defects in Human Cancer." (2) Levine AJ. Tumor suppressor genes. In: Mendelsohn., Howley, Israel, and Liotto, eds. The Molecular Basis of Cancer. Philadelphia: WB Saunders, 1995, pp 3–18.

Answer 1.57. **The answer is (e).**

Probing for loss of heterozygosity is a method of identifying areas on the genome where one of the two alleles for a given gene or genes is either mutated or deleted. If a given gene or gene area is consistently (i.e., clonally) lost for a given tumor, it is inferred that the area may contain a tumor suppressor gene (TSG) and that loss on the sister allele would result in tumorigenicity. Cytogenetically evident deletions are much larger than LOH areas, but if they occur consistently at a given location for a tumor, they also identify areas containing TSGs. Although originally described for retinoblastoma, the *Rb* gene has been found to be deleted in unrelated tumors (e.g., in 70% of patients who have small-cell lung carcinoma). In the more common adult epithelial tumors, *Rb* gene mutations may serve as one of the sequence of genetic changes required for tumorigenicity. A defective *Rb* gene (either through its absence or due to constitutive phosphorylation) cannot form a complex with free E2F proteins, which activate genes promoting entry into the DNA synthesis phase of the cell cycle.

For Detailed Discussion: (1) Chapter 6, "Tumor Suppressors and DNA Repair Gene Defects in Human Cancer."

Answer 1.58. **The answer is (c).**

The molecular control of the cell cycle is becoming increasingly understood. The control of transit through the cell cycle is mediated by cyclin-dependent kinases (CDK) along with their regulatory subunit cyclins. The CDK/cyclin system is under the regulatory control of inhibitors such as *Rb* and other tumor suppressor gene products. Phosphorylation by kinases activates many of these products. For example, the Rb gene product must become phosphorylated in order to open the restriction point gate and allow for transit of the cell into the S phase. Products of oncogenic viruses can bind and functionally deplete the cells of the *Rb gene product. p53,* another tumor suppressor gene, transcriptionally activates genes such as *WAF1/CIP/p21,* which regulates CDK activity.

For Detailed Discussion: (1) Chapter 1, "Cell Proliferation and Differentiation." (2) Hunter T, et al. Cyclins and cancer II: cyclin D and cdK inhibitors come of age. Cell 1994;79:573.

Answer 1.59.   **The answer is (d).**

The slow-growing ("dormant") micrometastases, such as those that occur in breast cancer, could result from multiple factors. If the tumor cells were "resting," that is, in G0 or not in cycle, or if the cycle time was very long, the metastases would either not grow or grow very slowly. A balanced rate of cell proliferation and death could explain kinetically active cells that are not expanding tumors such as in spheroids or those that occur before the production of angiogenesis factors. A low oxygen tension such as that which occurs with diminished blood supply can reduce the growth fraction and slow tumor growth.

For Detailed Discussion: (1) Chapter 9, "Invasion and Metastasis."

Answer 1.60.   **The answer is (a).**

Although the designation B referred to the bursa, a gut appendage in the chicken, recent studies indicate that B and T cells derive from pleuripotent stem cells in the marrow. B and T cells are indistinguishable by classical hematologic stains. Each specific antigen interacts with a clone of B cells, which along with T-cell helper products, results in monoclonal antibody production. T cells respond most vigorously to mitogens. Both B and T cells respond to alloantigens. Both the immunoglobulin molecules produced by B cells and the T-cell receptor protein are the result of somatic recombination of the relevant genetic segments. This recombinational event results in the ability of the immune system to respond to an incredibly diverse spectrum of antigens to which each T or B cell clone has unique specificity.

For Detailed Discussion: (1) Chapter 11, "Tumor Immunology."

Answer 1.61.   **The answer is (e).**

Cytokines may be produced by a variety of cells including endothelial cells, but T cells and macrophages produce the widest variety. Epitopes consist of the simplest forms of an antigenic determinant to which antibodies bind. Although proteins make up most antigens, glycoprotein, carbohydrates, and lipids may also play a role in the structure of epitopes. Antibody binding to the epitope depends on spatial complementation between the epitope and the antibody binding site. With repeated exposure to the antigen, the antibodies produced exhibit increasing affinity for the epitope.

For Detailed Discussion: (1) Chapter 11, "Tumor Immunology."

Answer 1.62.   **The answer is (b).**

Antibody diversity is extraordinary and occurs by somatic genomic mutations: Somatic recombination of immunoglobulin genes are fundamental to diversity generation. There may be association of different H and L chains. Hypermutable regions exist in which somatic mutations occur within complementarity-determining regions, thus promoting variation. Within the variable region of the H chain, for example, there are more than 100 variable areas joining diversity segments that can recombine in various ways. High-affinity, antibody-producing cells are selected through signals received following ligation of surface Ig by the appropriate antibody.

For Detailed Discussion: (1) Chapter 11, "Tumor Immunology."

Answer 1.63.   **The answer is (b).**

A revolution in the science of immunology occurred after the discovery of monoclonal antibody production. Within a few years, monoclonal antibodies were prepared against normal and neoplastic determinants that proved invaluable in the study of differentiation subsets and their function. These clusters of differentiation became known as CD. Tumor cells in contrast to normal cells commonly exhibited lineage infidelity. T cells assist B cells in the production of immunoglobulin by the production of certain cytokines. For example, IL-2, IL-4, and IL-5 drive IgM production; IL-2, IL-4, and IL-6 drive IgA production; IL-5 promotes IgG production; and IL-4 enhances IgG production.

For Detailed Discussion: (1) Chapter 11, "Tumor Immunology."

Answer 1.64.   **The answer is (b).**

Mature T-lymphocytes traffic through peripheral circulation and return through the venous and post-capillary venules to the skin and lymph nodes. T-lymphocytes recognize antigenic peptide only on the surface of antigen-presenting cells. Binding to tumor cell–receptor antigens generates a primary signal that traverses the lymphocyte membrane, which activates protein tyrosine kinase on the cytoplasmic extension of the receptor. This signal is then transduced through a series of protein phosphorylations, including activation of protein kinase C and the release of intracellular calcium. Full activation requires one or more co-stimulatory signals, such as B7.

For Detailed Discussion: (1) Chapter 11, "Tumor Immunology."

Answer 1.65.   **The answer is (b).**

Mature T cells express either CD4 helper or CD 8 cytotoxic and suppressor properties but not both. Mature T cells represent approximately 80% of normal blood lymphocytes, 35% of the lymph node cells, and only 25% of splenic lymphocytes. An immunologically functioning T-cell clone is produced by interaction with an appropriately processed and presented antigen in the presence of major histocompatibility complex molecules and co-stimulatory factors. When the antigen is cleared, the T-cell clone persists in small numbers (memory cells), which have the capacity for rapid expansion if again exposed to the antigen. Cytokine production is one basis for subdividing lymphocyte populations.

For Detailed Discussion: (1) Chapter 11, "Tumor Immunology."

Answer 1.66. **The answer is (d).**

Natural killer cells express the CD 56(NKH1) and IL-2 receptors, intracytoplasmic granules, and a binding site or surface receptor for the Fc region of IgG. They also have the ability to exercise antibody-dependent, cell-mediated cytotoxicity. NK cells have the ability to destroy tumor cells in the absence of specific immunoglobulin antibody. NK cell activity is increased by IL-2 , interferon, and TNF.

For Detailed Discussion: (1) Chapter 11, "Tumor Immunology."

Answer 1.67. **The answer is (b).**

Acute T-cell leukemia is caused by a retrovirus, human T-cell lymphotrophic virus (HTLV-III). Colon cancer is not known to be caused by a microorganism. Some cases of non-Hodgkin's lymphoma (especially in the immunosuppressed) and virtually all cases of nasopharyngeal carcinoma are associated with the Epstein-Barr virus. Cervical carcinoma is caused by the human papillomavirus. Recent evidence indicates that *Helicobacter* may play a role in the development of gastric cancer and gastric lymphoma. Finally, hepatitis B and C viruses can lead to chronic hepatitis, which increases the risk of hepatoma. Hepatitis C has been linked to non-Hodgkin's lymphoma with mixed cryoglobulinemia.

For Detailed Discussion: (1) Chapter 11, "Tumor Immunology."

Answer 1.68. **The answer is (e).**

Class I MHC antigens are expressed on the cell surface of almost all normal cells. These antigens contain β_2-microglobulin, which is released into the blood during cell turnover and, for many tumors (e.g., myeloma), correlates with tumor burden and growth. Class II antigens normally are expressed by lymphoreticular and endothelial cells. They may be induced on epithelial cells by inflammation or gamma interferon. Expression of class I gene products may be increased or decreased by neoplasia. Such changes may relate to immune surveillance and metastasis potential. It is interesting that tumor cells that express less MHC class I products are more resistant to cytotoxic T-lymphocytes, but conversely more sensitive to NK cell attack.

For Detailed Discussion: (1) Chapter 11, "Tumor Immunology."

Answer 1.69. **The answer is (b).**

Oncofetal antigens are expressed during fetal development but not in normal adult tissues. Such antigens are re-expressed during the neoplastic process, but this also occurs in benign, chronic diseases associated with normal cell turnover, such as infectious hepatitis, ulcerative colitis, and other inflammatory conditions. Human chorionic gonadotropin is the most sensitive oncofetal protein for monitoring microscopic tumor. For example, in patients who have gestational choriocarcinoma, this protein can detect as few as 1000 cells. Alpha-fetoprotein is useful in the diagnosis and monitoring of hepatoma, but this marker is also elevated in benign hepatic disease. CA-125 is an ovarian antigen that is commonly elevated in diseases that involve the peritoneal surface, such as ovarian cancer, as well as endometriosis, pelvic inflammatory disease, and a variety of carcinomas. Therefore, CA-125 is not sufficiently sensitive and specific enough for use alone or in combination in the detection of ovarian cancer.

For Detailed Discussion: (1) Chapter 11, "Tumor Immunology."

Answer 1.70. **The answer is (a).**

Human chorionic gonadotropin levels in patients who have gestational choriocarcinoma usually decline rapidly and exponentially toward normal values after chemotherapy. If the hCG level remains normal for several months, the likelihood that the patient is cured is approximately 90%. In patients who have non-Hodgkin's lymphoma, detectable levels of IL-10 predict for a poor prognosis. Serum levels of β_2-microglobulin predict response and allow for evaluation of response in myeloma and non-Hodgkin's lymphoma. Serum levels of IL-2 receptor correlate with disease activity in adult T-cell leukemia and in childhood non-Hodgkin's lymphoma. Finally, serum levels of an intracellular adhesion molecule, ICAM-1, correlate with disease activity for several childhood solid tumors.

For Detailed Discussion: (1) Chapter 11, "Tumor Immunology."

Answer 1.71. **The answer is (b).**

Large tumors, those with eccentric calcification, and particularly those with spiculated margins or endocrine-related syndromes are most always malignant. Lesions associated with endocrinopathies, such as inappropriate secretion of antidiuretic hormone or Cushing's syndrome, are usually due to lung cancer. Concentric calcification is somewhat reassuring. However, it is critically important to examine old radiographs for evidence of either change or stability.

For Detailed Discussion: (1) Chapter 35, "Imaging Neoplasms of the Thorax."

Answer 1.72. **The answer is (d).**

CT scanning cannot provide a specific explanation for lymphadeonopathy, cannot distinguish benign from malignant growth, and cannot visualize micrometastasis. The most useful information derives from hilar or mediastinal invasion or lympadenopathy. Although confirmation by invasive staging is required, the presence of mediastinal invasion is a contradiction to surgical resection.

For Detailed Discussion: (1) Chapter 35, "Imaging Neoplasms of the Thorax."

Answer 1.73. **The answer is (c).**

Although obviously a difficult situation, the patient, when alert, expressed a clear desire not to be maintained on mechanical ventilation. Patients have a constitutional right to refuse medical care. There is little difference between withholding an intervention and withdrawing the same intervention once it has begun. As such, the physician should honor the patient's wishes by discontinuing mechanical ventilation. Perhaps a "do not resuscitate" order should have been placed in the chart immediately upon the patient's admission.

For Detailed Discussion: (1) Chapter 91, "Ethical Aspects of Caring for Patients with Cancer."

Answer 1.74. **The answer is (a).**

Tumors with mutated *p53* respond to chemotherapy less well than those with the wild type gene, and animals and patients bearing *p53*–mutated tumors die faster. Bcl-2 expression inhibits apoptosis, but is not known to impair response to fludarabine in chronic lymphocytic leukemia. P-glycoprotein expression is associated with the multidrug resistance phenotype, and its absent expression would imply that the multidrug resistance pump is not the mechanism for resistance. Although mutated *ras* is common as a disease characteristic of alimentary tract and other cancers, and in itself is an attractive chemotherapeutic target, it is not specifically associated with a resistance. Mutation or loss of nm 23 predisposes to metastases. Its expression is the normal phenotype and not related to chemotherapy resistance.

For Detailed Discussion: (1) Chapter 4, "Signal Transduction in Cancer."

Answer 1.75. **The answer is (a).**

Tumor promoters, such as phorbol esters, activate protein kinases, which then initiate a cascade of biochemical events that result in signal transduction. Most tumor promoters stimulate growth cells with mutated DNA, which invites additional mutations that eventually promote autonomous proliferation. Protein phosphatases counterbalance this activity by catalyzing removal of phosphate bonds. Tumor promoters do not bring about reduced cellular calcium, direct activation of transcription factors, or amplification of surface receptors.

For Detailed Discussion: (1) Chapter 4, "Signal Transduction in Cancer."

Answer 1.76. **The answer is (c).**

The most important criterion for planning therapy is the histology of the tumor, together with knowledge of its origin. Thus, although radiology is indispensable, and may contribute to decisions on management, if the cancer is truly of an unknown primary site, the outcome will not be much changed. Thus, radiologic imaging may be most helpful to exclude a mass in the breast, for example, or disease in an unsuspected primary site, such as lung, pancreas, kidney, adrenal, stomach, or prostate, each of which might indicate different and distinct therapeutic approaches.

For Detailed Discussion: (1) Chapter 33, "Imaging Cancer of Unknown Primary Site."

Answer 1.77. **The answer is (c).**

Before undertaking treatment, the primary source must be known. Bilateral high neck nodes most often arise from cancers of the upper aerodigestive tract, or lymphomas. Endoscopy of the nasopharynx, oropharynx , and larynx, as well as MRI, are all useful, the latter often more so than CT scanning (which is indicated if bone involvement is present). Lung cancers would uncommonly spread to bilateral upper neck nodes without involving supraclavicular or lower cervical nodes on either side. Abdominal primary tumors would be even less likely to cause this scenario.

For Detailed Discussion: (1) Chapter 33, "Imaging Cancer of Unknown Primary Site."

CHAPTER 2

Treatment Principles

DIRECTIONS: Each question below contains five suggested responses. Select the best response to each question.

QUESTIONS

Question 2.1. **Which of the following phases of the cell cycle is the most radiosensitive?**

a) G0
b) G1
c) M
d) S
e) All phases of the cell cycle are equally radiosensitive.

Question 2.2. **Radiation dose is defined as the absorption of:**

a) Heat per unit mass (kcal/kg)
b) Heat per unit volume (kcal/cm^2)
c) Energy per unit mass (J/kg)
d) Energy per unit volume (J/cm^2)
e) None of the aforementioned

Question 2.3. **Which of the following isotopes is not currently used in either intracavitary or interstitial brachytherapy?**

a) Iridium 198
b) Cesium 137
c) Radium 226
d) Iodine 125
e) All are currently used in modern brachytherapy.

Question 2.4. **Which of the following chemotherapeutic agents enhances cell kill at elevated temperatures?**

a) Bleomycin
b) 5-fluorouracil (5-FU)
c) Methotrexate
d) Topoisomerase inhibitors
e) Vincristine

Question 2.5. **All of the following render cells more sensitive to hyperthermia EXCEPT:**

a) Low pH
b) High oxygen tension
c) Low glucose levels

d)   All of the aforementioned render cells more sensitive to hyperthermia.
e)   None of the aforementioned render cells more sensitive to hyperthermia.

Question 2.6.   **The development of thermotolerance in cells treated with heat (40 to 42°C) is accompanied by the preferential synthesis of a series of proteins referred to as:**

a)   Thermotolerance proteins
b)   Heat shock proteins
c)   Threshold proteins
d)   Heat-resistance proteins
e)   Heating does not result in protein synthesis.

Question 2.7.   **A 2-year-old child who has not previously had seizures is receiving treatment for a glioma with high-dose cyclophosphamide and intravenous (IV) 5% dextrose solution for hydration. Near the end of the infusion, the child has a seizure. A diagnostic technique likely to discover the cause would be:**

a)   A magnetic resonance image (MRI) of the head
b)   A complete neurologic examination
c)   Serum electrolyte determination
d)   Toxicology screen
e)   Cerebrospinal fluid (CSF) examination

Question 2.8.   **Alkylating agents are a usual component of high-dose therapy with stem cell support for breast cancer. This is because:**

a)   Alkylating agents are especially active against breast cancer.
b)   Alkylating agents have a steep dose-response curve, with bone marrow
     suppression being the usual dose-limiting toxicity.
c)   Alkylating agents are synergistic with 5-FU.
d)   Alkylating agents' most common toxicity is neurotoxicity.
e)   The usual resistance mechanism of breast cancer cells to alkylating agents is
     P-glycoprotein.

Question 2.9.   **A significant difference between cisplatin and carboplatin is:**

a)   The predominant toxicity of carboplatin is hematopoietic; renal and neurologic
     toxicity are less than that with cisplatin.
b)   Carboplatin is synergistic with alkylating agents, whereas cisplatin is not.
c)   Carboplatin is more active against lymphomas than is cisplatin.
d)   Tumors resistant to cisplatin are usually not cross-resistant to carboplatin.
e)   Carboplatin is a substrate for multidrug resistance (MDR), while cisplatin is not.

Question 2.10.   **A 45-year-old man who has chronic myeloid leukemia in the stable phase has a histocompatible sibling donor. In the course of discussions concerning potential allogenic bone marrow transplantation, certain issues regarding graft-versus-host disease are reviewed. All of the following statements about graft-versus-host disease are correct EXCEPT:**

a)   The likelihood of graft-versus-host disease is diminished if the donor's bone
     marrow is purged of some or all T cells before infusion into the patient.

b)   The most common sites affected are the skin, liver, and gastrointestinal tract.
c)   Graft-versus-host disease is more likely to occur in an allogenic rather than a syngeneic transplantation.
d)   Acute graft-versus-host disease is a risk factor for the eventual development of chronic graft-versus-host disease.
e)   The chief cause of mortality in a non–T-cell-depleted allogeneic bone marrow transplantation is leukemic relapse rather than graft-versus-host disease.

Question 2.11.   Which of the following statements regarding metabolic derangements involved in cancer cachexia is false?

a)   The enzyme hexokinase, which catalyzes the first step of the glycolytic pathway, is found to be highly overexpressed in tumor cells.
b)   The Cori cycle is the cyclic metabolic pathway in which glucose is converted to lactic acid by glycolysis in tumor tissue and then reconverted back to glucose in the liver.
c)   Tumors are effective nitrogen traps, and nitrogen is translocated from host to tumor, which produces nitrogen depletion of the host. Successful competition for nitrogen by tumors is not considered to be a major cause of cancer cachexia.
d)   The administration of recombinant tumor necrosis factor–α cachectin does not produce cachexia in humans.
e)   The metabolic manifestations of cachexia in cancer patients are similar to those of healthy subjects who are undergoing starvation.

Question 2.12.   A 56-year-old woman who has Stage IV breast cancer develops generalized headaches and trouble concentrating. She also complains of some tingling in her left forearm and hand. Neurologic examination is unremarkable except for absent reflexes in her left arm and right ankle, but she has normal strength and sensation. A cranial MRI scan with gadolinium is negative. The next step in the patient's evaluation should be:

a)   Electromyogram with nerve conduction studies
b)   An MRI of the cervical spine
c)   A lumbar puncture
d)   Corticosteroid therapy
e)   Careful observation

Question 2.13.   A 26-year-old man who has Stage IIA Hodgkin's disease completed mantle irradiation approximately 3 weeks ago. On a routine follow-up visit, he reports a new symptom. He develops intermittent electric shocklike feelings that travel down his back and arms into his hands. It seems that this sensation is precipitated by moving his head, particularly when he flexes his neck. The episodes last only seconds, and between episodes he is fine. The most likely cause of this symptom is:

a)   Epidural Hodgkin's disease compressing the cervical cord
b)   Lhermitte's sign
c)   Cervical disk disease
d)   Leptomeningeal metastases
e)   Psychosomatic complaint

Question 2.14.   **A 27-year-old man who has acute myelogenous leukemia in first remission has undergone allogeneic transplantation from a matched sibling donor 80 days ago. He developed moderately severe graft-versus-host disease and is still receiving cyclosporine and prednisone. He develops the rather rapid onset of cough and low-grade fever (38.2°C). Chest radiograph shows diffuse interstitial infiltrates throughout both lung fields. Complete blood count (CBC) and chemistries are unremarkable. Physical examination is unremarkable, except for mild tachycardia. Patient management should be:**

a)   Immediate increase in the steroid dose to 100 mg/d and observation

b)   Immediate open lung biopsy for diagnostic purposes

c)   Submission of blood and urine cytomegalovirus studies and immediate bronchoscopy with lavage; begin ganciclovir and intravenous immune globulin pending results of the aforementioned studies and hospitalize the patient

d)   Observation with no change in present management

e)   Administer intravenous trimethoprim-sulfamethoxazole

Question 2.15.   **A 42-year-old man completed treatment for a germ-cell tumor of the testis 1 year ago. He was treated with cisplatin, vinblastine, and bleomycin. The patient develops acute onset of abdominal pain, and laboratory study results are consistent with acute cholecystitis. A laparoscopic cholecystectomy is performed. During the immediate postoperative period, the patient becomes progressively hypoxic and requires re-intubation. Chest radiographs show diffuse interstitial abnormalities. A bronchoscopy and transbronchial biopsy is performed, which reveals moderate Type 2 pneumocyte atypia and mild interstitial fibrosis. Diagnosis and management should be:**

a)   Adult respiratory distress syndrome from sepsis secondary to cholecystitis; begin broad-spectrum antibiotics and intensive care unit support.

b)   Emphysema from prior smoking; begin a slow weaning process from the respirator.

c)   Excessive hydration by anesthesia; begin diuretic treatment.

d)   Probably bleomycin recall reaction following high oxygen concentrations during anesthesia; begin high-dose steroid treatment and reduce oxygen concentrations to the minimal required for adequate patient support.

e)   Perform open lung biopsy to rule out recurrent tumor; if present, then repeat cisplatin, vinblastine, and bleomycin chemotherapy.

Question 2.16.   **A 42-year-old woman who has Stage II breast cancer involving 23/26 axillary lymph nodes has recently undergone high-dose chemotherapy with cyclophosphamide, cisplatin, carmustine, and autologous hematopoietic progenitor cell support. She tolerated the treatment without difficulty and was returned to the care of her personal physician. Six weeks after the transplantation, she reports the onset over a 72-hour period of significant shortness of breath. The chest radiograph is unremarkable; the patient's temperature is 37.8°C, physical examination is unremarkable, and the CBC is normal. Pulmonary function tests reveal a carbon monoxide diffusing capacity 30% below pretreatment values. The patient's arterial oxygen satura-**

tion has decreased from 97% to 84% with exercise. The correct patient management would be:

a) Hospitalize the patient and perform an emergency open lung biopsy.
b) Observe the patient over a 72-hour period to confirm worsening symptoms.
c) Begin broad-spectrum antibacterial and antiviral therapy on an outpatient basis.
d) Begin high-dose steroid treatment and schedule a bronchoscopy with transbronchial biopsy and British anti-lewisite.
e) Administer trimethoprim-sulfamethoxazole.

Question 2.17. **A 26-year-old man is referred to you, an oncologist, for therapy of newly diagnosed Hodgkin's disease, diagnosed on cervical lymph node biopsy. Bone marrow biopsy also detects Hodgkin's disease. Which of the following statements are true?**

a) Semen cryopreservation at this point will be useless, because the patient has a high likelihood of having significant azoospermia.
b) Adriamycin, bleomycin, vincristine, and dacarbazine (ABVD) should be considered superior to Mustargen, Oncovin, procarbazine, and prednisone (MOPP) as a therapeutic option for this man.
c) Following 6 cycles of MOPP therapy, he will have a 50% risk of permanent infertility.
d) Following a curative course of ABVD, he should be advised that the risk of fathering defective children is high enough to warrant consideration of vasectomy.
e) Suppression of spermatogenesis before and during his chemotherapy will prevent long-term damage to his germinal epithelium and preserve his reproductive potential.

Question 2.18. **A 28-year-old woman is initially seen at your oncology practice with a new diagnosis of acute lymphoblastic leukemia. Her white blood count is 78,000, 90% blast forms; hematocrit is 34%, and her platelet count is 94,000. Her last menstrual period was 10 weeks ago; her pregnancy test is positive. For personal and religious reasons, the patient will not consider abortion. Which of the following statements are TRUE?**

a) The greatest risk to the fetus from the chemotherapeutic agents likely to be used in this woman's leukemia treatment occurs during the first trimester.
b) This woman's leukemia cannot be adequately treated as long as she is pregnant, and therapy should be delayed until the baby can be safely delivered.
c) High-dose methotrexate should be considered, because it is a good treatment for central nervous system leukemia in this woman, who is at high risk for this complication.
d) She should be strongly encouraged to keep the pregnancy, because it is quite likely that she will be rendered permanently infertile after she completes her therapy.
e) A therapeutic abortion would be contradicted due to the high complication rate.

Question 2.19. **The major mechanism by which nucleoside analogues enter cells uses which process for transport across the membrane?**

a) Passive diffusion
b) Carrier-mediated transport
c) Reduced folate binding protein
d) Nucleobase transport system
e) Endocytosis

Question 2.20. **The ability of cells to accumulate and retain cytosine arabinoside (ara-C) triphosphate is predictive of both cytotoxicity and clinical response to ara-C therapy for patients who have acute myelogenous leukemia. When ara-C is administered at dose rates that achieve >10 μmol ara-C in plasma, the rate-limiting step in the formation of ara-C triphosphate is:**

a) Transport of ara-C into the cell
b) Intracellular metabolism of ara-C by deoxycytidine deaminase
c) Metabolism of ara-C by large body organs
d) Phosphorylation to ara-C monophosphate by deoxycytidine kinase
e) Availability of deoxycytidine triphosphate

Question 2.21. **Knowledge of the pharmacokinetic characteristics of a drug can be useful in the design of treatment protocols. Which property characterizes a drug that exhibits linear pharmacokinetics?**

a) The half-life of elimination of the drug is independent of its plasma concentration.
b) Drug clearance is independent of the dose administered.
c) Clearance is not affected by the schedule of drug administration.
d) All of the aforementioned

Question 2.22. **Acrolein is the metabolite of ifosfamide principally responsible for which of the following toxicities?**

a) Hemorrhagic cystitis
b) Amenorrhea
c) Veno-occlusive disease
d) Alopecia
e) Myelosuppression

Question 2.23. **A 65-year-old man is found to have widely metastatic prostate cancer. Over the previous 2 months, he has had frequent episodes of angina and then developed increasing pain in the right hip and lower back. Neurologic examination is normal. His recent prostate specific antigen (PSA) level is 100 ng/mL, and a radioisotope bone scan showed increased radiotracer uptake in the lumbar spine, sacrum, pelvis, and both humeri. An MRI scan of the spine has been ordered. The patient has been taking nitrate, aspirin, and a β-blocker for 2 months, and recently an oral narcotic drug has been prescribed for his bone pain. Past medical history is significant for uncomplicated anterior non–Q-wave infarction 8 weeks ago, deep venous thrombosis 8 months ago, and mildly abnormal liver function for several**

years due to chronic alcoholism. What modality of treatment has the lowest risk for this patient?

a)   Diethylstilbestrol (DES)
b)   Surgical castration (orchiectomy)
c)   Luteinizing hormone-releasing hormone (LH-RH) agonist alone
d)   LH-RH agonist in combination with an anti-androgen (flutamide)
e)   LH-RH antagonist alone

Question 2.24.   **A 55-year-old man who has newly diagnosed prostate cancer is referred to you for medical treatment of his malignancy. He has increasing pain in the back and ribs. Neurologic examination is normal. PSA is 400 ng/mL; bone scan shows hot areas in the cervical spine, lumbar spine, and pelvis. MRI scan of the spine did not show extension of these lesions into the spinal canal. The patient has abnormal liver function due to chronic active hepatitis B and has declined surgical castration.**

At this point, the patient should be offered:

a)   Chemotherapy
b)   No specific therapy
c)   LH-RH antagonist
d)   DES
e)   Radiotherapy

Question 2.25.   **All of the following statements concerning the oncologic applications for somatostatin analogues are true EXCEPT:**

a)   Oncologic applications of somatostatin analogues are based on multiple effects, and several mechanisms of action are likely.
b)   Somatostatin analogues inhibit the growth of a variety of tumors in animals and various endocrine tumors in human patients.
c)   Somatostatin analogues are much less toxic than is adjuvant chemotherapy.
d)   The presence of somatostatin receptors in neuroendocrine and non-neuroendocrine tumors permits localization of primary tumors and metastases by scintigraphy with radiolabeled somatostatin analogues.
e)   Chronic administration of somatostatin analogues can produce medical castration.

Question 2.26.   **In a postmenopausal woman, the major source of plasma estrogen is:**

a)   Adrenal estrogens
b)   Red meat and dietary fats
c)   Enzymatic conversion of adrenal androgens
d)   Phytoestrogens
e)   Ovarian stromal tissue

Question 2.27.   **A 60-year-old woman who has metastatic breast cancer involving the chest wall, pleura, and bone received tamoxifen as the only therapy for 3 years. She experienced a complete remission of her disease, but recent evaluation now shows recurrence at previous sites of involvement.**

Tamoxifen was discontinued, but after 6 weeks there has been slight but definite progression of disease. Appropriate management now would be to:

a)   Increase the dose of tamoxifen to 40 mg/d.
b)   Administer systemic chemotherapy.
c)   Start megestrol acetate 800 mg/d.
d)   Refer for bilateral surgical adrenalectomy.
e)   Treat with an aromatase inhibitor.

Question 2.28.   **A 38-year-old previously untreated Hispanic woman is initially seen with a locally advanced, non-inflammatory, inoperable carcinoma of the breast with supraclavicular, bilateral axillary nodal and chest wall involvement. Biopsy reveals infiltrating duct carcinoma and estrogen receptor 75 and progesterone receptor 45 fmol/mg protein, respectively. She refuses both chemotherapy and radiotherapy. Which of the following therapies would be least effective?**

a)   Bilateral oophorectomy
b)   Goserelin (Zoladex)
c)   Tamoxifen
d)   An aromatase inhibitor
e)   A pure antiestrogen

Question 2.29.   **The most common cancer associated with antidiuretic hormone (ADH) production is:**

a)   Renal cell carcinoma
b)   Soft-tissue sarcoma
c)   Neuroblastoma
d)   Small-cell lung carcinoma
e)   Squamous cell lung carcinoma

Question 2.30.   **Which of the following paraneoplastic syndromes is the result of antibody production by the tumor?**

a)   Hypercalcemia
b)   Subacute cerebellar degeneration
c)   Hyponatremia
d)   Hypoglycemia
e)   None of the aforementioned

Question 2.31.   **Which of the following is (are) recommended by the Oncology Nursing Society in the event of an accidental exposure or spill of an antineoplastic agent?**

a)   Contaminated skin should be washed with soap and water.
b)   A medical evaluation should be obtained as soon as possible.
c)   In the event of a spill, personnel should have on double surgical latex gloves, eye protection, and disposable gowns with a closed front, long sleeves, and closed cuffs.
d)   The spill area should be cleaned three times with a detergent, followed by clean water.
e)   All of the aforementioned

Question 2.32. **All of the following statements regarding photodynamic therapy (PDT) are true EXCEPT:**

a) PDT involves the activation of dyes that are localized in target tissue.
b) The most studied light activated dye or sensitizer is photofrin.
c) The major side effect of PDT is cutaneous photosensitization.
d) Photofrin is not recommended in patients who have liver failure.
e) All of the aforementioned are true.

Question 2.33. **Which of the following statements is FALSE regarding nonproliferative cells?**

a) These cells may be permanently nonproliferative but may survive as long as the organism.
b) These cells may be permanently nonproliferative but may have a finite life span.
c) They may be recruited and proliferate on the proper extracellular signal.
d) Nonproliferative cells cannot be recruited and proliferate.
e) Examples of nonproliferative cells include neurons and stem cells.

Question 2.34. **An 81-year-old man is referred to the hospital with dehydration secondary to progressive dysphagia. He first developed dysphagia 18 months before admission. Evaluation at that time included an upper endoscopy that revealed a distal esophageal mass. Biopsy of the mass revealed squamous cell carcinoma. A computed tomography (CT) scan revealed hepatic and mediastinal metastases. The patient subsequently underwent two courses of chemotherapy with some improvement in dysphagia. During the 4 months before admission, the patient's dysphagia worsened, and he underwent several esophageal dilations. Each dilation provided relief of symptoms for no more than 7 days. Radiotherapy was attempted, but the patient refused further therapy because nausea and generalized debility ensued. On admission to the hospital, he was dehydrated, cachectic, and slightly icteric. Admission laboratory test results were notable for blood urea nitrogen, 35 mg/dL; creatinine, 1.3 mg/dL; total bilirubin, 4.4 mg/dL; and AST, 75 U/L. An esophagogastroduodenoscopy was performed, and the patient was found to have nearly complete obstruction of the esophageal lumen by tumor.**

The use of PDT with porfimer sodium (Photofrin) is considered. Which of the following is a correct statement?

a) The patient's jaundice precludes the use of PTD with porfimer sodium.
b) Age greater than 80 years is a contraindication for treatment with PDT with porfimer sodium.
c) Total obstruction of the esophagus makes PDT impossible.
d) The previous history of chemotherapy is a contraindication to PDT.
e) The history of radiotherapy is a contraindication to PDT.

Question 2.35. **You are asked to consult regarding a patient who has unresectable head and neck cancer recurrent after maximal radiotherapy; this patient has showed some evidence of response after receiving a single course of intra-arterial chemotherapy with cisplatin 50 mg/m^2 and doxorubicin 45 mg/m^2 administered into the external carotid artery. Your colleague asks for your suggestions about how to modify the regimen to take optimal advantage**

of the intra-arterial route of administration and increase the probability that the second cycle will produce a greater effect. Your recommendations would include all of the following EXCEPT:

a) Omit the doxorubicin, and increase the dose of cisplatin.
b) Give a second cycle of exactly the same regimen using the same technique.
c) Use a super-selective catheterization technique to infuse drug into an artery smaller than the external carotid.
d) Consider concurrent IV administration of a cisplatin neutralizing agent such as sodium bicarbonate.

Question 2.36. **All of the statements regarding cisplatin-induced ototoxicity are correct EXCEPT:**

a) Cisplatin ototoxicity is characterized by tinnitus and hearing loss.
b) Hearing loss is usually in the high-frequency range (>4000 Hz).
c) Hearing loss may not be symptomatic.
d) Vestibular toxicity usually does not occur.
e) The toxicity is idiosyncratic (equally likely to occur at any dose).

Question 2.37. **Which of the following is not recommended by the Oncology Nursing Society as a patient education outcome criteria for the patient and/or family?**

a) To describe the state of the disease and therapy at a level consistent with his or her educational and emotional status
b) To participate in the decision-making process pertaining to the plan of care and life activities
c) To identify appropriate community resources that provide information and services
d) To describe appropriate actions for highly predictable problems, oncologic emergencies, and major side effects of the disease and/or therapy
e) All of the aforementioned

Question 2.38. **A 52-year-old male patient who has advanced malignant fibrous histiocytoma of the nasal cavity complains of anorexia and a 16-lb weight loss. An evaluation reveals gastroparesis and delayed gastric emptying. The patients asks whether there are any medications that could improve his appetite and help him regain his body weight. You might offer which of the following remedy(ies)? Please note, for this question, that more than one answer may be correct.**

a) Cyproheptadine
b) Hydrazine sulfate
c) Megestrol acetate
d) Metoclopramide
e) Ranitidine

Question 2.39. **In which of the following condition(s) is total parenteral nutrition (TPN) indicated? Please note, for this question, that more than one answer may be correct:**

a) A 65-year-old man who has a diagnosis of laryngeal carcinoma and is receiving radiotherapy. He has dysphagia and has lost 15 lb over 3 months.

b)   A 70-year-old man with a 4-month history of dysphagia for solid food and a 12-pound weight loss has a diagnosis of squamous cell carcinoma in the middle one third of his esophagus.
c)   A 62-year-old woman with a diagnosis of pancreatic carcinoma is about to receive 5-fluorouracil infusion and local radiotherapy. She has frequent diarrhea and has lost 17 lb over 3 months.
d)   A 45-year-old woman who has ovarian carcinoma is seen with a large amount of ascites and evidence of partial intestinal obstruction.
e)   A 5-year-old boy with a diagnosis of Wilms' tumor who is about to undergo an intensive combined chemotherapy and radiotherapy program. He has a good appetite and is well nourished.

Question 2.40.   A 67-year-old man who has head and neck cancer was treated 7 years previously with a left radical neck dissection followed by 7000 cGy of radiotherapy to the neck. His cancer has been in remission, and his general health is good. He develops abrupt onset of an aphasia. MRI scan reveals a focal cortical infarction. He makes an excellent recovery from his stroke. An MR angiogram reveals >85% occlusion of the left internal carotid artery in the neck; the right carotid artery has only minimal atherosclerosis. The next step in this patient's management should be:

a)   Heparin followed by sodium warfarin
b)   One aspirin a day
c)   CT of the neck to look for tumor recurrence
d)   Endarterectomy of the left carotid artery
e)   Careful observation

Question 2.41.   Which level of the spine is the most common location for spinal cord compression in patients who have metastatic disease?

a)   Cervical spine
b)   Thoracic spine
c)   Lumbar spine
d)   Sacrum
e)   Spinal metastases and cord compression are seen equally throughout the vertebral spine

Question 2.42.   Extravasation of which of the following chemotherapeutic agents is the most likely to result in serious sequelae?

a)   5-Fluorouracil
b)   Doxorubicin
c)   Vincristine
d)   Melphalan
e)   Etoposide

Question 2.43.   Which of the following chemotherapeutic agents is LEAST likely to result in a radiation recall reaction?

a)   Actinomycin D
b)   Doxorubicin
c)   Cytarabine
d)   All of the aforementioned may result in a recall reaction.
e)   None of the aforementioned are associated with a recall reaction.

Question 2.44.   All of the following modalities have been clearly shown to reduce doxorubicin cardiotoxicity in human subjects EXCEPT:

a)   Reducing the total cumulative dose of doxorubicin to less than 300 mg/m^2
b)   Administration of doxorubicin after pretreatment with α-tocopherol (vitamin E)
c)   Modifying the administration schedule so as to give the doxorubicin in each cycle over 72 hours rather than as a rapid infusion
d)   Administration of doxorubicin in a liposomal delivery system
e)   Administration of doxorubicin with dexrazoxane

Question 2.45.   Which of the following akylators has been shown to produce permanent sterility in male rodents?

a)   Mechlorethamine
b)   Procarbazine
c)   Triethylene thiophosphoramide (Thio TEPA)
d)   Carmustine
e)   None of the aforementioned

Question 2.46.   Which of the following statements regarding the gonadal function of young male Hodgkin's disease patients is correct?

a)   Prior to therapy, approximately one third of young men with Hodgkin's disease are oligospermic.
b)   MOPP and ABVD are associated with comparable rates of post-treatment gonadal dysfunction.
c)   High radiation doses are necessary to impair spermatogenesis.
d)   Gonadal function returns to normal in the majority of men treated with MOPP.
e)   None of the aforementioned are true.

Question 2.47.   The frequency of permanent amenorrhea and infertility in women following chemotherapy depends upon all of the following factors EXCEPT:

a)   The type of chemotherapy
b)   The total dose of chemotherapy
c)   Concomitant radiation exposure
d)   Patient age
e)   All of the aforementioned are factors affecting the frequency of amenorrhea and infertility in women receiving chemotherapy.

Question 2.48.   All of the following represent measures for gonadal function preservation in patients undergoing cancer therapy EXCEPT:

a)   Hormonal manipulation
b)   Gonadal shielding
c)   Oophoropexy
d)   Lateral ovarian transposition
e)   Ovarian externalization

Question 2.49.   Which type of leukemia is most commonly observed in patients who survive cancer?

a)   Acute lymphoblastic leukemia (ALL)
b)   Acute myeloid leukemia (AML)

c)   Chronic lymphocytic leukemia (CLL)
d)   Chronic myelocytic leukemia (CML)
e)   Hairy cell leukemia (HCL)

Question 2.50.   **Which of the following statements is FALSE regarding the risk of breast cancer in female patients who have pediatric Hodgkin's disease?**

a)   The overall risk of breast cancer in female Hodgkin's disease patients is increased compared with the general population.
b)   The most important risk factor for the development of breast cancer in the pediatric Hodgkin's population is the use of mantle irradiation.
c)   The risk of breast cancer in female pediatric Hodgkin's disease patients treated before age 15 is greater than that for patients treated at an older age.
d)   Combined chemotherapy (MOPP or ABVD) is not associated with an overall increased risk of breast cancer in pediatric Hodgkin's patients.
e)   A greater than one-hundred-fold excess risk has been reported in young females receiving chest irradiation.

Question 2.51.   **What is the generally accepted reason for the failure of tumor necrosis factor alpha (TNF-α) to elicit in vivo activity against a wide variety of human tumors?**

a)   Limited doses of TNF-α can be safely administered systemically.
b)   TNF-α has limited efficacy in vitro against many tumor cell lines.
c)   Tumors are not inherently immunogenic.
d)   Tumors cannot elaborate the nitric oxide required for the effect of TNF-α.
e)   TNF-α is extruded by the multidrug resistance pump.

Question 2.52.   **Which of the following statements best describes the effect of tamoxifen on breast cancer cells?**

a)   Tamoxifen binds irreversibly to the estrogen receptor.
b)   Tamoxifen works equally well in estrogen receptor (ER)–positive and ER–negative patients.
c)   Tamoxifen competitively inhibits the binding of estradiol to the estrogen receptor.
d)   Tamoxifen directly inhibits the production of several kinds of proteins important for breast cancer cell proliferation.
e)   Tamoxifen is a pure estrogen antagonist.

Question 2.53.   **The ability of cells to accumulate and retain ara-C triphosphate (ara-CTP) is predictive of cytotoxicity and clinical response to ara-C therapy for patients who have acute myelogenous leukemia. When ara-C is administered at dose rates that achieve >10 μmol ara-C in plasma, the rate-limiting step in the formation of ara-C triphosphate is:**

a)   Transport of ara-C into the cell
b)   Intracellular deamination of ara-C by deoxycytidine deaminase
c)   Deamination of ara-C by large body organs
d)   Phosphorylation to ara-C monophosphate by deoxycytidine kinase
e)   Availability of deoxycytidine triphosphate

Question 2.54. **A 35-year-old woman with a history of diffuse large-cell lymphoma of the mediastinum who was treated with six cycles of cyclophosphamide, doxorubicin, vincristine, and prednisone as well as mediastinal radiotherapy 2 years previously is now seen with progressive dyspnea. The patient also has mild chest pain that is worse when she is recumbent. Examination is remarkable for blood pressure of 90/70, faint heart sounds, and mild confusion. The chest radiograph discloses an enlarged cardiac silhouette. Echocardiogram would likely reveal:**

a) Right atrial myxoma
b) Dilated cardiomyopathy
c) Right ventricular diastolic collapse
d) Wall motion abnormalities
e) Thickened myocardium due to tumor infiltration

Question 2.55. **A 7-year-old male, successfully treated 3 years previously for acute lymphocytic leukemia with a new induction regimen containing etoposide, is again seen with pancytopenia. Bone marrow aspiration study results reveal an acute myelomonocytic leukemia. The most likely cytogenetic abnormality would involve the following chromosome(s):**

a) Deletion of 5 and 7
b) 11q23
c) t(8;21)
d) t(9;22)
e) inv 3

Question 2.56. **You are about to treat a 60-year-old man for small-cell carcinoma of the lung. The patient has elevated liver enzymes (twice the upper limit of normal) and some mild renal insufficiency (serum creatinine, 1.7 mg/dL). You plan to use an etoposide-containing drug regimen. Which of the following is true?**

a) This patient should not be treated with etoposide.
b) The patient should definitely have a dose reduction because of hepatic dysfunction.
c) The patient is likely to experience an increased incidence of peripheral neuropathy.
d) The patient may have increased myelotoxicity because of hepatic and renal dysfunction.
e) The etoposide dose should be decreased by 50% because of renal insufficiency.

Question 2.57. **Which of the following statements concerning the use of interleukin-2 in renal cell carcinoma is true?**

a) The response rate is approximately 15%.
b) The United States Food and Drug Administration has deferred approval of this agent.
c) The most responsive metastatic site is the liver.
d) Interleukin-2 interacts with B cells.

e) Low-dose interleukin-2 and tumor infiltrating lymphocytes produce the best response in metastatic renal cell carcinoma.

Question 2.58.   **A 9-year-old boy undergoing chemotherapy for ALL develops an acute, Grade 3 hypersensitivity reaction to his third of six prescribed asparaginase doses. The asparaginase used was a native *Escherichia coli* asparaginase. The therapeutic decision for this child's therapy is:**

a) Hold all further asparaginase treatment
b) Switch to *Erwinia* asparaginase and maintain the schedule.
c) Switch to monomethoxypolyethylene glycol (PEG) asparaginase as a single dose.
d) Switch to PEG asparaginase on a monthly dose schedule.
e) Use high-dose prednisone and diphenhydramine and continue the asparaginase treatment.

Question 2.59.   **A 6-year-old girl who has ALL relapses after 18 months of conventional chemotherapy. Of note, during her initial induction therapy, she experienced a dose-limiting clinical hypersensitivity reaction to Elspar (*E. coli* asparaginase). The current re-induction regimen planned is prednisone, vincristine, daunorubicin, and asparaginase (PVDA). Asparaginase should be dosed as:**

a) Elspar, 12 doses (3 × weekly × 4)
b) PEG L-asparaginase (1 dose q 2 weeks)
c) PEG L-asparaginase (1dose q week)
d) Denatured asparaginase, 12 doses (3 × weekly for 4 weeks)
e) *Erwinia* asparaginase (bid for 7 days)

Question 2.60.   **A 16-year-old with T-cell ALL developed severe, acute pancreatitis during consolidation therapy that included asparaginase (Elspar) at 10,000 U/m^2 per dose every week for 20 weeks. The appropriate therapeutic maneuver for this patient is:**

a) Hold all further asparaginase treatment
b) Switch to *Erwinia*
c) Switch to PEG asparaginase
d) Continue asparaginase with somatostatin
e) Infuse asparaginase

Question 2.61.   **Randomized clinical trials involving the use of hematopoietic growth factors such as G-CSF as primary prophylaxis to support combination chemotherapy have documented each of the following EXCEPT:**

a) Shortening the duration of severe neutropenia by approximately 50%
b) Decreasing the incidence of fever with neutropenia
c) Prolonged survival
d) Decreasing utilization of parenteral antibiotics
e) Shortening hospitalization

Question 2.62.   **A 43-year-old woman who has metastatic breast cancer (two pulmonary nodules) undergoes high-dose alkylating agent therapy with infusion of previously harvested peripheral blood stem cells. She had initially**

been seen with Stage II breast cancer 3 years earlier and was treated with 6 cycles of cyclophosphamide, doxorubicin, and 5-FU chemotherapy. She has received four cycles of doxorubicin, methotrexate, and 5-FU since her metastasis was diagnosed approximately 6 months ago.

Ten days after receiving her stem cells, the patient has gained 4 kg in weight; developed ascites, as revealed by ultrasonographic examination; and has a serum bilirubin level of 8.0 mg/dL. The most likely reason for this set of clinical findings is:

a)   Vascular toxicity of chemotherapy
b)   Sepsis
c)   Myelosuppressive toxicity of chemotherapy
d)   Metastatic breast cancer
e)   Microangiopathic hemolytic anemia

Question 2.63.   **A 57-year-old man who has relapsed AML receives re-induction therapy with cytarabine at a dose of 3.0 g/m^2 given over 3 hours every 12 hours for six doses. He tolerates the therapy well, except for a fever of unclear etiology that occurs during profound neutropenia on the seventh day after the beginning of therapy. The patient was placed on broad-spectrum antibiotic therapy, defervesced, and experienced CBC recovery on Day 20 after the initiation of therapy. His antibiotic therapy was discontinued. However, on Day 22 after initiation of therapy, the patient developed daily fevers to 102°F, fatigue, and right upper quadrant pain. Although his CBC was essentially normal, his liver function test results were remarkable for an alkaline phosphatase level that was elevated to 5 times normal. Computed tomogram of the abdomen was unremarkable. The most likely diagnosis in this case is:**

a)   Gram-negative infection
b)   Cytomegalovirus infection
c)   Candidal infection
d)   Tuberculosis
e)   Cytarabine-mediated toxicity

Question 2.64.   **All of the following are properties of doxorubicin and related chemotherapeutic agents EXCEPT:**

a)   Interposition of the drug occurs between adjacent DNA bases, thereby altering DNA topology.
b)   The ability to intercalate between DNA bases correlates with the antitumor effect.
c)   These agents enhance topoisomerase-II–mediated DNA damage.
d)   These agents undergo metabolism to free radicals.
e)   Free radical–mediated damage is responsible for cardiotoxicity.

Question 2.65.   **All of the following approaches may limit anthracycline-mediated cardiotoxicity EXCEPT:**

a)   Limiting the total dose administered
b)   Measuring cardiac ejection fraction with radionuclide blood pool scan
c)   Coadministering a drug that is an active free radical scavenger
d)   Coadministering a drug that can be metabolized to an iron-chelating agent

e)   Limiting exposure to high peak drug levels by continuous infusion administration

Question 2.66.   All of the following have been described as mechanisms of methotrexate (MTX) resistance in experimental tumors EXCEPT:

a)   Amplification of target enzyme
b)   Mutation of target enzyme
c)   Decreased MTX uptake
d)   Decrease in MTX polyglutamation
e)   Increased expression of GP 170

Question 2.67.   All of the following neurologic toxicities have been associated with the use of either high-dose systemic or intrathecal methotrexate administration EXCEPT:

a)   Headache, fever, and meningismus
b)   Cranial nerve palsies and motor paralysis
c)   Seizures
d)   Demyelinating encephalopathy
e)   Purkinje's-cell dropout in the cerebellum

Question 2.68.   A 65-year-old widowed retired school teacher was admitted to the hospital for management of breast cancer that was metastatic to bone. She had been a previously well-adjusted woman who had adapted to her illness well. Recently, however, her daughter noted that she had become withdrawn and somnolent, and spoke less and looked depressed. The family felt that "the illness is finally getting to her." On examination, she spoke slowly with poor attention, and her orientation and general information was impaired. The most likely diagnosis is:

a)   Major depression related to her illness
b)   Suicidal behavior with depression
c)   Delirium secondary to hypercalcemia
d)   Anxiety/fear of death
e)   Paraventricular demyelination

Question 2.69.   A 45-year-old married art dealer was seen at her oncologist's office following a recent diagnosis of lung cancer with metastatic spread. Initial chemotherapy had no effect on the tumor. She complained of fatigue, weakness, anorexia, and insomnia. In addition, she stated that she has lost all interest in things she usually enjoyed. She was preoccupied with thoughts of death, was tearful several times a day, felt anxiety, and sometimes could not remain still, pacing the floor. She felt hopeless and guilty for the problems she was causing her husband. She had thoughts of suicide and of asking her doctor to help her. She looked depressed and distraught as she stated that she had always been a "worrier who saw the black side of every situation." She has lost a son to cancer 3 years earlier, which had left her depressed. The patient's psychiatric diagnosis is:

a)   Major depression related to her illness
b)   Anxiety and fear of death

c) Grief reaction
d) Existential crisis with normal response
e) Brain metastasis

Question 2.70. **Continued administration of a given antineoplastic treatment commonly results in resistance to that treatment. Which one of the following treatments is LEAST likely to result in a significant degree of resistance at the cellular level.**

a) Methotrexate
b) Cyclophosphamide
c) Etoposide
d) X-irradiation
e) Hydroxyurea

Question 2.71. **Which one of the following accounts for the linear relationship between dose and tumor response observed in some neoplasms?**

a) Tumor burden
b) Intrinsic tumor chemosensitivity
c) Type of tumor
d) Rapidity with which resistance develops
e) A linear relationship between dose and area of parent compound and active metabolites under the plasma curve (AUC)

Question 2.72. **The adjuvant chemotherapy strategy is increasingly influenced by our understanding of the cellular and molecular biology of metastases. With the understanding that much of this knowledge derives from experimental models, which one of the following is true?**

a) A long period of lack of growth (latent period) could result from sustained expression of tumor angiogenesis factors.
b) A failure of growth would necessarily be associated with a marked decrease in proliferation rate of the tumor cells.
c) Except for the lungs, the distribution of metastases is determined primarily by the magnitude of the blood supply to the various organs.
d) The relationship between adhesion molecules on the surface of the circulating tumor cells and the endothelium and basement membrane of the organ is the major determinant of the distribution of metastases.
e) Although primary tumors are clonal, metastases are not.

Question 2.73. **All of the following in vitro observations distinguish neoplastic from normal cells EXCEPT:**

a) Short (1–2 days) generation time (Tc, time of cell cycle)
b) Loss of ability to decrease proliferative thrust when contact is made in a crowded culture (so-called contact inhibition)
c) Ability to grow in agar; that is, no direct contact with a solid surface is required.
d) Tumor cells in culture may be immortal.
e) Increased telomerase activity

Question 2.74. **The growth rate (volume doubling time) of human tumors varies substantially. For example, diffuse large-cell lymphoma is a fast-growing tumor, whereas follicular lymphoma and breast cancer are slow growing. Major contributory cytokinetic factors associated with and often responsible for this difference include all the following EXCEPT:**

a)   A longer generation or cell cycle time in the more slow-growing tumors
b)   A slower rate of programmed cell death in the rapidly growing tumors
c)   A higher growth fraction in the fast-growing tumors
d)   Tumor cell surface expression of growth factor receptors
e)   Resting cells (G0) are clonogenic, that is, may re-enter cycle, and are therefore important from the therapeutic perspective.

Question 2.75. **Experimental and clinically evident solid tumors commonly cause hypoxia, often to severe degree (less than 5 mm Hg). All of the following represent reasons why such hypoxia may limit, or be associated with, a reduced effect of chemotherapy EXCEPT:**

a)   Hypoxia is a co-variable with decreased blood supply.
b)   Hypoxia is associated with a low growth fraction.
c)   Molecular oxygen is essential for the activity of therapeutic modalities such as irradiation and certain chemotherapeutic agents.
d)   Tumor hypoxia may limit genetic instability, including gene amplification, with resultant decrease in the production of drug resistance.
e)   Hypoxia may prevent or limit programmed cell death.

Question 2.76. **All of the following statements regarding therapy with methotrexate (MTX) are correct EXCEPT:**

a)   In contrast to standard-dose MTX, 10-fold higher doses may provide therapeutic concentrations in the central nervous system and be effective for prophylaxis of CNS leukemia.
b)   Leukovorin rescue should be instituted within 24 hours after the administration of MTX.
c)   The duration of exposure to MTX makes a greater contribution than the peak concentration.
d)   MTX excretion is determined primarily by hepatic metabolism.
e)   A pleural effusion may significantly affect the pharmacokinetics of MTX.

Question 2.77. **All of the following statements regarding MTX pharmacodynamics are correct EXCEPT:**

a)   The discovery of gene amplification resulted from studies of MTX resistance.
b)   The amplified dihydrolate reductase (*DHFR*) gene may be present in cytoplasmic episomes known as double minutes.
c)   The amplified *DHFR* gene may be integrated into the cellular genome, which is recognized by homogenously staining regions.
d)   Reversible resistance is more likely to be associated with double minutes than with homogenous staining regions.
e)   The production of the MTX resistance in vitro has been found to be schedule independent.

Question 2.78. **All of the following statements regarding the schedule dependence of chemotherapy are correct EXCEPT:**

a) For a given total dose, MTX given by continuous infusion is less toxic than when given by bolus.
b) Intermittent MTX (once or twice per week) is more effective than daily MTX for remission maintenance in treating acute lymphocytic leukemia.
c) Doxorubicin given by continuous infusion over 4 days is less cardiotoxic than bolus administration.
d) Doxorubicin delivered in low doses weekly is less cardiotoxic than bolus doxorubicin given every 21 days at the same dose intensity.
e) The schedule of administration for alkylating agents does not have a major impact on tumor response or toxicity.

Question 2.79. **The kinetics of cancer treatment can be considered zero-order (100% of tumor cells treated are destroyed) or first-order (a fraction of tumor cells are destroyed by each treatment). Which of the following best describes the kinetics of each treatment modality?**

a) Surgery = zero-order; radiotherapy = first-order; chemotherapy = first order
b) Surgery = zero-order; radiotherapy = first-order; chemotherapy = zero-order
c) Surgery = zero=order; radiotherapy = zero-order; chemotherapy = first-order
d) Surgery = first order; radiotherapy = first-order; chemotherapy = zero-order
e) Surgery = first-order; radiotherapy = first-order; chemotherapy = first-order

Question 2.80. **Which of the following best describes our understanding of surgery for metastatic disease?**

a) Once cancer has spread to a distant site, surgery should be considered as an option of last resort.
b) Surgery is indicated for a solitary metastasis, but not for multiple metastases to a single organ system.
c) The growth rate of a tumor has no bearing on the decision for operative intervention.
d) Most patients who have colon cancer metastatic to the liver are candidates for hepatic resection and postoperative radiotherapy.
e) Resection of a solitary pulmonary metastasis may provide a higher survival rate than resection of primary bronchogenic carcinoma of the lung.

Question 2.81. **Which of the following is true of adjuvant therapy for cancer?**

a) Presently, there is no effective postoperative adjuvant therapy for American Joint Commission on Cancer stage III melanoma.
b) Combination therapy for melanoma with cisplatin-based agents and tamoxifen is restricted to postmenopausal women.
c) Adjuvant chemotherapy is based on zero-order cell killing.
d) Neoadjuvant chemotherapy is based on zero-order cell killing.
e) Adjuvant chemotherapy improves the survival of patients undergoing surgical resection of breast cancer, ovarian cancer, and colon carcinoma.

Question 2.82. **The tumor, nodes, and metastases (TNM) system has four chronologic classifications. Which of the following is true?**

a) The clinical classification (cTNM) represents the extent of disease at the completion of definitive treatment.
b) The cTNM represents the preoperative (preTNM) and pathologic (pTNM) classification.
c) The final classification at autopsy (aTNM) is based on postmortem examination.
d) TNM changes with each encounter, but only the last measurement is considered when estimating prognosis.
e) Staging TNM is identical to therapeutic TNM.

Question 2.83. **The schedule of fluoropyrimidine administration substantially influences the biologic effects. All of the following are correct EXCEPT:**

a) 5-flurouracil given by intravenous push daily for 5 days is twice as potent as when given by continuous infusion for 5 days.
b) 5-fluorodeoxyuridine (FdUrd) given by continuous IV infusion is at least 10-fold more potent than 5-FU given in any schedule.
c) FdUrd is 10-fold more potent when given by continuous IV infusion than when given by push.
d) The fluoropyrimidines affect both DNA synthesis and the quality and synthesis of RNA.
e) The mechanism of resistance to fluoropyrimidines is the same regardless of schedule.

Question 2.84. **A 49-year-old registered nurse complains of retrosternal chest pain. She is undergoing adjuvant chemotherapy for T1N1M0 breast carcinoma treated by lumpectomy and axillary dissection, with 9 of 19 nodes containing cancer. She has just completed her third cycle of chemotherapy with doxorubicin, cyclophosphamide, and fluorouracil at doses of 75, 750, and 750 mg/m^2 cycle, respectively. On Day 6, she becomes febrile, with a leukocyte count of 230 K/μL, hemoglobin 11.2 g/dL, and platelet count of 90,000 K/μL. She vomits twice, the second time with tinges of blood, and has sustained exacerbation of her chest pain. She has pharyngeal ulcers. A chest radiograph is normal, and an electrocardiogram is read as sinus tachycardia. After giving her 2 mg of morphine intravenously for her chest pain and intravenous ceftazidime, your correct course of action would be:**

a) Prescribe amphotericin B
b) Prescribe acyclovir
c) Prescribe amphotericin B and acyclovir
d) Undertake esophagogastroscopy
e) Undertake double-contrast barium esophagram

Question 2.85. **Video-assisted thoracic surgery (VATS) is best used for:**

a) Pneumonectomy
b) Lobectomy
c) Nodulectomy

d) Pleural inspection
e) Pleurodesis

Question 2.86. **In a patient with neurologically complete thoracic paraplegia due to metastatic disease of the spine, the primary functional goal is to:**

a) Obtain spinal stability by application of the thoracolumbar sacral orthosis
b) Provide electrical stimulation of the spinal cord to encourage neural regeneration
c) Restore neurologic function by prompt surgical decompression
d) Obtain independence in the activities of daily living by an interdisciplinary rehabilitation approach
e) Provide personal assistance at home or at a nursing facility as early as possible in order to reduce the length of stay and cost of care

Question 2.87. **In a metastatic disease of the femur, the person LEAST likely to suffer a pathologic fracture would be an individual who:**

a) Has a cortical bone lesion that affects 25% of the bony circumference as seen on an imaging study
b) Has a large single lytic lesion in the proximal femur
c) Is a woman
d) Has persisting or increasing pain
e) Has metastatic disease in other bones and organs

Question 2.88. **Successful prosthetic use following above-the-knee amputation for a sarcoma in the distal femur depends on all of the following factors EXCEPT:**

a) Surgical techniques
b) Preoperative counseling
c) Length and shape of residual limb
d) Absence of phantom pain
e) Emotional adjustment

Question 2.89. **A 66-year-old patient who has chronic lymphocytic leukemia is about to begin chemotherapy with chlorambucil and prednisone. Which of the following antiemetics would you recommend?**

a) Intravenous metoclopramide (1–2 mg/kg)
b) Oral tetrahydrocannabinol (Dronabinol) (10 mg/m^2)
c) Intravenous granisetron (10 mcg/kg)
d) Oral ondansetron (8 mg)
e) No antiemetic

Question 2.90. **Which of the following anticancer drugs is most likely to cause significant nausea and vomiting?**

a) Cisplatin
b) Bleomycin
c) Tamoxifen
d) Vinblastine
e) Fluorouracil

Question 2.91.   Ondansetron and granisetron have been proved to be safe and effective for which of the following vomiting syndromes?

a)   Delayed emesis
b)   Motion sickness
c)   Anticipatory emesis
d)   Bowel obstruction
e)   Radiation-induced

Question 2.92.   A 50-year-old woman is seen with a pathologic fracture through a large lytic lesion in the humerus. Bone scan demonstrates no other lesions and only peripheral uptake around this lesion. The most likely diagnosis is:

a)   Metastatic breast carcinoma
b)   Plasmacytoma
c)   Malignant lymphoma of the bone
d)   Metastatic renal cell carcinoma
e)   Fibrous dysplasia of the bone

Question 2.93.   A 50-year-old woman who had a cold lesion on bone scan complained about generalized weakness, nausea and vomiting, polyuria, dehydration, and confusion. This clinical presentation suggests:

a)   Diabetes mellitus
b)   Hypercalcemia of malignancy
c)   Meningeal metastases with diabetes insipidus
d)   Adrenal metastases with addisonian crisis
e)   Renal failure

Question 2.94.   Measurement of the estrogen receptor content of a breast cancer specimen can provide, among other information, a highly reliable indication of whether:

a)   The patient will respond favorably to endocrine manipulation.
b)   The patient will respond favorably to combined cytotoxic chemotherapy.
c)   The patient will not respond favorably to endocrine manipulation.
d)   The patient is premenopausal or postmenopausal.
e)   The patient comes from a familial background at high risk for breast cancer.

Question 2.95.   A 32-year-old man developed fever and a dry cough 9 days after receiving an allogeneic bone marrow transplantation for chronic myeloid leukemia. Physical examination revealed the presence of a few respiratory rales in the right upper lung field. Laboratory evaluation revealed severe pancytopenia, with a neutrophil count of $<100/mm^3$. The initial radiograph was read as "unremarkable." The patient was placed on a broad-spectrum antibacterial regimen (vancomycin 1 g every 12 hours + imipenem 500 g every 6 hours). He remained febrile, and his cough worsened. On Day 12, amphotericin B (1.0 mg/kg) was added. Repeat chest radiograph showed a rounded, nodular density in the right upper lung field. On Day 17, the patient was still febrile but showed a trend toward defervescence. He was still neutropenic (<500 PMN/mm^3) and now complained of occasional hemoptysis. Chest radiograph revealed cavitation in the nodular density in the right upper lobe.

Computerized tomography confirmed these findings and revealed no other areas of involvement. Further management should consist of:

a) Continuation of the same dose of amphotericin B
b) Increase dose of amphotericin B (3.0 mg/kg/d)
c) Amphotericin B lipid complex (5 mg/kg/d)
d) Amphotericin B plus surgical excision
e) Amphotericin B plus itraconazole

Question 2.96. **A 43-year-old woman complains of "a lump in her throat." She had received external beam radiotherapy for acne during her teenage years. She has no other complaints, and she specifically denies dysphagia, dyspnea, and hoarseness. On examination, the thyroid is enlarged bilaterally, with several nodules from 0.5 to 1.0 cm in diameter and a 2-cm nodule in the midportion of the right thyroid lobe. There is no cervical adenopathy. The remainder of her physical examination is unremarkable. Which of the following is the most appropriate at this time?**

a) Perform fine needle aspiration of the dominant nodule
b) Reassure the patient that thyroid nodules associated with radiation exposure are nearly always benign
c) Refer the patient for a radioiodine scan of the thyroid
d) Refer the patient for a radioiodine ablation of the thyroid
e) Refer the patient for thyroidectomy

Question 2.97. **A 52-year-old man was found to have recurrence of a previously resected non-secreting pituitary tumor, and he has just completed a course of conventional radiotherapy (total dose: 45 Gy in 25 fractions). Serum testosterone, thyroid-stimulating hormone, free thyroxine, and cortisol following stimulation were normal before radiotherapy. What treatment should be recommended.**

a) Testosterone enanthate IM monthly: follow-up in 2 months
b) Cortisone 25 mg/d po: follow-up in 1 month
c) No treatment: follow-up in 3 months
d) Triiodothyronine 150 μg/d: follow-up in 1 month
e) Sodium chloride 2 g/d: follow-up in 1 month

Question 2.98. **A 62-year-old man who was treated with 60 Gy of radiation for a squamous cell carcinoma of the floor of the mouth is seen 9 months following the completion of therapy with a lesion of his lower jaw. On examination, the lesion is foul smelling, appears to involve bone, and has a grayish, necrotic surface. Antibiotic treatment and local debridement cause improvement, but ulceration persists. The next therapy should be:**

a) Surgical resection of the involved area
b) Hyperbaric oxygen
c) 2000 cGy of radiation
d) Corticosteroids and pamidronate
e) Change of antibiotics

Question 2.99. **A 24-year-old woman receiving chemotherapy for lymphoma complains of dental pain. Unfortunately, the patient was not**

screened before the initiation of chemotherapy, so a carious maxillary pre-molar was undetected. The patient is febrile, neutropenic, and thrombocy-topenic (platelet count of 40,000 cells per cubic millimeter). The optimum treatment would be:

a) Intravenous antibiotic therapy until her white blood cell count and platelet recover, and then extraction of the tooth

b) Intravenous antibiotic therapy, filgrastim treatment, and immediate tooth extraction

c) Intravenous antibiotics and palliation for discomfort and delayed root canal therapy

d) Intravenous antibiotics, platelet transfusion, and immediate extraction

e) Intravenous antibiotics, filgrastim granulocyte transfusion, platelet transfusion, and immediate extraction

Question 2.100.   An 18-year-old man is receiving induction therapy for acute myelogenous leukemia. Ten days following the administration of chemother-apy, the patient complains of mouth sores, and you note multiple oval ulcers of the cheek and lip mucosa. The most important diagnostic step is:

a) Additional diagnostic testing is indicated, because the patient has mucositis caused by stomatotoxicity of chemotherapy.

b) Determination of HSV antibody status

c) Fungal and viral cultures

d) Blood culture

e) Biopsy ulcer margin

Question 2.101.   On recall examination of a 55-year-old man who has had ra-diotherapy for a parotid tumor, you note brown discoloration of the teeth close to the gum line. The most likely reason for this change is:

a) Caries secondary to radiation-induced xerostomia

b) Exogenous pigmentation associated with radiation-induced salivary changes

c) Intrinsic pigmentation-induced changes in tooth microvasculature

d) Poor oral hygiene due to failure to brush teeth during radiotherapy

e) Melanocyte activation by radiation

Question 2.102.   In addition to altered topoisomerase II activity, the biochem-ical basis of tumor cell resistance to etoposide is likely to involve which of the following mechanisms?

a) Increased expression of P-glycoprotein (P-170, MDR)

b) Increased topoisomerase I activity

c) Decreased expression of P-glycoprotein (P-170, MDR)

d) Increased adenosine deaminase

e) Increased cyclic AMP

Question 2.103.   Based on known mechanisms of cellular resistance and cross resistance to anticancer drugs, which of the following pairs of drugs are LEAST likely to exhibit cross-resistance?

a) Doxorubicin and mitozantrone

b) Vincristine and vinorelbine

c) Cytarabine and daunorubicin

d) Methotrexate and trimetrexate
e) Chlorambucil and melphalan

Question 2.104. **A 70-year-old man is referred for possible chemotherapy. He had a hemicolectomy 3 years earlier for a carcinoma of the colon. A CT scan of the abdomen shows multiple lesions in the liver. Liver biopsy reveals adenocarcinoma. Which of the following is the most appropriate treatment?**

a) Hepatectomy followed by a liver transplantation
b) A doxorubicin-paclitaxel regimen
c) Irinotecan treatment
d) Recombinant interferon three times per week
e) High-dose IL-2 for 3 weeks

Question 2.105. **Drugs active against topoisomerase I impair the ability of the enzyme to incise and religate a single strand of DNA because they stabilize the reversible cleavable complex. Which drugs have this property?**

a) Docetaxel (Taxotere)
b) Topotecan (hycamtin)
c) Gemcitabine (Camptosar)
d) Paclitaxel (Taxol)
e) Vinorelbine (Navelbine)

Question 2.106. **A 60-year-old man is admitted to the hospital with lethargy and somnolence. His serum calcium level is found to be 18 mg/dL. Chest radiograph shows a 2-cm mass in the right upper lung field. The most likely histology of the lung mass is:**

a) Epidermoid carcinoma
b) Adenocarcinoma of the lung
c) Metastatic gastric carcinoma
d) Anaplastic carcinoma of the lung
e) Metastatic colon cancer

Question 2.107. **The most effective treatment for the 60-year-old man with hypercalcemia of malignancy described in the previous question is:**

a) Subcutaneous calcitonin injections: 100 units q 12 h
b) Intravenous saline at 200 mL/h and furosemide 80 mg IV
c) Pamidronate 90 mg intravenously over 12 to 24 hours
d) Emergency irradiation treatment of the primary cancer along with IV saline and furosemide as in answer (2)
e) Dexamethasone 20 mg IV and 2000 mL normal saline in 4 hours

Question 2.108. **A 45-year-old woman has Cushing's syndrome. Twenty-four-hour urinary cortisol level is 190 μg/d; 8:00 AM plasma level ACTH is 150 pg/mL; cortisol level is 25 μg%. She fails to suppress AM cortisol with a single 1-mg dose of dexamethasone given at 11:00 PM, but decreases AM cortisol to 1 μg% after 8 mg of dexamethasone is given at 11:00 PM. MRI of the hypothalamus/pituitary shows no abnormality. Petrosal venous catheterization shows no ACTH gradient over peripheral blood ACTH, and the patient is sus-**

pected of having ectopic ACTH syndrome. The most likely neoplasm to account for these findings is:

a)   Oat cell carcinoma of the lung
b)   Carcinoma of the thymus
c)   Carcinoma of the colon
d)   Carcinoid of the bronchus
e)   Medullary carcinoma of the thyroid

Question 2.109.   Which minimally invasive surgical (MIS) procedure is LEAST likely to be useful in the gynecologic oncology patient?

a)   Biopsy of enlarged left aortic lymph nodes in a patient with clinical stage IB squamous cell carcinoma of the cervix
b)   Diaphragmatic biopsies in a patient with metastatic ovarian carcinoma of low malignant potential
c)   Oophoropexy in a young patient with stage IB vaginal cancer before pelvic irradiation
d)   Debulking of a 14-cm omental implant in a patient with epithelial ovarian cancer that is otherwise amenable to complete surgical cytoreduction
e)   Total hysterectomy, bilateral salpingo-oophorectomy, pelvic cytology, omental biopsy, pelvic and aortic lymph node biopsies for a patient who has endometrial carcinoma

Question 2.110.   Which of the following neoplasms is the least likely to cause superior vena cava syndrome (SVCS)?

a)   Small-cell lung cancer
b)   Non–small-cell lung cancer
c)   Hodgkin's disease
d)   Diffuse large-cell lymphoma
e)   Breast cancer

Question 2.111.   A 67-year-old woman with a 35-year, 2½ pack-per-day history of cigarette smoking is seen with a 1-month history of dyspnea and cough, and 1 day of new-onset periorbital edema and face and arm swelling. No other findings are noted on examination. Chest radiograph reveals right hilar adenopathy and mediastinal widening. A CT scan of the chest shows a superior mediastinal mass. The initial diagnostic test to obtain a pathologic diagnosis should be:

a)   Fiberoptic bronchoscopy
b)   Cervical lymph node biopsy
c)   Fine needle aspiration (FNA) biopsy
d)   Mediastinoscopy
e)   Sputum cytology

Question 2.112.   All of the following statements concerning SVCS are correct EXCEPT:

a)   SVCS is rarely a true oncologic emergency.
b)   A poor clinical response of SVCS to therapy suggests the possibility of superimposed thrombosis.

c)   Treatment of SVCS due to small-cell lung cancer with radiotherapy results in faster and more complete resolution than treatment with chemotherapy.
d)   SVCS caused by chronic indwelling venous access lines or catheters may be effectively treated with thrombolytic agents.
e)   The use of anticoagulation therapy in SVCS does not improve survival.

Question 2.113.   A 57-year-old man with metastatic renal cell carcinoma who is receiving infusional IL-2 develops hematemesis and melena. His blood pressure is noted to have fallen from 110/80 mm Hg to 90/60 mm Hg, with orthostatic changes. Hematocrit is 23%, which is down from 33% the day before, and his serum creatinine is 2.9 mg/dL. The most likely cause for the patient's clinical syndrome is:

a)   Erosive gastritis
b)   Mallory-Weiss syndrome
c)   Mucosal metastases
d)   Esophageal varices
e)   IL-2–induced thrombocytopenia

Question 2.114.   All of the following statements concerning spontaneous carotid artery rupture in the patient with head and neck cancer are correct EXCEPT:

a)   Preoperative radiotherapy and development of orocutaneous fistulas are the most common predisposing risk factors.
b)   Carotid artery rupture is often preceded by transient minor bleeding episodes.
c)   Definitive treatment requires double ligation and excision of the necrotic artery segment while maintaining control of the bleeding site.
d)   Carotid artery rupture carries a low risk of neurologic compromise.
e)   Digital pressure should be applied to control the bleeding.

Question 2.115.   A 47-year-old woman receiving adjuvant cyclophosphamide, doxorubicin, and 5-fluorouracil (CAF) for 4-node positive stage II breast cancer complains of pain and discomfort at her IV site during administration of chemotherapy. The appropriate response should be:

a)   Administer analgesics and continue the chemotherapy
b)   Immediate plastic surgery consultation
c)   Test the IV site with another injection of chemotherapy. If no further discomfort occurs, continue with the treatment as planned.
d)   Inject corticosteroids
e)   Immediately discontinue chemotherapy, aspirate and remove the IV, apply cold compresses to the site, document the event, and closely follow up the patient.

Question 2.116.   All of the following statements concerning pleural effusions in the cancer patient are correct EXCEPT:

a)   Drainage of a symptomatic malignant pleural effusion without pleurodesis or effective systemic therapy will lead to reaccumulation of the effusion in the majority of patients.
b)   Pleural effusions may result from the effects of chemotherapy drugs.

c) Pleural effusions may be caused by chemotherapy drugs.
d) Malignant mesothelioma is associated with a high frequency of cytologically non-diagnostic malignant pleural effusions on thoracentesis.
e) Mediastinal adenopathy with bilateral pleural effusion virtually eliminates the diagnosis of lymphoma.

Question 2.117. **A 23-year-old man is seen with fevers, weight loss, increasing abdominal girth, and lymphadenopathy. Lymph node and bone marrow biopsy are diagnostic of Burkitt's (high-grade) lymphoma. CT scan shows hepatosplenomegaly with bulky retroperitoneal adenopathy. Appropriate management of this patient before initiating chemotherapy includes all of the following EXCEPT:**

a) IV hydration
b) Sodium bicarbonate administration
c) Allopurinol
d) Corticosteroids
e) Close monitoring of fluids and electrolytes

Question 2.118. **A 54-year-old man with stage III large-cell undifferentiated lung carcinoma complains of increasing dyspnea, cough, dizziness, and ankle swelling. On physical examination his pulse is 140 per minute and thready. Blood pressure is noted to be 90/60 mm Hg, with a pulsus paradoxus of 15 mm Hg. He is noted to be mildly cyanotic, and has distended neck veins, dull lung bases, and 2–3+ pedal edema. Electrocardiogram shows sinus tachycardia, and chest radiograph shows bilateral pleural effusions and an enlarged cardiac silhouette. His blood pressure fails to improve after a fluid challenge. Your next intervention should be:**

a) Continue fluid administration and observation
b) Pericardiocentesis
c) Vasopressors
d) Right heart catheterization
e) Heparin anticoagulation

ANSWERS

Answer 2.1. **The answer is (c).**

Radiation survival curve analysis has demonstrated that radiation sensitivity is not constant throughout the cell cycle. The most radiosensitive phases of the cell cycle are M (mitoses) and G2. In contrast, cells in G0, G1, and S (DNA replication) are less radiosensitive.

For Detailed Discussion: (1) Chapter 48, "Biologic and Physical Basis of Radiation Oncology."

Answer 2.2. **The answer is (c).**

The quantification of radiation dose for therapeutic purposes has evolved over time. Previously, units of skin erythema and the roentgen, a measure of ionization produced in air, were used to quantify the given dose. Today, dose—the energy absorbed per unit mass—is much more precisely measured. The unit of absorbed dose is the gray (Gy), which is equivalent to the absorption of 1 joule per kilogram of tissue. One gray is equivalent to 100 centigray (cGy), or 100 rad.

For Detailed Discussion: (1) Chapter 48, "Biologic and Physical Basis of Radiation Oncology."

Answer 2.3. **The answer is (c).**

Brachytherapy involves the use of sealed radioactive sources placed in proximity to the tumor (intracavitary) or within the tumor volume (interstitial treatment). Because the sources are placed in direct contact with the tumor, the dose falls off rapidly, and the dose distribution is more localized than with external beam radiotherapy. Brachytherapy has been applied either alone or in combination with external beam therapy in the curative treatment of tumors in a variety of sites, including the cervix, head and neck, bladder, and breast. Naturally occurring radioisotopes, that is, radium and radon, were initially used; today, artificially produced isotopes are in use, including cesium 137, iridium 198, and iodine 125. The main role of brachytherapy today is in conjunction with external beam radiotherapy, that is, as a boost, or in sites previously treated with conventional radiotherapy techniques, for example, recurrent soft-tissue sarcomas, cervical tumors, and lung tumors.

For Detailed Discussion: (1) Chapter 48, "Biologic and Physical Basis of Radiation Oncology."

Answer 2.4. **The answer is (a).**

Preclinical data suggest that a variety of chemotherapeutic agents demonstrate increased antitumor activity at elevated temperatures. Drugs whose rate-limiting step is primarily chemical would, on thermodynamic grounds, be expected to be more efficient at higher temperatures. The rates of alkylation of DNA, or the rates of conversion of a nonreactive to a reactive species, can be expected to increase as temperature increases. This is true for the nitrosoureas and cisplatin. Other drugs show a threshold at 43°C, at which drug activity is greatly enhanced. Two such drugs are bleomycin and doxorubicin. The antimetabolites (5-FU, methotrexate) and vincristine do not demonstrate enhanced cell kill at higher temperatures. Among other drugs, including the topoisomerase inhibitors, drug activity may be reduced at elevated temperatures. Although theoretically appealing, combinations of hyperthermia and chemotherapy have been the subject of very few trials.

For Detailed Discussion: (1) Chapter 49, "Principles of Hyperthermia."

Answer 2.5. **The answer is (b).**

Although hyperthermia as a methodology to treat cancer has a long history, hyperthermia is not commonly used today. The most common setting in which hyperthermia is used is in the treatment of small superficially located, recurrent, or metastatic tumors, for example, chest wall locoregional breast cancer recurrences. Locoregional hyperthermia alone is rarely administered today. Instead, hyperthermia is usually given as an adjunct to radiotherapy. There is no documented difference in the inherent heat sensitivity between normal and malignant cells. The microenvironment of cells in solid tumors is particularly conducive to heat sensitivity. The combination of low pH, low oxygen tension, and lack of glucose and other nutrients tends to make cells extremely responsive to elevated temperatures.

For Detailed Discussion: (1) Chapter 49, "Principles of Hyperthermia."

Answer 2.6. **The answer is (b).**

Hyperthermia involves the use of elevated temperatures in the treatment of malignant tumors. The ideal tumors are superficially located. Superficial tumors allow the greatest chance of adequate heating; temperatures can be readily monitored, and tumor response and complications can be easily followed up. The phenomenon of thermotolerance must be taken into account in patients whose tumors are treated with hyperthermia. Thermotolerance is the induction of a temporary resistance to elevated temperatures when cells are exposed to heat in the range of 40 to 41°C for extended periods of time. The development of thermotolerance is accompanied by the preferential synthesis of a series of proteins known as heat shock proteins, which are proteins involved in a variety of normal cellular functions and other disease states.

For Detailed Discussion: (1) Chapter 49, "Principles of Hyperthermia."

Answer 2.7. **The answer is (c).**

Cyclophosphamide can produce free water retention with marked hyponatremia. This phenomenon is exacerbated by hypotonic fluids, and seizures have been reported in children under these conditions. The condition can be avoided and also reversed by avoiding hypotonic fluids and using diuretics that promote free water clearance.

For Detailed Discussion: (1) Chapter 62, "Alkylating Agents and Platinum Antitumor Compounds."

Answer 2.8. **The answer is (b).**

The steep dose-response curve of tumors to alkylating agents makes it possible to obtain significantly more effect from the feasible increases of the dose of these agents. Because the usual dose-limiting toxicity of alkylating agents is hematopoietic, stem cell support allows this toxicity to be bypassed, and a significant dose and effect increment can be achieved before nonhematopoietic dose-limiting toxicities are encountered.

For Detailed Discussion: (1) Chapter 62, "Alkylating Agents and Platinum Antitumor Compounds."

Answer 2.9. **The answer is (a).**

Carboplatin has predominantly hematopoietic toxicity and much less neurotoxicity and renal toxicity. This fact makes it the platinum drug of choice in patients who are at particular risk from renal or neurologic toxicity.

For Detailed Discussion: (1) Chapter 62, "Alkylating Agents and Platinum Antitumor Compounds."

Answer 2.10. **The answer is (e).**

Graft-versus-host disease occurs due to activation of lymphocytes that react against alloantigens present on host tissues. Cytokines generated by these activated T cells further contribute to the pathologic process. The most common clinical manifestations include skin rash, hepatitis, and gastroenteritis (particularly involving the colon and small bowel). Pathologic changes tend to be nonspecific, but generally involve a mononuclear cell infiltrate in the affected tissue. The greater degree of allodisparity that exists between the donor and the recipient, the more likely that severe, acute graft-versus-host disease will occur. Graft-versus-host disease is nonexistent in syngeneic transplantations and is very frequent in partially mismatched or matched unrelated donor transplantations. T-cell depletion of the donor bone marrow results in a reduced instance of acute and chronic graft-versus-host disease. This procedure also makes the likelihood of leukemic relapse more likely by diminishing any associated graft-versus-leukemia effect. Chronic graft-versus-host disease, manifested by scleroderma-like changes of the skin and possible joint contractures, occurs most frequently in patients who have antecedent acute graft-versus-host disease. Graft-versus-host disease, particularly common in older adults receiving sibling marrow grafts and individuals receiving transplants from matched unrelated donors, is the chief cause of mortality in patients who have non–T-cell-depleted bone marrow grafts.

For Detailed Discussion: (1) Chapter 86, "Allogeneic Transplantation."

Answer 2.11. **The answers are (c) and (e).**

Tumor cells have high rates of glucose use with production of lactic acid. Hexokinase, the enzyme that catalyzes the first step in the glycolytic pathway, is highly overexpressed in tumor cells. Cancer cells act as energy parasites. The conversion of glucose to lactate in cancer cells yields two molecules of adenosine triphosphate (ATP), whereas the conversion of lactate to glucose in the liver requires 6 ATP molecules. The cyclic metabolic pathway in which glucose is converted to lactic acid in tumor tissue and then reconverted back to glucose in the liver is referred to as the Cori cycle. Although tumors are effective nitrogen traps, successful competition for nitrogen is not considered to be a major cause of cancer cachexia. The role of TNF-α cachectin in the development of cancer cachexia has not been established. The metabolic manifestations of cancer cachexia are similar to those of healthy subjects undergoing starvation. Cancer patients do not exhibit increased resting energy expenditure or elevated basal metabolic rates. Several studies show that most cancer patients are not hypermetabolic.

For Detailed Discussion: (1) Chapter 173, "Anorexia and Cachexia." (2) Knox LS, Crosby LD, Feurer ID, Buzby GP, Miller CL, Mullen JL. Energy expenditure in malnourished cancer patients. Ann Surg 1983;197:152.

Answer 2.12. **The answer is (c).**

Leptomeningeal metastases are common in breast cancer and can cause the multifocal symptoms and signs present in this patient. The patient has both cranial (headache and cognitive impairment) and radicular (sensory symptoms in the arm and absent ankle jerk) symptoms. In leptomeningeal metastases, symptoms are usually more prominent than signs, and neuroimaging may be unrevealing. Definitive diagnosis requires the demonstration of malignant cells in the CSF. Corticosteroid therapy is unlikely to help, and institution of early treatment with radiotherapy and chemotherapy offers the only opportunity for disease control.

For Detailed Discussion: (1) Chapter 175, "Neurologic Complications."

Answer 2.13. **The answer is (b).**

Lhermitte's sign is probably due to transient demyelination induced by the radiotherapy that included the cervical cord in its port. This is a relatively common occurrence after mantle irradiation and is completely benign. In the presence of a normal neurologic examination, further work-up is not necessary. This sign usually resolves within weeks to a few months and rarely persists for periods up to a year. It has no prognostic significance for the development of late delayed radiation myelopathy.

For Detailed Discussion: (1) Chapter 175, "Neurologic Complications."

Answer 2.14. **The answer is (c).**

In the 1- to 3-month period after allogeneic transplantation, cytomegalovirus is a common cause of diffuse interstitial pneumonitis. It is particularly common among patients who either have had prior cytomegalovirus exposure or have received blood or marrow products from donors with such exposure. Newer studies, particularly blood polymerase chain reaction studies for cytomegalovirus, are useful in monitoring for the risk of cytomegalovirus pneumonitis. Although the use of this test and other preventative strategies have significantly reduced the risk of cytomegalovirus pneumonitis, this infection is still a common cause of death among allogeneic bone marrow transplantation patients. It is mandatory that the infection be diagnosed rapidly by bronchoscopy and that appropriate treatment be instituted.

For Detailed Discussion: (1) Chapter 182, "Respiratory Complications."

Answer 2.15. **The answer is (d).**

High oxygen concentrations administered during anesthesia can synergize with several drugs, most notably bleomycin, to produce pulmonary injury. The bleomycin exposure can have occurred years before the anesthesia. Any patient who has received bleomycin should receive lowered oxygen concentrations during anesthesia to help prevent this syndrome. If it develops, early bronchoscopy diagnosis is desirable, particularly to rule out adult respiratory distress syndrome secondary to interoperative sepsis. If there is substantial Type 2 pneumocyte atypia without major fibrosis seen, a trial of steroids is useful to try and reverse what otherwise may be a fatal outcome.

For Detailed Discussion: (1) Chapter 182, "Respiratory Complications."

Answer 2.16. **The answer is (d).**

The cyclophosphamide, cisplatin, and carmustine regimen produces a 30 to 40% risk of pulmonary lung injury occurring 1 to 3 months after transplantation. At the time this patient was seen, her immune system was largely reconstituted and, unlike allogeneic transplantation patients who often have impaired immunity, was at low risk for opportunistic infection. The normal chest radiograph largely rules out a focal infectious processes. The decreased DLCO and exercise oxygen desaturation are classic findings for BCNU–induced pulmonary lung injury. A high-dose steroid taper will produce rapid improvement (within 72 hours) if this is the etiology of the problem. In the meantime, nonemergent bronchoscopy can be performed to rule out the small possibility of an infectious or neoplastic process.

For Detailed Discussion: (1) Chapter 182, "Respiratory Complications."

Answer 2.17. **The answer is (b).**

Significant numbers of young men with newly diagnosed Hodgkin's disease have severely deficient sperm counts and motility, but recent technology has allowed concentration of cryopreserved germ cells, and there are increasing reports of successful inseminations from these specimens. Despite improving odds of recovering spermatogenesis after ABVD administration, preserving semen should at least be considered for every young man about to undergo cytotoxic chemotherapy. Although the antitumor efficacy of MOPP compared with ABVD suggests similar activity, the side-effect profile is distinctly different. In this instance in which preservation of reproductive function is clearly important, ABVD is the treatment of choice. Numerous series have documented the incidence of total and permanent azoospermia to be essentially 100% in young men who receive as few as three cycles of MOPP therapy. From a number of series collected over the past 2 decades, the congenital defects in offspring of cancer survivors appears to be essentially that of the general population. Patients should be reassured that children conceived following completion of chemotherapy and/or radiotherapy are overwhelmingly likely to be normal, have normal intelligence, and grow normally. We do not know what the cancer risk is for these children, however. Although administration of gonadotropin releasing hormone analogues can temporarily suppress spermatogenesis, there are no convincing data that this is an effective technique for the maintenance of fertility.

For Detailed Discussion: (1) Chapter 186, "Gonadal Complications."

Answer 2.18. **The answer is (a).**

In general, the literature supports the observation that in utero exposure to cytotoxic agents during the second and third trimesters is relatively safe. First-trimester exposure during the period of organogenesis is the highest risk time, but even then many agents can be given safely, although low-birth-weight infants are common. Many small series and case reports of women undergoing antileukemic therapy during pregnancy suggest that this therapy can be performed safely and successfully, and that postponement in most cases is not an ideal strategy. This woman is early in her pregnancy and already has significant hematologic compromise; waiting another 6 to 7 months would not be considered appropriate management. Antimetabolites, the most clearly documented drugs with associated teratogenesis, should not be administered in the first trimester and should be used with caution afterward. Abortion would greatly simplify her management; the risk of permanent infertility is difficult to assess from the literature, but there are many case reports of women conceiving and delivering normal infants after therapy for leukemia.

For Detailed Discussion: (1) Chapter 186, "Gonadal Complications."

Answer 2.19. **The answer is (b).**

The translocation of nucleosides across the plasma membrane occurs by carrier-mediated transport. Considered generally as facilitated diffusion, the receptors that mediate the process may exhibit specificity for different nucleosides and their analogues. Furthermore, the process may be equilibrative, or concentrative. In the former case, the intracellular concentration of the transported nucleoside will not exceed the extracellular concentration. Energy, generally in the form of ATP hydrolysis, is required to actively concentrate nucleoside inside the cell.

For Detailed Discussion: (1) Chapter 58, "Pharmacology." (2) Cass CE. In: Georgopapadakou NH, ed. Drug Transport in Antimicrobial and Anticancer Therapy. New York: Marcel Dekker, 1994.

Answer 2.20. **The answer is (d).**

The dose rate of ara-C infusion is critical to the intracellular metabolism of this pro-drug. At dose rates less than 20 mg/m^2/h, the plasma ara-C concentration is unlikely to exceed 1 μM, a concentration at which transport into the cell limits the availability of ara-C for anabolism to the active triphosphate. At dose rates that achieve plasma concentrations of ara-C up to 10 μM, ara-cytidine triphosphate formation is a function of the transport of ara-C by deoxycytidine kinase and becomes saturated when plasma ara-C is in excess of 10 μM. Because ara-C enters the cell by an equilibrative transport system, this limit is reached at an ara-C dose rate of 250 mg/m^2/h, which produces 10 μM of ara-C in plasma.

For Detailed Discussion: (1) Chapter 58, "Pharmacology." (2) Plunkett, et al. Saturation of 1-beta-D-arabinofuranosylcytosine 5-triphosphate accumulation in leukemia cells during high-dose 1-beta-D-arabinofuranosylcytosine therapy. Cancer Res 1987;47:3005.

Answer 2.21. **The answer is (d).**

Linear pharmacokinetics are characterized by plasma clearance and an elimination half-life that are independent of dose. Furthermore, the schedule of administration does not influence clearance. Although there may be exceptions to these somewhat idealized predictions, an understanding of the pharmacokinetic behavior of a drug that exhibits linear pharmacokinetics is valuable for protocol design.

For Detailed Discussion: (1) Chapter 58, "Pharmacology." (2) Gibaldi M. Biopharmaceutics and Clinical Pharmacokinetics. Philadelphia: Lea & Febiger, 1991.

Answer 2.22. **The answer is (a).**

Ifosfamide, cyclophosphamide, and the oxazosphorines result in bladder toxicity not seen with the other alkylating agents. The toxicity is hemorrhagic cystitis, which may progress to massive bleeding. The toxicity is principally caused by the metabolite acrolein, which is excreted in the urine. Other metabolites, including phosphoramide mustard and chloracetaldehyde, may also contribute to the hemorrhagic cystitis. Although hemorrhagic cystitis is more commonly seen after ifosfamide therapy than cyclophosphamide therapy, the difference is probably caused by the use of higher doses of ifosfamide in clinical practice. The systemic administration of thiols, notably

2-mercaptoethane sulfonate (Mesna), can prevent or ameliorate the bladder damage from the oxidative metabolites of ifosfamide and cyclophosphamide.

For Detailed Discussion: (1) Chapter 62, "Alkylating Agents and Platinum Antitumor Compounds."

Answer 2.23. **The answer is (e).**

Palliative endocrine therapy is indicated for this patient who has symptomatic advanced prostate cancer. The inhibition of testicular androgen secretion can induce a high degree of initial response; up to 80% of such patients benefit from endocrine therapy and experience a reduction in bone pain, decrease in PSA levels, and objective evidence of tumor regression. The aim of endocrine therapy is to improve quality of life and prolong survival.

DES should not be used in this patient because he has a history of deep venous thrombosis, cardiac disease, and liver dysfunction. Surgical castration should be avoided, if possible, because this patient, who has a recent (less than 3 months) non–Q-wave infarction and post-infarction angina, is at high risk for cardiac complications from noncardiac surgery and epidural anesthesia. Patients who have prostate cancer with metastases to the spine should not begin treatment with LH-RH agonists alone because of the following reasons: During the first few days of administration of LH-RH agonists, plasma testosterone rises. This initial rise in testosterone may be responsible for the elevation in prostatic acid phosphatase, and the increase in bone pain. The flare-up of disease, which is usually transient, may occur in the first 2 weeks of treatment in approximately 10% of patients. The expanding tumor may cause spinal cord compression with damage to the cauda equina as well as irreversible neurologic loss (paraplegia). Severe fatal reactions have been observed in patients.

Administration of antiandrogens such as flutamide, together with LH-RH agonists, can prevent disease flare-up. However, because of the side effects of antiandrogens, especially liver toxicity, the use of the combination of LH-RH agonists with antiandrogens is contraindicated in this patient, who has abnormal liver function.

For Detailed Discussion: (1) Chapter 71, "Hypothalamic and Other Peptide Hormones."

Answer 2.24. **The answer is (c).**

This patient with chronic active hepatitis and symptomatic disseminated prostate carcinoma who declines surgical castration may benefit from appropriate hormonal treatment. The aim of endocrine therapy is to improve the quality of life and prolong survival. Approximately 80% of such patients can benefit from endocrine treatment, with improvement in bone pain, decreases in tumor marker levels such as PSA and acid phosphatase, and objective evidence of tumor regression. These beneficial effects last an average of 2.5 years, and then most patients who have advanced prostate carcinoma relapse and finally die, apparently of androgen-independent prostate cancer. Chemotherapy for prostate cancer is associated with poor response rates and significant toxicity. Radiotherapy would not be helpful because of the diffuse nature of the patient's disease. Diethylstilbestrol is contraindicated for this man who has chronic active hepatitis. Recent work with the LH-RH antagonist

Cetrorelix in patients who have advanced prostate cancer and paraplegia due to metastatic invasion of the spinal cord suggests that LH-RH antagonists could be indicated for patients with extensive metastases in whom the LH-RH agonists cannot be used as single agents because of the possibility of flare-up.

For Detailed Discussion: (1) Chapter 71, "Hypothalamic and Other Peptide Hormones."

Answer 2.25. **The answer is (e).**

Oncologic applications of somatostatin analogues are based on multiple effects, and several mechanisms of action are likely. It is probable that somatostatin analogues, by virtue of having a wide spectrum of activities (which include suppression of the secretions of the pituitary, pancreas, stomach, and gut; interference with growth factors; and direct antiproliferative effects on some tissues), inhibit various tumors through multiple mechanisms. Somatostatin analogues are much less toxic than adjuvant chemotherapy.

With the use of scanning techniques, the presence of somatostatin receptors may permit the localization of some tumors and metastases. Radioiodinated analogues of somatostatin, such as [indium 111-DTPA-D-Phe[1]]-octreotide (OctreoScan) and [iodine 123-tyrosine 3]-octreotide have been used clinically for the localization of tumors containing receptors for somatostatin. Technetium 99m–labeled RC-160 or ^{111}In-DTPA-RC-160 could also be used. Scintigraphy with radiolabeled somatostatin analogue octreotide has been used with success for detection of both neuroendocrine or non-neuroendocrine tumors. Non-neuroendocrine tumors containing somatostatin receptors that can be localized in vivo with radiolabeled somatostatin analogue octreotide include non–small-cell lung carcinoma, meningiomas, breast cancer, and astrocytomas, but not exocrine pancreatic tumors. Other radiolabeled somatostatin analogues such as RC-160 have yet to be evaluated clinically. Administration of somatostatin analogues inhibits the levels of growth hormone, IGF-I, insulin, glucagon, and other gastrointestinal hormones, but not the secretion of LH, follicle-stimulating hormone, and sex steroids.

For Detailed Discussion: (1) Chapter 71, "Hypothalamic and Other Peptide Hormones."

Answer 2.26. **The answer is (c).**

In postmenopausal women, negligible amounts of estrogen are made in the ovary; the contribution to plasma estrogens from dietary sources is minor and of doubtful biologic significance. In these women, the major source of estrogen is the result of the conversion of androgen precursors to estrone through the activity of the aromatase enzyme complex. The major substrates are androstanedione, and to a lesser extent, testosterone, which are both produced primarily in the adrenal glands. However, the actual conversion of androgens to estrone, which is catalyzed by aromatase, takes place not in the adrenal gland but at peripheral sites such as fat, muscle, liver, and tumor tissue.

For Detailed Discussion: (1) Chapter 74, "Clinical Use of Aromatase Inhibitors in Breast Carcinoma."

Answer 2.27. The answer is (e).

The patient's disease is now refractory to tamoxifen, and there has been no evidence of a "withdrawal response." Nevertheless, this patient remains an excellent candidate for further hormonal therapy. Her previous good response to tamoxifen and the sites of her metastatic disease make her an excellent candidate for treatment with an aromatase inhibitor such as anastrozole. Bilateral surgical adrenalectomy has been abandoned as therapy for breast cancer. Megestrol acetate would be a reasonable choice, but the dose indicated is that used in management of anorexia. The standard dose for treating breast cancer is 160 mg daily, and there is now no evidence that higher doses are any more effective.

For Detailed Discussion: (1) Chapter 74, "Clinical Use of Aromatase Inhibitors in Breast Carcinoma."

Answer 2.28. The answer is (d).

Aromatase inhibitors have not been shown to effectively lower estrogens in premenopausal women, presumably because of the activity of feedback loops between the ovary and pituitary axis and the very high levels of ovarian aromatase in the premenopausal state.

For Detailed Discussion: (1) Chapter 74, "Clinical Use of Aromatase Inhibitors in Breast Carcinoma."

Answer 2.29. The answer is (d).

The syndrome of ADH overproduction in patients who have cancer was first described in 1957. ADH production has been reported in a wide spectrum of histologic carcinoma types as well as Hodgkin's disease. The most common cancer that is associated with ADH production is lung cancer, predominantly small-cell or oat cell carcinoma. As many as 40% of patients who have oat cell carcinoma have inappropriate ADH production.

For Detailed Discussion: (1) Chapter 77, "Paraneoplastic Syndromes."

Answer 2.30. The answer is (b).

In contrast to the majority of paraneoplastic syndromes that result from the production of a substance that circulates in the blood and produces symptoms, the neurologic syndromes generally are produced through the stimulation of antibody production by the tumor. The antibody initially may impair tumor growth, but it also circulates and cross-reacts with one or more antigens in normal tissues to produce symptoms. Cerebellar cortical degeneration most often is associated with carcinoma of the lung or ovary. The etiology is believed to be the production of antibodies reacting with cerebellar Purkinje's cells.

For Detailed Discussion: (1) Chapter 77, "Paraneoplastic Syndromes."

Answer 2.31. The answer is (e).

The Oncology Nursing Society (ONS) provides guidelines for safe handling and disposal of antineoplastic agents. All of the listed choices are recommended guidelines in the event of an accidental exposure. In addition, ONS guidelines recommend that all contaminated gloves or gowns be immediately removed and discarded. An eye that is accidentally exposed should be washed with water or isotonic eye wash for at least 5 minutes. Small amounts of liquid should be cleaned up with gauze pads, whereas larger spills require absorbent pads. Broken glassware should be placed in a leak-proof, puncture-proof container, placed in a sealable polyethylene or polypropylene bag, and marked with a distinctive warning label.

For Detailed Discussion: (1) Chapter 88, "Principles of Oncology Nursing."

Answer 2.32. **The answer is (e).**

Photodynamic therapy involves light activation of certain dyes that have been previously localized in target issues. The most explored dyes are the porphyrins, particularly Photofrin. Side effects are infrequent. However, prolonged phototoxicity may occur and last up to 4 to 6 weeks. Because Photofrin is metabolized and excreted via the liver, its use in patients who have compromised hepatic function is not recommended. A number of new non-Photofrin photosensitizers have been developed, including mono-aspartyl chlorine, zinc phthalocyanine, and the porphycenes. There are currently more than 30 photosensitizers. Clinical trials have revealed promising results in patients who have a variety of cutaneous tumors, including breast cancers on the chest wall, basal and squamous cell skin cancer, melanoma, mycosis fungoides, and Kaposi's sarcoma.

For Detailed Discussion: (1) Chapter 50, "Photodynamic Therapy of Cancer."

Answer 2.33. **The answer is (d).**

There are three types of nonproliferative cells in the body. Neurons are an example of cells that are permanently nonproliferative and survive as long as does the organism. Polymorphonuclear lymphocytes never proliferate but have a limited life span. The third type of nonproliferative cell is in the unstable G0 stage, which means that it may be recruited into G1 with the proper extracellular signal. Stem cells are examples of this last type of nonproliferative cell.

For Detailed Discussion: (1) Chapter 52, "Cytokinetics."

Answer 2.34. **The answer is (a).**

A bilirubin level greater than 4.0 mg/dL or an AST level greater than three times normal is generally considered a contraindication to the use of porfimer sodium. However, advanced age alone is generally not a contraindication to the use of PDT, nor is prior chemotherapy and/or radiotherapy. An advantage of PDT is that it is capable of treating tumors that completely obstruct the esophagus. An interstitial fiber is available that can be inserted directly into the tumor under endoscopic guidance.

For Detailed Discussion: (1) Chapter 50, "Photodynamic Therapy of Cancer."

Answer 2.35. **The answer is (b).**

The relative advantage of an intra-arterial infusion is greater for the use of drugs that are rapidly cleared from the plasma; this relative advantage increases markedly as the flow rate in the injected artery decreases. Thus, cisplatin is a better choice for intra-arterial infusion than is doxorubicin because the former drug has a shorter plasma half-life, and its plasma half-life can be shortened further by administration of a complexing agent such as thiosulfate. Likewise, superselective catheterization of the arteries feeding the tumor is likely to improve the therapeutic index further.

For Detailed Discussion: (1) Chapter 55, "Regional Chemotherapy."

Answer 2.36.   **The answer is (e).**

Ototoxicity is a significant problem with cisplatin. This toxicity is characterized by both hearing loss and tinnitus. The hearing loss is usually in the high-frequency range (4000 to 8000 Hz), and thus it may not be symptomatic. Although vestibular toxicity may occur, it is unusual. The ototoxicity is dose-related and cumulative. Concomitant or prior radiotherapy appears to enhance the toxicity, but this additive effect may be less if the cisplatin therapy precedes the radiotherapy.

For Detailed Discussion: (1) Chapter 62, "Alkylating Agents and Platinum Antitumor Compounds."

Answer 2.37.   **The answer is (e).**

The oncology nurse is a fundamental member of the oncology team. The nurse is in a unique position to spend the necessary time with patients and their families to develop the required rapport for effective patient and family education. The Oncology Nursing Society recommends specific patient education outcome criteria for the patient and/or family. Nurses should describe the patient's disease and therapy at a level consistent with his or her educational and emotional status. In addition, nurses should participate in the decision-making process pertaining to the plan of care and identify appropriate community resources. Finally, the nurse should describe potential side effects of treatment and the treatment schedule.

For Detailed Discussion: (1) Chapter 88, "Principles of Oncology Nursing."

Answer 2.38.   **The answers are (c) and (d).**

Cyproheptadine is a serotonin antagonist. A randomized study of patients who had various malignancies showed that cyproheptadine decreased nausea and mildly enhanced appetite, but it did not abate progressive weight loss in these patients.

Two randomized studies by a cooperative study group assessing the effects of hydrazine sulfate failed to demonstrate that the compound improved appetite, body weight, quality of life, or survival. Several randomized studies showed that megestrol acetate produced appetite stimulation and increased food intake and weight gain. Although there has been no evidence that megestrol increases lean body mass, it has been argued that the gain of adipose tissue should not be considered inherently negative, because depletion of body fat is generally an undesirable outcome of cancer. Patients who have advanced cancer often have symptoms of delayed gastric emptying and gastroparesis. In these patients, oral administration of metoclopramide, a prokinetic agent, produces improvement in appetite and relieves other dyspeptic symptoms associated with anorexia. Ranitidine has not been improved to

have any activity in patients who have anorexia or in individuals who have documented tumor-associated gastroparesis.

For Detailed Discussion: (1) Chapter 173, "Anorexia and Cachexia." (2) Kardinal
CG, et al. A controlled trial of cyproheptadine in cancer patients with anorexia
and/or cachexia. Cancer 1990;65:2657. (3) Loprinzi CL, et al. Placebo controlled
trial of hydrazine sulfate in patients with newly diagnosed non-small-cell lung cancer. J Clin Oncol 1994;12:1126. (4) Creagan ET, et al. A prospective, randomized
controlled trial of megestrol acetate among high-risk patients with resected malignant melanoma. Am J Clin Oncol 1989;12:152. (5) Loprinzi CL, et al. Controlled
trial of megestrol acetate for the treatment of cancer anorexia and cachexia. J Natl
Cancer Inst 1990;82:1127. (6) Loprinzi CL, et al. Phase III evaluation of four doses
of megestrol acetate as therapy for patients with cancer anorexia and/or cachexia.
J Clin Oncol 1993;11:762. (7) Nelson KA, et al. Metoclopramide in anorexia
caused by cancer-associated dyspepsia syndrome (CADS). J Palliat Care 1993;
9:14. (8) Shivshanker K, et al. Tumor-associated gastroparesis: correction with
metoclopramide. Am J Surg 1983;145:221.

Answer 2.39.   **The answers are (d) and (e).**

For patients who have laryngeal carcinoma and esophageal carcinoma with dysphagia, insertion of a gastrostomy feeding tube should be considered before institution of TPN.

Diarrhaea in the patient who has pancreatic carcinoma may be due to the lack
of pancreatic enzymes in the gastrointestinal tract. The patient should first be treated
with pancreas enzyme preparation. TPN has not beeen proved to enhance effects
of chemotherapy and/or radiotherapy or to improve survival in these patients. With
debulking surgery and combination chemotherapy, the patient who has ovarian carcinoma is expected to do well. Therefore, TPN should be indicated in this patient to
maintain/improve nutritional status, until the obstruction has resolved. Because of
limited nutritional reserve, children who have cancer develop malnutrition more often than do adult cancer patients. Therefore, combined chemotherapy-radiotherapy
protocols for children who have neuroblastoma and Wilms' tumor routinely incorpo-
rate parenteral nutritional support. Prolonged parenteral nutrition given concurrently
with chemotherapy and radiotherapy have resulted in significant improvements in
arm muscle area and increases in serum albumin levels.

For Detailed Discussion: (1) Chapter 173, "Anorexia and Cachexia." (2) Richard
KA, et al. Integration of nutrition support into oncologic treatment protocols for high
and low nutritional risk children with Wilms' tumor. Cancer 1989; 64:491.

Answer 2.40.   **The answer is (d).**

This patient has accelerated atherosclerosis occurring within a previously irradiated
field. This represents a focal process and does not necessarily indicate widespread
vascular disease. Patients who have high-grade carotid occlusions have a superior
outcome with endarterectomy compared with medical management. Prior radiotherapy is not a contraindication to endarterectomy, and outcome is comparable to
patients who have not undergone irradiation.

For Detailed Discussion: (1) Chapter 175, "Neurologic Complications."

Answer 2.41. **The answer is (b).**

Vertebral spinal metastases are common in patients who have metastatic disease. Spinal metastases may occur in all regions of the spine. However, the thoracic spine is the most common location of spinal metastases that result in spinal cord compression, followed by the lumbosacral and cervical spines; the ratio of occurrence is approximately 4:2:1, respectively. Spinal metastases typically occur when cancer spreads hematogeneously to the vertebral column. Spinal cord compression may alternatively occur without vertebral body involvement in the case of tumors that invade the epidural space through the neural foramen. Approximately one quarter of patients have involvement of one or more continuous bodies. Subclinical non-contiguous involvement occurs in 8 to 22% of patients.

For Detailed Discussion: (1) Chapter 175, "Neurological Complications."

Answer 2.42. **The answer is (b).**

Extravasation of a chemotherapeutic drug into the skin and/or subcutaneous tissue may result in a serious chemical cellulitis. Of the drugs listed, extravasation injury from doxorubicin is the most serious. Approximately one third of patients develop ulcerations after extravasation of doxorubicin. These lesions heal poorly and often cause necrosis that requires surgical debridement and grafting. Numerous studies have focused on the development of pharmacologic antidotes, but few studies have demonstrated any significant impact of these antidotes on the risk of extravasation injury.

For Detailed Discussion: (1) Chapter 176, "Dermatologic Complications."

Answer 2.43. **The answer is (c).**

Several chemotherapeutic agents are radiosensitizing or "radiomimetic" and can cause reactivation of tissue in areas previously irradiated. Radiation recall reactions are inflammatory reactions marked by erythema and desquamation within the previously irradiated field. Such reactions have also been reported in areas of previous drug infiltration. The esophagus is one site associated with a particularly severe recall reaction. Actinomycin D and doxorubicin are the usual chemotherapeutic agents associated with radiation recall reactions.

For Detailed Discussion: (1) Chapter 176, "Dermatologic Complications."

Answer 2.44. **The answer is (b).**

Cardiac sequelae are important side effects of doxorubicin. Cardiac sequelae have included acute side effects, for example, pericarditis and electrophysiologic aberrations, and a chronic cardiomyopathy. Cardiomyopathy from doxorubicin is dose dependent. At total doses below 500 mg/m^2, the incidence of cardiomyopathy is less than 1%. In contrast, at total doses above 600 mg/m^2, the incidence is approximately 30%. Multiple measures have been attempted to reduce the risk of cariomyopathy in patients receiving doxorubicin. Restriction of the total cumulative dose, modification of the administration schedule, the use of dexazoxane, and a liposomal delivery system have all been clearly shown to reduce cardiotoxicity. Vitamin E has been studied in animal models but has not been shown to be clinically useful in humans for preventing doxorubicin cardiotoxicity.

For Detailed Discussion: (1) Chapter 181, "Cardiac Complications." (2) Speyer, et al. ICRF-187 permits longer treatment with doxorubicin in women with breast cancer. J Clin Oncol 1992;10:117.

Answer 2.45. **The answer is (b).**

In the majority of animal models, male infertility is reversible. In contrast to the other alkylators, procarbazine, when administered long term, can produce permanent sterility in male rodents. Although every akylating agent is potentially toxic to the human gonads, the very high frequency of long-term infertility seen in survivors of Hodgkin's disease who are treated with MOPP regimens suggests that procarbazine may be particularly toxic in humans as well.

For Detailed Discussion: (1) Chapter 186, "Gonadal Complications."

Answer 2.46. **The answer is (a).**

Gonadal dysfunction is an important sequela in male Hodgkin's disease patients who are treated with chemotherapy and/or radiotherapy. Chemotherapeutic regimens differ greatly in their effect on gonadal function. Unlike patients who are treated with MOPP, the majority of patients who are treated with the ABVD regimen regain gonadal function after treatment. The testes are exquisitively sensitive to radiation, and even low doses are associated with profound and prolonged oligospermia. Before any therapy, approximately 30% of young male Hodgkin's disease patients are oligospermic and have disorders in both sperm motility and morphology. The high level of oligospermia before therapy complicates the interpretation of published reports regarding the gonadal toxicity of treatment with either chemotherapy, radiotherapy, or combined therapy.

For Detailed Discussion: (1) Chapter 186, "Gonadal Complications."

Answer 2.47. **The answer is (e).**

Amenorrhea and infertility are important problems in cancer patients who are receiving chemotherapy. The specific type and total dose of chemotherapy are major determinants of the frequency of both amenorrhea and infertility in women who are treated with chemotherapy. The alkylators are the chemotherapeutic drugs most frequently associated with premature ovarian failure. Cyclophosphamide is probably the best studied of all the alkylators in this regard. Multiple trials have shown that the toxic effect of the alkylators on the ovaries shows a striking age-dependent susceptibility, with younger patients less sensitive and more likely to regain function after completion of therapy.

For Detailed Discussion: (1) Chapter 186, "Gonadal Complications."

Answer 2.48. **The answer is (e).**

Gonadal dysfunction is an important sequela in cancer patients who are treated with chemotherapy and/or radiotherapy. In an attempt to preserve gonadal function, numerous protective measures have been explored in both male and female patients. The use of hormonal manipulation, for example, gonadotropin releasing hormone analogues, is based upon data suggesting that the toxic effect on the male gonads secondary to chemotherapy is a function of the brisk mitotic rate seen in spermatogenesis. Unfortunately, a number of animal and human studies have failed to demonstrate a protective benefit of hormonal manipulation. Numerous techniques are available to the radiation oncologist to limit treatment to the gonads. Gonadal shielding is possible in male patients who are undergoing pelvic irradiation. In addition, surgical techniques, including oophoropexy (central placement of the ovaries) and lateral ovarian transposition, have been used. Oophoropexy with central blocking is used in Hodgkin's disease patients. Lateral ovarian transposition is useful in patients with early stage cervical carcinoma in whom ovarian preservation is desired. The ovaries are placed laterally or superiorly above the pelvic brim outside the radiation portal.

For Detailed Discussion: (1) Chapter 186, "Gonadal Complications."

Answer 2.49. **The answer is (b).**

Leukemia was the first malignancy that was recognized to be a consequence of treatment for an initial primary malignancy. It is not surprising that the occurrence of leukemia was first noted in Hodgkin's disease patients because of the sizable number of survivors available for study. AML is the most common type of leukemia observed in cancer survivors. Overall, the risk of leukemia in Hodgkin's survivors ranges from 16 to 90 times than expected, with the excess rate varying from 8 to 20 cases per 100,000 person-years of follow-up. The vast majority of individuals who have so-called secondary AML have stereotypical chromosome abnormalities (deletion of all or part of chromosomes 5 and/or 7) due to alkylating agent exposure. The wide range of risk estimates reported likely reflects differences in treatment intensity and distribution of patient stage and age, as well as methodologic study differences.

For Detailed Discussion: (1) Chapter 188, "Secondary Cancers."

Answer 2.50. **The answer is (c).**

In the past, radiotherapy occupied an important position in the treatment of pediatric Hodgkin's disease patients. Currently, combination chemotherapy has assumed a primary role, whereas low-dose radiotherapy is used as an adjunct. Although the overall risk of the development of breast cancer is higher in Hodgkin's disease patients (1.3–4-fold excess risk), the most important risk factor in the pediatric Hodgkin's disease group is the use of mantle irradiation. A mantle field is used to encompass the cervical, supra- and infraclavicular, axillary, mediastinal, and axillary lymph nodes. The treatment volume routinely includes the breast region. The risk of breast cancer development in patients who are treated with radiotherapy is age dependent. The highest risk is in patients under the age of 15. In one study, patients who were treated with mantle irradiation before age 15 had a 136-fold excess risk of breast cancer.

For Detailed Discussion: (1) Chapter 188, "Secondary Cancers." (2) Bhatia S, et al. Breast cancer and other second neoplasms after childhood Hodgkin's disease. N Engl J Med 1996; 334:745.

Answer 2.51. **The answer is (a).**

TNF-α is a 17-kd polypeptide produced by activated monocytes, macrophages, and natural killer cells, among others. TNF-α has multiple biologic effects, including direct tumor cell killing in 30 to 50% of tumor cell lines; immunostimulation; induction of cachexia; induction of nitric oxide synthesis, which leads to hypertension; and overactivation of the immune system. Humans are highly sensitive to TNF-α. Phase 1 trials have found dose-limiting toxicities to be profound constitutional symptoms, including fever and significant hypotension. At clinically tolerable doses, there was limited activity against a wide variety of common tumors in both Phases 1 and 2 clinical trials. When combined with other cytokines or chemotherapy, this agent seems to have minimal antitumor activity. It may be that isolation-perfusion therapy will be required to capitalize on the profound antitumor effects of this agent without eliciting any significant systemic toxicity.

For Detailed Discussion: (1) Chapter 81, "Cytokines: Biology and Applications in Cancer Medicine."

Answer 2.52. **The answer is (c).**

Tamoxifen competitively inhibits the binding of estradiol, which is required for the proliferation of ER–positive breast cancer cells, to the estrogen receptor. Estrogens cause an increase in stimulatory growth factors such as tumor growth factor alpha (TGF-α) and a decrease in inhibitory growth factors such as TGF-β; antiestrogens such as tamoxifen interrupt these estrogen stimulatory effects, thereby causing the cell to be held in the G1 phase.

The dose schedule of choice is 10 mg bid. Tamoxifen is a partial agonist as well as being a competitive antagonist, thereby producing weak estrogen-like effects in postmenopausal women. Tamoxifen is generally prescribed (1) to treat metastatic breast cancer in those who have ER tumors or primary bony disease, and (2) as adjuvant therapy for older patients and/or those who have ER–positive tumors.

For Detailed Discussion: (1) Chapter 73, "Estrogens and Antiestrogens."

Answer 2.53. **The answer is (d).**

The dose rate of ara-C infusion is critical to the intracellular metabolism of this prodrug. At dose rates less than 20 mg/m²/h, the plasma ara-C concentration is unlikely to exceed 1μmol, a concentration at which transport into the cell limits the availability of ara-C for anabolism to the active triphosphate. At dose rates that achieve plasma concentrations of ara-C up to 10 μmol, ara-CTP formation is a function of both the transport of ara-C by deoxycytidine kinase and becomes saturated when plasma ara-C is in excess of 10μmol. Because ara-C enters the cell by an equilibrative transport system, this limit is reached at an ara-C dose rate of 250 mg/m²/h, which produces 10 μmol ara-C in plasma.

For Detailed Discussion: (1) Chapter 58, "Pharmacology." (2) Plunkett et al, Cancer Res 1987;47:3005.

Answer 2.54. **The answer is (c).**

A patient who has a history of malignant neoplasm, particularly carcinoma of the lung, breast, esophagus, lymphoma, or melanoma, may develop fluid accumulation in the pericardium, with ultimate development of pericardial tamponade. Initial symptoms of pericardial tamponade, which results in obstruction to flow in both ventricles, may be shortness of breath or fatigue. Chest pain may be positional or vary with respiration; cough or hoarseness may also occur. Physical examination typically reveals hypotension with a pulsus paradoxus (decrease in the auditory systolic pressure during inspiration) of more than 10 mm Hg. Echocardiography would reveal biventricular diastolic collapse that is diagnostic of tamponade physiology. If a right heart catheterization were performed, it would show equalization of pressure in the right atrium and the right ventricle; a left ventricular catheter would also demonstrate equal pressures in the left ventricle. Six cycles of the regimen of cyclophosphamide, hydroxydaunorubicin, Oncovin, and prednisone chemotherapy is unlikely to yield a high enough cumulative doxorubicin dose to be associated with significant left ventricular failure; severe congestive heart failure is not likely with the dose that the patient received. Right atrial myxoma typically mimics subacute bacterial endocarditis with systemic symptoms, including fever.

Patients presenting with hemodynamically significant pericardial tamponade require emergency decompression with pericardiocentesis. It is important to send the aspirated cells to cytology to be sure that a recurrent neoplasm accounts for the clinical findings. It is also possible, particularly in the patient described, that pericardial disease may be secondary to prior radiotherapy.

For Detailed Discussions: (1) Chapter 190, "Oncologic Emergencies."

Answer 2.55.   The answer is (b).

Secondary leukemia has been described in patients treated with etoposide or teniposide. This leukemia is predominantly monocytic (French-American-British classification M4/M5) and is usually characterized by the absence of a preleukemic syndrome, a shorter latency period, and frequent cytogenetic abnormalities involving 11q23.

For Detailed Discussion: (1) Chapter 64, "Epipodophyllotoxins." (2) Whitlock JA, et al. Epipodophyllotoxin-related leukemia: identification of a new subset of secondary leukemia. Cancer 1991;68:600.

Answer 2.56.   The answer is (d).

Approximately 30 to 50% of etoposide is recovered in the urine as unchanged drug. Etoposide is highly protein bound and is metabolized by the liver. There are no specific dose reductions that are recommended in the event of hepatic and/or renal dysfunction. Patients who have hepatic dysfunction and/or impaired renal function do tend to exhibit increased neutropenia. It has been suggested that the etoposide dose be decreased by 30% in patients who have serum creatinine levels of >1.4 mg/dL because of decreased drug clearance. There is no evidence of increased peripheral neuropathy in this particular situation.

For Detailed Discussion: (1) Chapter 64, "Epipodophyllotoxins."

Answer 2.57.   The answer is (a).

Interleukin-2 (IL-2) is an immunoregulatory protein secreted by helper T cells that plays a central role in the maturation and development of T cells. Interleukin-2 has multiple biologic effects, including the induction and proliferation of antigen-stimulated T cells and natural killer cells. In vivo studies have demonstrated that IL-2 could stimulate murine leukocytes to kill a large variety of malignant tumor cells. Interleukin-2 has been approved by the United States Food and Drug Administration for the treatment of patients with metastatic renal cell cancer who have good performance status. The approval was based on results from 255 patients who received a regimen developed at the National Cancer Institute. The regimen is considered to represent high-dose IL-2 (600,000–720,000 units per kilogram by a bolus every 8 hours for Days 1–5 and 15–19). Approximately 14% of patients who have metastatic renal cell sarcoma will respond to this regimen. Only approximately 4% of patients experience a complete response, although some of these responses may be quite prolonged. Although responses occurred in all treated sites, those patients who had lung or lymph node metastases were most likely to respond. Despite the approval using this high-dose approach, many oncologists select a less aggressive subcutaneous daily schedule. Preliminary data suggest that the response rate using a lower dose of interleukin-2 may be similar to that achieved with the higher approved dose.

For Detailed Discussion: (1) Chapter 81, "Cytokines: Biology and Applications in Cancer Medicine." (2) Fyfe G, et al. J Clin Oncol 1995;13:688.

Answer 2.58.   The answer is (b).

Asparaginase is an important antileukemic agent that should not be omitted. A single dose of PEG-asparaginase is inadequate. *Erwinia* and *E. coli* proteins are not cross-reactive. PEG-asparaginase is safe even after hypersensitivity to free protein, but should be given weekly after a reaction to *E. coli* asparaginase. Prednisone and diphenhydramine do not guarantee against anaphylaxis.

For Detailed Discussion: (1) Chapter 67, "Asparaginase."

Answer 2.59.   The answer is (c).

Resumed use of Elspar would evoke hypersensitivity again. The use of asparaginase every 2 weeks is inadequate to maintain suppression of serum asparagine levels at zero. Denatured asparaginase is not used in medicine. *Erwinia* asparaginase should be given in a dose schedule similar to that for Elspar.

For Detailed Discussion: (1) Chapter 67, "Asparaginase."

Answer 2.60.   The answer is (a).

Continuation or switch to other asparaginases will increase duration of asparaginase and is contraindicated. Asparaginase infusions have not been studied, but would not be expected to restore pancreatic structural damage.

For Detailed Discussion: (1) Chapter 67, "Asparaginase."

Answer 2.61.   The answer is (c).

G-CSF therapy after myelosuppressive chemotherapy represents an important advance in supportive care for cancer patients. In randomized trials in patients who have acute leukemia, non–small-cell lung cancer, and other tumors, G-CSF use was associated with a lower incidence of neutropenia and fevers and lower hospitalization duration compared with controls who were not receiving a growth factor. Approximately 4 to 6 fewer days of neutropenia were noted in patients who received G-CSF. However, none of these benefits have been translated into a survival advantage, probably because the aforementioned benefits are not of sufficient magnitude to allow significant enough increases in doses to provide a major effect on antitumor efficacy.

For Detailed Discussion: (1) Chapter 82, "Hematopoietic Growth Factors."

Answer 2.62. **The answer is (a).**

Although the pathogenesis of vascular toxicities associated with chemotherapy is not well understood, it is known that high-dose alkylating agents can produce endothelial cell injury. Such injury may be a partial explanation for the pulmonary toxicity induced by bleomycin, Raynaud's phenomenon seen in patients who receive cisplatin, and certainly for the veno-occlusive disease of the liver, which is a major complication of bone marrow transplantation. Approximately one in five patients who undergo allogeneic transplantation and one in ten patients who undergo autologous transplantation in which high doses of alkylating agents are used in the ablative regimen experience this complication, which is manifested by third-spacing, ascites, and intrahepatic cholestasis. The clinical course of this syndrome may range from mild to fatal. Biopsy of the liver, if carried out, would reveal marked microcapillary damage. Anticoagulation therapy and thrombolytic therapy have each been tried, with mixed success.

For Detailed Discussion: (1) Chapter 179, "Coagulopathic Complications." (2) Dulley FL, et al. Veno-occlusive disease of the liver after chemoradiotherapy in autologous bone marrow transplantation. Transplantation 1984;43: 870.

Answer 2.63. **The answer is (c).**

Although disseminated candidiasis may be a fulminant infection, with hypertension and shock as well as metastatic lesions in the eyes, skin, and central nervous system, there is also a chronic form of candidal infection known as hepatosplenic candidiasis. This syndrome typically occurs in patients with acute leukemia who are undergoing profoundly myelosuppressive chemotherapy. Fevers occur during the period of neutrophil recovery and may be associated with right upper quadrant pain, hepatosplenomegaly, and an elevated serum alkaline phosphatase level. The diagnosis is difficult; attempts to identify *Candida*-related products have been largely unsuccessful. Radiographic studies such as ultrasonography or computed tomography may be helpful, but there is a high false-negative test result rate. Percutaneous liver biopsy or biopsy under laparoscopic guidance may be necessary to firmly establish the diagnosis. Paitents will respond slowly, if at all, to amphotericin B. Prolonged treatment is required. Fluconazole may be useful in this condition as well.

For Detailed Discussion: (1) Chapter 189, "Infections in Patients with Cancer."

Answer 2.64. **The answer is (b).**

Anthracyclines, such as doxorubicin, have a wide range of antitumor activity. Because of their polar-planar ring structure, these compounds intercalate between adjacent DNA bases in the DNA helix. Such intercalation disrupts DNA topology and causes an unwinding of the DNA strand. However, compounds in this class that have a greater ability to distort DNA strands in this fashion are not necessarily more cytotoxic. Moreover, DNA intercalation may not occur at clinically achievable concentrations. Instead, much recent data support the notion that anthracyclines enhance the stabilization of the topoisomerase-II/DNA complex, which leads to increased numbers of strand breaks. Cell lines that have developed altered topoisomerase-II structure are likely to become resistant to doxorubicin and related agents. These drugs undergo metabolism to free radicals that are capable of altering biologic membranes and even participating in the covalent modification of the DNA strand itself. Although the role of free radicals in the actual antitumor effect of the anthracyclines is unclear, oxidant-mediated damage is important in the production of cardiotoxicity, a side effect common to all the drugs in this class. Oxygen radicals generated by anthracycline metabolism attack the fatty acid component of membrane phospholipids.

For Detailed Discussion: (1) Chapter 63, "Anthracyclines and DNA Intercalaters."

Answer 2.65. **The answer is (c).**

There are two patterns of anthracycline-mediated cardiotoxicity. The first is an acute myocarditis-pericarditis syndrome in which the patient experiences rapidly progressive heart failure and arrhythmias that usually appear within the time of administration of one of the first three doses of doxorubicin. The second, and more commonly recognized manifestation of cardiotoxicity, is a gradual loss of pump function secondary to high cumulative doses of the anthracycline. Each antracycline derivative may be given to different maximum cumulative doses. For example, a 550 mg/m^2 cumulative dose of doxorubicin or a 900 mg/m^2 cumulative dose of daunorubicin each have an approximate risk for heart failure of 5%. Because the propensity to develop cardiotoxicity can vary widely among individuals, some investigators have performed serial endocardial biopsies; a more accepted and commonly used technique is to obtain a nuclear medicine estimation of left ventricle ejection fraction when patients have received significant cumulative doses of these drugs. In the presence of cardiac oxidases, doxorubicin free-radical formation occurs. However, such oxidase enzymes are common in all tissues; cardiac tissue is unusual in that it contains a relatively low level of enzymes, such as glutathione, which is responsible for detoxifying such oxidants. However, agents that are active free-radical scavengers such as N-acetylcysteine do not block chronic cardiotoxicity. It appears that doxorubicin-mediated cardiotoxicity requires iron to mediate the local free-radical damage. A successful approach is to make the iron unavailable to the anthracycline by administration of dexrazoxane, which undergoes hydrolysis in the presence of the doxorubicin-iron complex. The product of this reaction is a carboxylamine molecule that can accept the iron and thereby allow the regeneration of free doxorubicin, thus preventing iron-mediated, free-radical damage. Another clinical approach that can decrease the severity of anthracycline-mediated cardiotoxicity is to limit exposure to peak serum levels by infusing the agent via a lower dose weekly bolus or a 96-hour infusion schedule.

For Detailed Discussion: (1) Chapter 63, "Anthracyclines and DNA Intercalaters."

Answer 2.66. **The answer is (e).**

Methotrexate inhibits the enzyme dihydrofolate reductase (DHFR). DHFR is responsible for regenerating reduced folates (specifically tetrahydrofolate), which is required for the formation of thymidylate, an obligate requirement for DNA synthesis. The inhibition of DHFR causes a shutdown of pyrimidine synthesis and rapid cell death. Therefore, if gene amplification leads to increased levels of DHFR, or if a mutation in a gene encoding DHFR results in decreased ability to bind methotrexate, then resistance may result. A critical step in the metabolism of methotrexate is its polyglutamation by the enzyme folylpolyglutamate synthetase. The enzyme may add up to seven or eight glutamate residues to MTX. Polyglutamation is required for appropriate interaction of MTX with DHFR. In addition to decreased levels of folylpolyglutamate synthetase, increased levels of an enzyme that removes glutamate residues from MTX, gamma-glutamyl hydrolase, may result in acquired resistance. MTX is not one of the chemotherapeutic agents known to be pumped out of cells by the pleiotrophic resistance molecule GP170, the product of the *mdr* gene. DHFR gene amplification may be associated with so-called double minute or centromereless chromosomes.

For Detailed Discussion: (1) Chapter 60 "Folate Antagonists."

Answer 2.67. **The answer is (e).**

Intrathecal methotrexate is commonly used to treat leukemic or carcinomatous meningitis. The most common side effect of intrathecal methotrexate is presumably a chemical arachnoiditis that is manifested by severe headache, fever, meningismus, vomiting, and a cerebrospinal fluid pleocytosis. Another possible mechanism for the phenomenon may be the release of adenosine, which is a central nervous system neurotransmitter. If such symptoms persist, switching to an alternative agent for intrathecal use such as cytarabine may be helpful. Approximately 5% of patients receiving intrathecal methotrexate at a dose of 12 to 15 mg/m^2 may develop a more serious form of neurotoxicity consisting of motor paralysis of the extremities, cranial nerve palsies, seizures, and even coma. This syndrome may arise during the second or third week of intrathecal treatment and may be difficult to distinguish from the effects of the cancer itself. A white matter degenerative disease of the brain has been observed in patients, particularly children, who have received intrathecal or high-dose methotrexate alone or particularly in addition to prophylactic cranial irradiation. This dreaded complication results in dementia and limb spasticity, which can occur months or years after the antineoplastic therapy has been delivered. Intrathecal overdoses of methotrexate (greater than 100 mg) have been reported and may be fatal. Intrathecal doses of carboxypeptidase may ameliorate this complication.

For Detailed Discussion: (1) Chapter 60, "Folate Antagonists."

Answer 2.68. **The answer is (c).**

A marked change in mental status in a previously high functioning individual is rarely due to psychological decompensation in coping with illness. The etiology is more likely related to disease or treatment effects. Hypercalcemia commonly presents first with an unexplained change in mental status, with mild confusion and somnolence.

In such a patient, one should also rule out a metastasis to brain or meninges, and side effects of narcotic analgesics. When the cause cannot be corrected, low-dose haloperidol 0.5 to 1.0 mg bid is helpful, especially when behavior or agitation is a problem.

For Detailed Discussion: Chapter 87, "Principles of Psycho-Oncology."

Answer 2.69. **The answer is (a).**

The patient has classical symptoms of depression that are superimposed on her illness. Despite the diagnosis of a life-threatening illness, most patients, after a transient period of turmoil, cope with the reality without major depressive symptoms. This patient has two risk factors for depression, personality and grief. One must depend on the psychological symptoms, not the physical symptoms of depression, which can also be caused by advanced cancer. The patient should be treated with supportive psychotherapy and psychotropic drugs aimed to reduce her insomnia.

For Detailed Discussion: (1) Chapter 87, "Principles of Psycho-Oncology."

Answer 2.70. **The answer is (d).**

High levels of resistance can be rapidly induced experimentally with antimetabolites such as methotrexate, and to a lesser degree, hydroxyurea. Etoposide resistance can also be readily induced by repetitive treatment. Resistance develops less readily to cyclophosphamide and the other alkylating agents. On the other hand, X-irradiation in vitro does not commonly result in significant resistance. When the surviving fraction of tumor cells is plotted against dose, the result is a straight line for irradiation, but curvilinear for alkylating agents and antimetabolites. Radiation resistance in vivo would appear to relate to tumor hypoxia. Methotrexate resistance can occur at the level of membrane transport, cytoplasmic activation, or change in target enzyme (dihydrofolate reductase) levels or mutation. Cyclophosphamide resistance has been reported to occur on the basis of aldehyde dehydrogenase induction, or increases in glutathione and its conjugating enzymes in the glutathione transferase isozyme system. Etoposide resistance may occur at the level of the target enzyme topoisomerase II or at the multidrug (P-170 transporter) level, and hydroxyurea resistance may be due to changes in ribonucleotide reductase. In general, there are multiple active processes (membrane transport, enzyme activation or inactivation) that affect chemotherapeutic agents and may form the basis for resistance development. These processes are much less prominent with irradiation, which perhaps explains the low level of resistance development.

For Detailed Discussion: (1) Chapter 48, "Biological and Physical Basis of Radiation Oncology."

Answer 2.71. **The answer is (b).**

Although multiple factors contribute to the impact of dose on tumor response, the largest impact relates to the intrinsic sensitivity to the agent involved. At a clinical level, the tumors that are most sensitive to chemotherapy, such as the hematologic malignancies and embryonal cancers, are those that respond best with high-dose bone marrow protection therapy. If one assumes that the same fraction of tumor cells are killed by each repetitively administered chemotherapy cycle, then a highly effective agent produces, at standard dose, a three log tumor cell kill; and doubling of dose may reduce viable cells to $1/10^6$. On the other hand, for a chemo-insensitive tumor where a given agent produces a less than half log kill, doubling the dose produces little additional meaningful effect. Tumor burden will impact on the dose effect in that blood supply; low growth fraction, hypoxia, and other factors accompany increasing tumor burden and are associated with diminished response. Clearly, the type of tumor, such as whether it is leukemia or lung cancer, will affect sensitivity, but such tissue differences are outweighed by intrinsic tumor chemosensitivity. The rapidity with which resistance develops could affect the impact of dose when repeated treatments are involved. Finally, a linear relationship between dose and AUC is a common finding and is consistent with the aforementioned variables' impact on dose. A steep dose effect could occur if inactivating enzymes are saturated and the AUC increases disproportionately to dose.

For Detailed Discussion: (1) Chapter 54, "Combination Chemotherapy, Dose, and Schedule."

Answer 2.72.   The answer is (d).

A long latent period could indeed result from failed, not sustained, activation, and expression of tumor angiogenesis factor genes. Tumors up to 0.5 mm in diameter can survive by diffusion of oxygen and metabolites, but growth beyond this requires angiogenesis. A long latent period might indeed be associated with G0 (resting) cells, but at least some experimental models, including the aforementioned angiogenesis model, suggest that cytokinetic activity may be prominent in small microscopic tumors and that growth does not occur because cell death and cell differentiation are in equilibrium with cell proliferation. Metastases require the ability of cancer cells to break through the basement membrane, travel through lymphatics of blood vessels, and bind to a distant organ, presumably via adhesion molecules. Metastases may exhibit clonal evolution impaired with the primary, but are not polyclonal.

For Detailed Discussion: (1) Chapter 51, "Principles of Medical Oncology."

Answer 2.73.   The answer is (a).

Most tumor cells in culture have a short (1–2 days) generation time, which is not different from normal, nontransformed cells. In vitro surrogates for neoplasia include lack of contact inhibition, ability to grow in soft agar, and immortalization. These qualities do not apply to normal cells. Telomerase produces telomeres, required for continued proliferation, which are essential for neoplasia and whose lack contributes to senescence of normal cells.

For Detailed Discussion: (1) Chapter 52, "Cytokinetics." (2) Murikami MS, Strobel MC, and Vander Woude G. Cell cycle regulation, oncogenes, and antineoplastic drugs. In Mendelsohn, Howley, Israel, and Liotto, eds. The Molecular Basis of Cancer. Philadelphia: WB Saunders, 1995, pp 3–18.

Answer 2.74. **The answer is (a).**

The volume doubling time for different tumors may vary substantially. For example, the volume doubling time for Burkitt's lymphoma may be as little as 2 weeks, whereas it can be as long as 6 months for some types of breast or bowel cancer. The cell cycle time is not a major determinant of the volume doubling time. In general, programmed cell death is enhanced in the more slow- growing tumors. The growth fraction, that is, the proportion of tumor cells in active cycle, is a major determinant of volume doubling time. In general, the number of growth factor receptors on the surface of tumor cells will effect growth rates as measured by volume doubling times. Finally, therapeutic tactics must consider resting (clonogenic) cells, because such cells are generally less susceptible to chemotherapy but capable of re-entering cycle.

For Detailed Discussion: (1) Chapter 52, "Cytokinetics."

Answer 2.75. **The answer is (d).**

Experimental and clinical solid tumors are commonly hypoxic; in general, the larger the tumors, the greater the degree of hypoxia. Such hypoxia may, in part, be the result of the diminished blood supply as well as increased metabolic activity on the part of the tumor cells. Hypoxia may limit tumor growth rate and thus affect the cell cycle. It may adversely affect response to therapeutic intervention with modalities such as x-irradiation and bleomycin, and perhaps other chemotherapeutic agents that require oxygen or other mechanisms of action. Hypoxia increases with "stress" on tumor cells, thus increasing genetic instability that is associated with an increased production of drug resistance.

For Detailed Discussion: (1) Chapter 48, "Biological and Physical Basis of Radiation Oncology." (2) Vaupel P. Oxygenation of solid tumors. In Teicher B, ed. Drug Resistance in Oncology. New York: Marcel Dekker, 1993, pp 53–86.

Answer 2.76. **The answer is (d).**

MTX enters the CSF with a 1% CSF/blood ratio at equilibrium. However, the marked increase in dose and blood levels made possible by leukovorin rescue does provide therapeutic concentrations in the CSF. It is crucial to begin rescue 24 hours after MTX; if leukovorin is delayed beyond 36 hours, toxicity is unacceptable. The biologic effect of MTX, as is true for many other cell cycle selective agents, correlates more with duration of exposure than with peak serum concentration. MTX is primarily cleared by the kidney, although hepatic catabolism to the inactive hydroxylated moiety plays a small role. Pleural effusions (or other third spacing) increase the volume of distribution of MTX, which decreases the plasma clearance.

For Detailed Discussion: (1) Chapter 60, "Folate Antagonists." (2) Chu E, Allegra CJ. Antifoles. In Chabner BA, Longo DL, eds. Cancer Chemotherapy and Biotherapy. Philadelphia: JB Lippincott, 1996, pp 109–148.

Answer 2.77. **The answer is (e).**

Studies have demonstrated that methotrexate resistance is associated with high levels of the target enzyme of DHFR due to extra gene copies or amplification. The amplified

DHFR gene was found to be present in the cytoplasm in episomes known as double minutes, and later, at greater levels of methotrexate resistance, as homogeneous staining regions (HSRs) evident on cytogenetic preparation. Reversion of resistance occurred more rapidly with double minutes than with HSRs. The production of resistance in vitro to methotrexate was found to be schedule dependent. Gene amplification was more likely to occur with sustained, continuous exposure to methotrexate than with higher peak concentrations of methotrexate.

For Detailed Discussion: (1) Chapter 60, "Folate Antagonists." (2) Chu E, Allegra CJ. Antifolates. In Chabner BA, Longo DL, eds. Cancer Chemotherapy and Biotherapy. Philadelphia: JB Lippincott, 1996, pp 109–148.

Answer 2.78.   The answer is (a).

The schedule of cancer chemotherapy administration frequently influences the biologic effect. Thus, methotrexate and most cell cycle–specific agents have a greater biologic effect for given total dose when given continuously as compared with intermittently. An important early study was the demonstration that intermittent methotrexate was superior to daily administration of methotrexate in the maintenance of complete remissions in children who have acute lymphocytic leukemia. The avoidance of peak concentrations of chemotherapeutic agents may diminish nausea and vomiting. Four-day continuous infusion of doxorubicin is less cardiotoxic than the same dose given by bolus. Similarly, weekly administration of doxorubicin is less cardiotoxic than the same dose given every 3 weeks. In contrast, the administration schedule of alkylating agents, which are not S-phase specific (independent of total dose) appears not to have a major impact on biologic effect.

For Detailed Discussion: (1) Chapter 54, "Combination Chemotherapy, Dose, Schedule."

Answer 2.79.   The answer is (a).

Surgery is the most frequent treatment for cancer. As a single modality, more patients are cured by surgery than any other treatment option. The success of surgery is based on 100% killing of all tumor cells that are excised. Thus, surgery is curative for local/regional disease. In contrast, chemotherapy and radiotherapy work by successive treatments that fractionally reduce the tumor burden, allowing adjacent normal cells or other susceptible normal tissues an interval for recovery. Often, these treatments are complementary, a phenomenon that is the basis for treatment protocols combining surgery with nonsurgical adjuvant or neoadjuvant therapies.

For Detailed Discussion: (1) Chapter 45, "Principles of Surgical Oncology."

Answer 2.80.   The answer is (e).

Certain patients who have a variety of solid neoplasms metastatic to distant sites (lung, liver, brain, etc) may enjoy prolonged survival following surgical resection. Slow-growing tumors, whether solitary or multiple, may be successfully resected with the result of long-term survival, especially when limited to one organ system. In fact, growth rates of pulmonary metastases (as measured by tumor doubling time) have been used to stratify patients into survival groups and thereby select those most likely to benefit from pulmonary resection. Patients who are candidates for hepatic resection are a minority, and postoperation radiotherapy is not indicated. The 5-year survival rate following resection of a solitary pulmonary metastasis for some cancers can exceed the 5-year survival for resectable primary bronchogenic carcinoma of the lung.

For Detailed Discussion: (1) Chapter 45, "Principles of Surgical Oncology."

Answer 2.81.   **The answer is (e).**

Results of the Eastern Cooperative Oncology Group trial 1684 have shown a statistically significant increase in the overall and relapse-free survival of AJCC stage III melanoma patients receiving interferon alpha-2b. Use of tamoxifen for treatment of melanoma is not restricted by gender. Chemotherapy and radiotherapy work by first-order cell killing, whereas surgery is based on zero-order kinetics. Neoplasms that respond to adjuvant chemotherapy include breast cancer, osteosarcoma, Ewing's sarcoma, Wilms' tumor, ovarian carcinoma, and colon carcinoma.

For Detailed Discussion: (1) Chapter 45, "Principles of Surgical Oncology."

Answer 2.82.   **The answer is (c).**

The TNM system has four subclassifications; cTNM, the clinical classification, represents the extent of disease before first definitive treatment; pTNM, the pathologic classification, incorporates prior biopsy results with those of the specimen resected during definitive surgery; rTNM, the retreatment classification, is used when restaging a cancer after recurrence and can include both clinical and pathologic evidence; and aTNM, the autopsy classification, is based on the postmortem examination. There is no pre-TNM or therapeutic TNM. The first classification by TNM is used in calculating survival, for example, not the last TNM.

For Detailed Discussion: (1) Chapter 45, "Principles of Surgical Oncology."

Answer 2.83.   **The answer is (e).**

When 5-FU is given by continuous infusion, higher doses are required to sustain adequate steady-state drug levels. In contrast, FdUrd by continuous IV infusion is at least 10-fold more potent than FU given in any other schedule. FdUrd can be relatively easily converted to the actual inhibitor of thymidylate synthase, 5-fluorodeoxyuridine monophosphate. If FdUrd is given by continuous infusion, it is not cleaved as rapidly to 5-FU. The fluoropyrimidines affect both DNA and RNA synthesis; the mechanism of resistance may differ according to the schedule; however, the reason for this remains unclear.

For Detailed Discussion: (1) Chapter 61, "Pyrimidine and Purine Antimetabolites."

Answer 2.84.   **The answer is (d).**

Empiric chemotherapy with a single agent in the presence of symptomatic esophagitis possibly due to *Candida, Aspergillus,* herpes simplex, herpes zoster, cytomegalovirus, bacterial infection, or chemotherapeutic necrosis may fall short of the mark. Esophagoscopy is more sensitive than a barium swallow. The patient should have cultures and smears performed of obvious ulcerative lesions in the oral cavity and esophagus that should be managed with parenteral medications, pain relief, and with a myelostimulatory hormone. Although empiric use of amphotericin B and acyclovir, together with parenteral hydration and pain control, might produce a satisfactory outcome, the diagnosis of cytomegalovirus could be missed. CMV esophagitis could respond more favorably to gancyclovir than acyclovir.

For Detailed Discussion: (1) Chapter 184, "Gastrointestinal Complications."

Answer 2.85. The answer is (c).

Lobectomy and pneumonectomy performed by VATS are attended by almost as much morbidity as open procedures. Removal of nodules, however, is highly successful if needed for diagnosis, and sometimes for therapy. Pleural inspection and pleurodesis are seldom undertaken without an intent to perform biopsy.

For Detailed Discussion: (1) Chapter 47, "Minimally Invasive Surgery."

Answer 2.86. The answer is (d).

Independence in the activities of daily living is the most important goal. After complete paraplegia, there is no basis to anticipate neural recovery despite the surgery, spine stabilization, or electrical stimulation. Personal assistance is not a satisfactory substitute for independence.

For Detailed Discussion: (1) Chapter 89, "Principles of Cancer Rehabilitation Medicine."

Answer 2.87. The answer is (a).

Pathologic fractures most often occur with large lesions in weightbearing bones, more often in women than men, and when widespread metastatic disease is present, more bones are put at risk. Pain, particularly when increasing, may signal impending fracture. A lesion that affects only 25% of cortical bone rarely fractures.

For Detailed Discussion: (1) Chapter 89, "Principles of Cancer Rehabilitation Medicine."

Answer 2.88. The answer is (d).

Phantom pain does not preclude successful use of a prosthetic limb. Inadequate performance status, emotional adjustment, stamina, motivation, family support—all can compromise successful prosthetic use. The surgical approach should provide an adequately shaped and sized stump.

For Detailed Discussion: (1) Chapter 89, "Principles of Cancer Rehabilitation Medicine."

Answer 2.89. The answer is (d).

Daily chlorambucil by mouth is only mildly emetogenic. It is reasonable to offer oral ondansetron and then to withdraw it after 1 or 2 days. If chlorambucil is being given as a single large dose at infrequent intervals, oral ondansetron may need to be repeated with each dose of chemotherapy.

For Detailed Discussion: (1) Chapter 174, "Chemotherapy-Induced Nausea and Vomiting."

Answer 2.90.   The answer is (a).

Cisplatin is the most emetogenic chemotherapeutic agent, causing predictable and severe vomiting. Young adults are particularly susceptible during the first 4 to 6 hours after administration. It is recommended that prophylactic antiemetics be given before the chemotherapy. The other drugs listed, especially vinblastine, tamoxifen, and bleomycin, rarely cause vomiting.

For Detailed Discussion: (1) Chapter 174, "Chemotherapy-Induced Nausea and Vomiting."

Answer 2.91.   The answer is (e).

Ondansetron and granisetron are potent and specific antagonists of the serotonin receptor, which exists in both central and peripheral sites. These drugs are the most effective agents for suppression of chemotherapy-induced or radiotherapy-induced emesis. Unfortunately, these safe drugs have limited effectiveness in non-cytotoxic therapy–induced vomiting.

For Detailed Discussion: (1) Chapter 174, "Chemotherapy-Induced Nausea and Vomiting."

Answer 2.92.   The answer is (d).

Metastatic neoplasms to bone usually produce significant technetium uptake. Only pure osteolytic lesions such as myeloma are cold, with a possibility of peripheral uptake around the margins. One would expect a different description of the bone scan and films in metastatic carcinomas or lymphomas. Fibrous dysplasia of bone in the humerus at age 50 is a remote possibility.

For Detailed Discussion: (1) Chapter 177, "Skeletal Complications."

Answer 2.93.   The answer is (b).

The description is one of calcinuric diabetes, which may occur in the course of hypercalcemia. Nausea, vomiting, torpor, confusion, polyuria, dehydration, and weakness are cardinal signs. Diabetes mellitus could produce all of these symptoms if the patient were becoming acidotic. Polyuria and dehydration could occur with diabetes insipidus, but this does not accompany meningeal metastases. Adrenal metastases can produce addisonian crisis, but polyuria is less prominent. Uremia could mimic this state, and the differential diagnosis would clearly depend on emergency blood chemistry tests that measure electrolytes, calcium, and osmolality of plasma and urine.

For Detailed Discussion: (1) Chapter 177, "Skeletal Complications."

Answer 2.94. **The answer is (c).**

Not all patients who are estrogen positive respond well to tamoxifen or to oophorectomy. Alternatively, patients who are ER negative have very low response rates. Chemotherapeutic response is not dependent on ER status.

For Detailed Discussion: (1) Chapter 69, "Steroid Hormone Binding and Hormone Receptors."

Answer 2.95. **The answer is (d).**

A profoundly neutropenic patient who has a nodular density in the upper lung field that cavitates, which leads to hemoptysis, suggests *Aspergillus* infection. In a fungal cavity, slight hemoptysis can change to massive blood loss and asphyxiation. Surgical excision is the conservative therapy, but continuation of amphotericin is needed to prevent dissemination. There are no data that support combining amphotericin B with itraconazole.

For Detailed Discussion: (1) Chapter 189, "Infections in Patients with Cancer."

Answer 2.96. **The answer is (e).**

The association of thyroid cancer with thyroid irradiation is well established. The multiplicity of nodules in an irradiated thyroid precludes biopsy of all. The dominant nodule may be falsely negative. Fine needle aspiration entails considerable sampling error that is reduced by larger bore surgical biopsy needles. Radioiodine scanning does not exclude malignancy. Radioiodine ablation may not affect a neoplasm without high uptake. Thyroidectomy is the procedure of choice.

For Detailed Discussion: (1) Chapter 187, "Endocrine Complications."

Answer 2.97. **The answer is (c).**

Substitution therapy should not be given before a recognized need for it. Observation alone is appropriate, and the radiation effect on the pituitary and nearby hypothalamus should not cause significant alteration, if any, before 3 months. The incidence of panhypopituitarism approaches 90% at 10 years. Pituitary function should be reassessed at 1 year after radiotherapy.

For Detailed Discussion: (1) Chapter 187, "Endocrine Complications."

Answer 2.98. **The answer is (b).**

The rapid reappearance of ulceration involving necrotic bone suggests radionecrosis. Mucosal biopsy (but not bone biopsy) excludes the unlikely diagnosis of recurrent carcinoma. Because antibiotic coverage should have included anaerobic and gram-positive coverage, there is little basis to change antibiotics. Most radionecrotic mouth ulcers heal with hyperbaric oxygenation, and surgical intervention is not required.

For Detailed Discussion: (1) Chapter 185, "Oral Complications." (2) Mansfield MJ, et al. Hyperbaric oxygen as an adjuvant in the treatment of osteoradionecrosis of the jaw. J Oral Surg 1981;39:585.

Answer 2.99.   **The answer is (b).**

Delay until spontaneous recovery of granulocyte or platelet count is too dangerous, because of the possibility of infection. Local control eventually will require extraction, because root canal therapy will be inappropriate in this situation. Antibiotic treatment should cover all possible organisms: gram-positive, gram-negative, and anaerobic. Granulocyte transfusions are unnecessary, and major blood loss should not be expected from a wound where tissue clotting factors abound. Because filgrastim may elevate the granulocyte count rapidly, extraction ideally should be delayed until the granulocyte count is high enough to defend against bacteria. If the prospect is for significant delay, however, extraction should be performed with the recognition that granulocytosis will soon occur.

For Detailed Discussion: (1) Chapter 185, "Oral Complications."

Answer 2.100.   **The answer is (c).**

Chemotherapy can enhance herpes simplex ulcerations that are usually discrete. Stomatitis from chemotherapy is most typically a field phenomenon with focal ulceration. Fungal infection ordinarily is indicated by white punctuate lesions. Antibody titers do not indicate present infection status, and blood culture would be uninformative. Viral (and fungal) culture is important, because an established diagnosis would not only allow proper treatment for the present attack, but also for prophylactic administration of acyclovir with the next chemotherapy cycle.

For Detailed Discussion: (1) Chapter 185, "Oral Complications."

Answer 2.101.   **The answer is (a).**

Xerostomia following parotid irradiation (usually the contralateral parotid is in the exit portal too) predisposes to caries. None of the other statements is true. Loss of saliva secondary to radiotherapy is associated with a decrease in oral flushing and diminished oral IgA levels, which predispose the patient to infections and caries; post-radiotherapy prophylaxis could involve secretion replacement (salivary substitute), pilocarpine HCl, and topical fluoride.

For Detailed Discussion: (1) Chapter 185, "Oral Complications."

Answer 2.102.   **The answer is (a).**

Increase in P-glycoprotein expression results in amplification of the MDR pump, thereby diminishing intracellular drug concentration and exposure time to etoposide. No known effects on etoposide resistance occur from altered topoisomerase I activity or change in cyclic AMP or adenosine deaminase.

For Detailed Discussion: (1) Chapter 53, "Drug Resistance and its Clinical Circumvention."

Answer 2.103.   **The answer is (c).**

Doxorubicin and mitozantrone, even though synthetic, are both planar polycyclic molecules susceptible to the MDR pump and usually show cross-resistance. Vincristine and vinorelbine have chemical substituent changes on different halves of the complex *Vinca* molecules. Nonetheless, their mechanisms of action are the same, and cross-resistance would doubtless be encountered shortly after the second drug was started. Methotrexate and trimetrexate have some difference in cellular uptake, but both inhibit dihydrofolic reductase, and if used successively, on a clinical basis would doubtless display cross-resistance. Chlorambucil and melphalan are similar alkylating agents whose use results in every expectation of cross-resistance. Ara-C, as a precursor for Ara-CTP and DNA incorporation (with chain termination), works differently from daunorubicin, which has activities on topoisomerase II and on DNA directly, probably as a quinone.

For Detailed Discussion: (1) Chapter 53, "Drug Resistance and its Clinical Circumvention."

Answer 2.104.　The answer is (c).

Liver transplantation for multiple colonic metastases is of dubious value at best, and certainly inappropriate for a patient who is 70 years old. Doxorubicin-paclitaxel, although active in treating breast and lung cancers, has not been favorably reported on for metastatic colon cancer. rhIFNa has been used with fluorouracil in treating metastatic colon cancer, but is not known to show activity alone. Although anecdotal reports have appeared that show benefit of IL-2 for patients with colon carcinoma, a high-dose regimen every 3 weeks is not a treatment of choice. The relative merits of irinotecan, fluorouracil, or a combination of these drugs with other agents or with each other have not yet been established.

For Detailed Discussion: (1) Chapter 65, "DNA Topoisomerase I Inhibitors."

Answer 2.105.　The answer is (b).

Topotecan and irinotecan exert their activity against topoisomerase I. Docetaxel and paclitaxel are active against microtubule. Gemcitabine is a nucleotide analogue of a DNA constituent and acts as an antimetabolite. Vinorelbine is a *Vinca* alkaloid that impairs tubular polymerization.

For Detailed Discussion: (1) Chapter 65, "DNA Topoisomerase I Inhibitors."

Answer 2.106.　The answer is (a).

Hypercalcemia occurs in approximately one in eight patients with lung cancer, especially those who have squamous cell histology. Epidermoid carcinoma is by far the most likely diagnosis for this patient of those listed. Secretion of PTH–like hormone by the tumor can be detected in serum. Other mechanisms of hypercalcemia include direct bony destruction due to metastatic tumors or the secretion of local substances (eg, osteoclast activating factor).

For Detailed Discussion: (1) Chapter 77, "Paraneoplastic Syndromes."

Answer 2.107.　The answer is (c).

The effects of calcitonin are short-lived. Saline infusion should certainly be used in addition to other treatment to replete the plasma volume (required for adequate output) often diminished by calcinuric diabetes. Furosemide diminishes Na+ reabsorption but not Ca++. Pamidronate binds tightly to the ATP binding site on the osteoclast, which inhibits further bone resorption. Dexamethasone has weak if any activity on calcium resorption in the renal tubule. Radiotherapy to the tumor would take weeks to have an effect. The patient is too ill for surgery with a serum calcium of 18 mg/dL.

For Detailed Discussion: (1) Chapter 77, "Paraneoplastic Syndromes."

Answer 2.108.   **The answer is (d).**

Oat cell carcinoma is by far the most common tumor cause of Cushing's syndrome. Cortisol levels are not suppressed by 8 mL of dexamethasone, however, as they were in this woman. The MRI of the brain stem and petrosal venous sampling showing no ACTH gradient over the periphery effectively eliminate primary Cushing's disease. The most likely diagnosis then is carcinoma of the thymus or bronchial carcinoid. The latter is favored on the basis of prevalence, although a CT scan of the chest would be definitive.

For Detailed Discussion: (1) Chapter 77, "Paraneoplastic Syndromes."

Answer 2.109.   **The answer is (d).**

Surgical cytoreduction is of primary importance in the patient found to have primary ovarian carcinoma; a cytoreductive procedure like that described is technically not feasible with current technology. Despite the possible advantages MIS may offer some patients, any diminution in survival based on the surgical approach is not generally acceptable.

For Detailed Discussion: (1) Chapter 47, "Minimal Invasive Surgery".

Answer 2.110.   **The answer is (c).**

SVCS is commonly caused by invasion of the superior mediastinum and obstruction of the SVC by tumor (78–97%). Small-cell lung carcinoma is the most common neoplasm causing SVCS (27–50%), followed by non–small-cell lung carcinoma. Lymphoma accounts for 2 to 20% of cases of SVCS, but these are almost exclusively lymphoblastic and diffuse large-cell non-Hodgkin's lymphomas. SVCS as a result of Hodgkin's disease is extremely rare, accounting for 0 to 1% of cases. Breast cancer, by its high prevalence, is the most metastatic "extrathoracic" cancer to cause SVCS, representing approximately 5% of cases reported.

For Detailed Discussion: (1) Chapter 190, "Oncological Emergencies."

Answer 2.111.   **The answer is (e).**

This patient has the characteristic findings of SVCS. Unfortunately, less than half of patients at preservation have a histologic diagnosis of cancer. The evaluation should proceed from the least invasive to the most invasive to achieve a pathologic diagnosis. Small-cell lung carcinoma (SCLC) is the most common cause, accounting for 27 to 50% of cases of SVCS. SCLC primary tumors tend to be large and involve the larger, more central bronchi. The diagnosis can be made by sputum cytology in more than 60% of cases when the cause is SCLC. If cytology is nondiagnostic, progressively more invasive procedures up to and including open thoracotomy and biopsy may be safely performed in patients with SVCS. Only those patients with neurologic findings due to increased intracranial pressure or airway obstruction require emergency radiotherapy without a tissue diagnosis. Once stabilized, these patients should then rapidly undergo an appropriate biopsy to establish the diagnosis.

For Detailed Discussion: (1) Chapter 190, "Oncological Emergencies."

Answer 2.112.   The answer is (c).

The use of chemotherapy as a single modality or in combination with radiotherapy is as effective as radiotherapy alone in sensitive neoplasms such as small-cell lung carcinoma or lymphoma. Resolution of both subjective complaints and physical findings of SVCS occur equally as rapidly and completely with chemotherapy for these diseases as with radiotherapy. A poor response of SVCS to initial treatment suggests the possibility of superimposed SVC thrombosis, which may be seen in 30 to 50% of patients. However, the use of anticoagulation therapy in this circumstance does not appear to improve survival and may be associated with an increased risk of intracerebral hemorrhage. SVCS caused by indwelling venous access catheters may be safely and effectively treated with a low dose of a thrombolytic agent such as urokinase. Despite older literature to the contrary, SVCS is rarely life-threatening. In large series, 20 to 30% of patients with SVCS survived for 2 years. Those who do succumb do so because of progression of the underlying cancer, and not the SVCS. Only patients who have neurologic findings due to increased intracranial pressure or airway obstruction are at risk for serious acute morbidity or mortality.

For Detailed Discussion: (1) Chapter 190, "Oncological Emergencies."

Answer 2.113.   The answer is (a).

In cancer patients who have serious acute upper gastrointestinal bleeding, the most frequent cause found on endoscopy is acute erosive gastritis or stress ulceration, which accounts for 32 to 48% of cases. Risk factors include use of nonsteroidal anti-inflammatory drugs, corticosteroids, and ethanol, as well as concurrent sepsis and renal or hepatic failure. The Mallory-Weiss syndrome, which develops from uncontrolled emesis, although reported, is rare. Mucosal metastases as a cause of serious GI bleeding are also uncommon, but have been reported with metastatic melanoma and lung and breast carcinoma. IL-2–induced thrombocytopenia is rarely severe or long-lasting and does not usually cause bleeding without a pre-existing structural abnormality of the gastrointestinal tract. Esophageal varices are usually indicative of pre-existing liver disease and may be a source of bleeding.

For Detailed Discussion: (1) Chapter 190, "Oncological Emergencies."

Answer 2.114.   The answer is (d).

The incidence of spontaneous carotid artery rupture ("blowout") has declined precipitously, even in patients with advanced head and neck cancers, as a result of improved surgical and radiotherapy techniques. Preoperative radiotherapy and tissue necrosis, with the development of orocutaneous fistulas and necrosis of the wall of the carotid artery, are the most common predisposing events. The blowout is often preceded by minor bleeding episodes or "sentinel" bleeds. Once the rupture occurs, it is essential that control of the bleeding be obtained by firm digital pressure to occlude the carotid artery. The patient should then be stabilized and taken to the operating room for ligation and excision of the necrotic segment of the artery. Carotid artery rupture carries up to a 50% risk of serious neurologic sequelae.

For Detailed Discussion: (1) Chapter 190, "Oncological Emergencies."

Answer 2.115. **The answer is (e).**

Doxorubicin is a powerful vesicant which, if extravasated, can result in severe tissue necrosis. Because of its frequent use in treating breast cancer and many other common malignancies, doxorubicin probably has the greatest risk of serious extravasation injury. Once an extravasation is suspected, all drug administration should be stopped, and the IV line should be aspirated of any drug and then removed. Cooling of the extravasation site with an ice pack reduces the risk of tissue necrosis as a result of doxorubicin extravasation from 50% to approximately 10%. Because necrosis may not be evident for 10 to 14 days, close follow-up is mandatory. Good quality assurance and medicolegal intervention mandates complete documentation of the event and interventions taken. Photographs should be taken, if possible. Local injections of corticosteroids or other commercially available agents have not been proved to be beneficial and may increase the risk of ulceration. A plastic surgery consultation should be obtained for consideration of excision and grafting if there is necrosis or ongoing inflammation 48 hours after the extravasation has occurred.

For Detailed Discussion: (1) Chapter 190, "Oncological Emergencies."

Answer 2.116. **The answer is (e).**

Without pleurodesis or definitive systemic therapy, more than 70% of symptomatic malignant pleural effusions will reaccumulate within 30 days of drainage. Several commonly used chemotherapeutic agents, including interleukin-2, methotrexate, bleomycin, procarbazine, cyclophosphamide, and mitomycin have been associated with the development of non-malignant pleural effusions in cancer patients. More than 50% of pleural effusions reported in modern series are cytologically positive for malignant cells; when the effusion is massive, as defined by a volume ≥ 200 mL, the probability that it is due to a neoplasm is almost 100%. Although the frequency of pleural effusion in malignant mesothelioma is as high as 95%, cytologic examination of pleural fluid is diagnostic of mesothelioma in only 3 to 16% of patients. Lymphomas can cause bilateral effusions, as can any other metastatic disease.

For Detailed Discussion: (1) Chapter 190, "Oncological Emergencies."

Answer 2.117. **The answer is (d).**

This young male patient with bulky high-grade non-Hodgkin's lymphoma is at increased risk for urate nephropathy and tumor lysis syndrome (TLS). The approach to TLS should be prophylactic by maintaining hydration, good urine output, an alkaline urine pH (7.5), and inhibition of the enzyme xanthine oxidase by allopurinol. This decreases the production of relatively insoluble uric acid. Additionally, close monitoring of electrolytes and renal function is required. The expectant management and early institution of hemodialysis has decreased the mortality from TLS significantly. If possible, therapy should be delayed until the patient has received adequate TLS prophylaxis. Use of corticosteroids in patients who have lymphoma has been associated with tumor necrosis and induction of TLS because of these agents' lympholytic activity.

For Detailed Discussion: (1) Chapter 190, "Oncological Emergencies."

Answer 2.118.   **The answer is (b).**

The history and physical examination is entirely consistent with acute hemodynamically significant pericardial tamponade, most likely from involvement of the pericardium by lung cancer. The patient has not responded to intravascular volume expansion, which indicates that he is on a critical limb of his cardiac work-function curve and cannot compensate any further. It is unlikely that vasopressors will improve blood pressure, and they may only serve to induce serious arrhythmias. Right heart catheterization is reserved for stable patients in whom the diagnosis is unclear after echocardiography. Two-dimensional echocardiography is a noninvasive, safe, rapid, and accurate diagnostic technique for pericardial tamponade; however, in the patient who is hemodynamically unstable and may not have easy access to echocardiography, emergency pericardiocentesis or pericardiotomy (pericardial "window") is the appropriate treatment. An emergency pericardiocentesis can be performed safely at the bedside with a 3% risk of morbidity and a less than 1% risk of mortality. Anticoagulation therapy plays no role in the treatment of malignant pericardial tamponade and may worsen the tamponade by increasing intrapericardial bleeding.

For Detailed Discussion: (1) Chapter 190, "Oncological Emergencies."

CHAPTER 3

Specific Neoplasms

DIRECTIONS: Each question below contains five suggested responses. Select the best response to each question.

QUESTIONS

Question 3.1.   **A 34-year-old woman has a right thyroid lobectomy and isthmusectomy to remove a suspicious mass found by fine needle aspiration. Permanent section of the specimen demonstrates medullary carcinoma. The patient has no family history of thyroid cancer. The next step in her management is:**

a)   Calcitonin and carcinoembryonic antigen (CEA) serum level markers are monitored to predict recurrence.
b)   A computed tomography (CT) scan of the neck and chest are performed to rule out local or distant metastases.
c)   External beam radiation of the remaining thyroid tissue is performed.
d)   Reoperation and completion of thyroidectomy are done.
e)   Reoperation, completion of thyroidectomy, and ipsilateral cervical node dissection are performed.

Question 3.2.   **A 55-year-old man has a thyroid lobectomy and isthmusectomy for a 2-cm papillary carcinoma. At the time of surgery, the patient is found to have one of five nodes that contain metastases. Which one of the following is a poor prognostic indicator:**

a)   Age
b)   Size of the tumor up to 5 cm
c)   Papillary carcinoma histology
d)   Lymph node metastases
e)   Remaining thyroid gland after lobectomy and isthmusectomy

Question 3.3.   **Patients who have differentiated thyroid carcinoma may be managed with less than total thyroidectomy. Arguments that support this statement include all EXCEPT:**

a)   Any multifocality of the tumor will be microscopic and insignificant.
b)   Postoperative radioiodine is rarely necessary for diagnosis or therapy.
c)   High-risk patients can be accurately determined by clinical criteria.
d)   Papillary carcinoma never converts to anaplastic carcinoma.
e)   The incidence of hypoparathyroidism is less with subtotal thyroidectomy.

Question 3.4.   **A 68-year-old woman, a widow of a smoker, was initially seen with a 3-month history of persistent cough. A chest radiograph showed a 4-cm midlung mass. Further work-up confirmed the initial suspicion of lung** cancer. What percent increase in lung cancer incidence is seen when a non-smoker living with a smoker is compared with a nonsmoker living with a non-smoker?

a)   3%
b)   15%
c)   30%
d)   75%
e)   100%

Question 3.5.   Multiple co-carcinogens in the work environment are noted to contribute to carcinogenesis. Which of the following elements is not a documented occupational carcinogen for lung cancer?

a)   Beryllium
b)   Nickel
c)   Chromium
d)   Cadmium
e)   Arsenic

Question 3.6.   A 66-year-old insulation worker was initially seen with a 6-month history of anorexia and fatigue and was found to have Stage II lung cancer. The tumor was biopsied. The surgeon called the pathology department after the procedure to find out whether c-myc was expressed in the specimen. ***C-myc*** amplification in small-cell lung carcinoma is shown to be significant for which of the following parameters?

a)   Early metastasis
b)   Chemotherapy resistance
c)   Radiation resistance
d)   Early relapse
e)   None of the aforementioned

Question 3.7.   A 71-year-old uranium miner recently migrated to the United States and visited a doctor with a 4-month history of hemoptysis. Subsequent work-up included a bronchoscopy and a specimen sent to a research labora-tory to check for presence of the ***k-ras*** oncogene. How are ***ras*** family onco-genes activated?

a)   Point nucleotide mutation
b)   Signal transduction
c)   Receptor amplification
d)   Gene integration
e)   Autocrine hormonal stimulation

Question 3.8.   A 55-year-old tobacco industry executive developed hoarse-ness and subsequently was found to have an apical tumor that was causing vocal cord paralysis. Subsequent biopsy showed squamous cell carcinoma. Which of the following is a tobacco-specific nitrosamine that might be in-volved in the development of lung cancer in this patient?

a)   Nitrosodimethylamine
b)   Ethyl nitrosamine

c)   Tyrosine
d)   Suramin
e)   Tetranitromethylamine

Question 3.9.   **A 50-year-old pesticide manufacturer developed shortness of breath and subsequently was found to have small-cell lung carcinoma. Which of the following growth factors is produced by most small-cell lung carcinoma cell lines?**

a)   Epidermal growth factor
b)   Bombesin
c)   Transforming growth factor alpha
d)   Keratinocyte growth factor
e)   Endothelial growth factor

Question 3.10.   **A 53-year-old fisherman who smoked a pipe for more than 30 years developed dysphagia and was found to have Stage II laryngeal cancer that was completely resected and subsequently treated with adjuvant therapy. Other than metastasis, which of the following would be the most likely type of cancer in this patient?**

a)   Adenocarcinoma of the lung
b)   Bladder cancer
c)   Cancer of the esophagus
d)   Squamous cell carcinoma of the lung
e)   Gastric cancer

Question 3.11.   **A 72-year-old retired man was admitted because he was experiencing recent dyspnea on exertion. Chest radiograph revealed a right pleural effusion. Physical findings were otherwise unremarkable, and he was afebrile. Thoracentesis yielded 1200 mL of clear exudate. Cytology test results were negative for malignant cells. Pleural needle biopsy showed "reactive fibrosis." The patient had a 20 pack-year history of cigarette smoking and quit smoking 30 years previously. Prior history revealed that he worked for 10 months as a pipe-fitter in a naval shipyard during World War II. CT scan of the chest showed minimal residual pleural fluid and thickening. Bronchoscopy was entirely normal. The most appropriate course of action for this patient is:**

a)   Injection of a sclerosing agent into the pleural cavity
b)   A short trial of oral corticosteroid therapy
c)   Careful follow-up, including chest radiograph every 3 months
d)   Thoracoscopy
e)   Exploratory thoracotomy

Question 3.12.   **A 35-year-old man was initially seen with a 2-week history of bleeding gums and easy bruising. A complete blood count reveals: white blood cells (WBC), 1500/μL; hematocrit (HCT), 25%; and platelet count, 16,000/μL. WBC differential includes 20% neutrophils, 10% bands, 20% lymphocytes, 5% metamyelocytes, 5% myelocytes, 20% blasts, and 20% promyelocytes. Partial thromboplastin time is 45 seconds, and prothrombin time is 18 seconds. Bone marrow aspiration discloses infiltration with heavily granulated**

"promyelocytes." Which of the following represents the best antineoplastic management for this patient?

a) Cytosine arabinoside (ara-C) 3 g/m^2 intravenously over 3 hours, twice daily on Days 1, 3, and 5
b) Ara-C 400 mg/m^2 by continuous intravenous (IV) infusion on Days 1 through 5
c) Idarubicin 12 mg/m^2 intravenous bolus daily for 3 days, plus ara-C 100 mg/m^2 per day by continuous intravenous infusion for 7 days
d) All-*trans*-retinoic acid 45 mg/m^2 orally per day for 30 days
e) 13-*cis*-retinoic acid 45 mg/m^2 orally per day for 30 days

Question 3.13.　A 7-year-old girl was treated at age 4 for medulloblastoma. The tumor was totally resected, and following surgery the child received 3600 cGy of craniospinal irradiation and local boost radiotherapy to a total dose of 5500 cGy. The parents come to your office complaining that the child is not doing well in school and is not growing well. Do you:

a) Suggest to the family that this is an emotional problem and refer the child to a child psychiatrist.
b) Immediately begin an extensive work-up for tumor recurrence, including chest radiograph and bone marrow biopsy.
c) Explain that this a normal occurrence after posterior fossa surgery, so further tests are not needed.
d) Reassure the parents that the majority of children spontaneously improve, and tell them that this is a transient finding after surgery and radiotherapy.
e) Explain to the family that these are known sequelae after radiotherapy, and inform them that means should be employed to try to remediate the problems.

Question 3.14.　A 6-year-old boy has a 2-month history of headaches and a 1-week history of unsteadiness and double vision. Magnetic resonance imaging (MRI) scan demonstrates a large mass filling the fourth ventricle and causing hydrocephalus. Surgery is performed, and a large posterior fossa mass abutting the brain stem is removed; this mass is pathologically comprised of small undifferentiated cells. The next step in management should be:

a) Immediate local site irradiation to a total dose of 4000 cGy
b) Reassurance that the tumor has been surgically cured, so no further treatment is indicated
c) Performance of tests to determine a systemic primary tumor
d) Performance of staging studies, including MRI of the spine and cerebrospinal fluid cytology before initiation of further treatment delivery
e) Delivery of intra-arterial chemotherapy

Question 3.15.　A 7-year-old girl is initially seen with a 2-month history of nonspecific mild headaches, double vision, and unsteadiness. On examination, the child has a right sixth nerve palsy, right-sided peripheral facial weakness, left-sided weakness of the arm and leg, and right upper extremity dysmetria. The child has had difficulty swallowing for the last week, and on examination has a decreased gag response. MRI of the brain demonstrates a diffusely enlarged brain stem, which is of decreased signal intensity on T1-weighted images and of increased signal intensity on T2-weighted images. There is no contrast enhancement. The lateral and third ventricle are normal

in size; the fourth ventricle is somewhat effaced and pushed posteriorly. The next step in management would be to:

a) Attempt to surgically remove the lesion
b) Obtain cerebrospinal fluid to make a specific diagnosis; if the cerebrospinal fluid is normal, observe the patient for further changes before initiating management
c) Begin definitive therapy without histologic confirmation
d) Begin an extensive work-up for systemic metastases
e) Withhold all treatment, because the likelihood of benefit is low

Question 3.16.   A 13-month-old girl is initially seen with right eye leukocoria. She is otherwise well, and the physical examination is otherwise unremarkable. You refer her to an ophthalmology consultant whose clinical diagnosis is unilateral retinoblastoma. Which of the following would not be appropriate considerations as part of the initial treatment plan?

a) Ophthalmologic examination under general anesthesia
b) MRI imaging of the head and orbit
c) Biopsy of the intraocular mass
d) Enucleation of the eye without prior pathologic confirmation of the diagnosis
e) Consultation with the radiation oncologist

Question 3.17.   A 12-year-old boy has a 3-day history of right-sided frontal headache. History reveals that he was diagnosed with bilateral retinoblastoma as an infant and was treated with external beam radiotherapy only. He has subsequently done well until the current problem began. Which of the following is the LEAST likely diagnosis?

a) Recurrent retinoblastoma
b) Right ethmoid sinus osteosarcoma
c) Migraine headache
d) Right frontal glioblastoma multiforme
e) Right maxillary sinusitis

Question 3.18.   A 55-year-old woman who has known metastatic breast cancer to multiple skeletal areas has shown an excellent response to tamoxifen, as monitored by bone scans. She now develops bilateral decreasing visual acuity and is sent for an ophthalmic examination. Findings at that examination include multiple choroidal metastases in the posterior region of each eye, with associated serious detachments. The next step in this patient's management should be:

a) Biopsy of one of these lesions with a fine needle aspiration
b) Discontinuation of the tamoxifen treatment and initiation of adriamycin-containing multidrug chemotherapy
c) Obtaining an MRI or CT scan of the head and initiating external beam radiotherapy to the eyes
d) Cryotherapy of the lesions with a specially designed posterior segment cryotherapy probe
e) Discontinuation of tamoxifen therapy and starting treatment with megestrol acetate

Question 3.19. **A 2½-year-old girl is initially seen with a "cat's eye" reflex in her right eye noted by her parents in looking at a photograph taken with flash photography. The child is referred to an eye tumor specialist who diagnoses bilateral retinoblastoma. After an extent-of-disease work-up reveals that the disease is limited to both eyes, the parents are advised that radiotherapy is the treatment of choice. Because of the extent of disease in both eyes, the other alternative is bilateral enucleation. The parents of this child are leaning strongly toward a decision to conserve both eyes and treat with radiotherapy. The most serious side effect for the girl's parents to consider is:**

a)   Permanent loss of eyelashes and eyebrows
b)   Increase in the relative risk of a second malignancy
c)   Pronounced and disfiguring temporal bone hypoplasia
d)   Dry eyes, with subsequent corneal abrasion and possible loss of vision
e)   Learning disability

Question 3.20. **Lung cancer epidemiology is changing. Which cell type of lung carcinoma is decreasing in frequency?**

a)   Small-cell
b)   Large-cell
c)   Squamous cell
d)   Adenocarcinoma
e)   Adenosquamous cell

Question 3.21. **A 76-year-old retired worker from a Mustard gas plant developed fatigue and was found to have anemia. Subsequent work-up revealed Stage IV adenocarcinoma of the right lung. The most frequent site of metastases for this tumor is the:**

a)   Spleen
b)   Bone
c)   Brain
d)   Heart
e)   Retroperitoneum

Question 3.22. **A 44-year-old waiter had a 3-month history of flushing, wheezing, and diarrhea and was found to have a carcinoid tumor of the left lung. From the biopsy specimen, all of the following criteria were used to distinguish an atypical carcinoid from a typical one EXCEPT:**

a)   Increased mitotic activity
b)   Nuclear pleomorphism, hyperchromatism
c)   Disorganization of architecture
d)   Tumor necrosis
e)   Cytologic pleomorphism

Question 3.23. **A 56-year-old retired nuclear engineer had several weeks' history of cough and recently worsening dyspnea. A radiograph showed a right midlung mass. The patient underwent an open lung biopsy. Which of the following immunohistochemistry stains would be appropriate to use to differ-**

entiate small-cell lung carcinoma (SCLC) from non–small-cell lung carcinoma (NSCLC) in this patient?

a) Keratin
b) Myeloperoxidase
c) nM-23 tumor suppressor gene expression
d) Terminal deoxynucleotidyl transferase (TdT)
e) S100 or HMB-45 immunohistochemistry staining

Question 3.24. **A 56-year-old engineer from the refining industry was seen with a complaint of worsening dyspnea. A chest radiograph showed a large pleural effusion on the right side and a right hilar mass of indeterminate size. Malignant cells were detected on sputum cytology. All of the following factors relating to this patient will significantly influence survival in lung cancer EXCEPT:**

a) Size of the tumor
b) Location in relation to the carina
c) Precarinal lymph node involvement
d) Thoracentesis fluid showing malignant cells
e) Performance status

Question 3.25. **A 56-year-old technician working in the aerospace industry developed fevers up to 102°F as well as dyspnea. Examination showed distention of neck veins and inspiratory crackles. Subsequent echocardiogram showed pericardial thickening and effusion. Which of the following neoplasms would be the most likely to produce pericardial involvement?**

a) Lung cancer
b) Colon cancer
c) Melanoma
d) Breast cancer
e) Esophageal cancer

Question 3.26. **A 58-year-old television repairman who is undergoing adjuvant chemotherapy for Stage II SCLC was observed to have seizure activity by his co-workers. In the emergency room, his serum sodium level was 110 mEq/dL, and results of CT scan of his head were negative for an acute process. Which of the following disorders needs to be ruled out before determining that a tumor has caused syndrome of inappropriate antidiuretic hormone (SIADH)?**

a) Volume depletion
b) Pneumonia
c) Drug effect from vincristine
d) Adrenal insufficiency
e) Cirrhosis

Question 3.27. **A 56-year-old railroad worker smoked one to two packs of cigarettes up until 2 years ago. He comes into his internist's office with complaints of gynecomastia. An endocrine work-up showed a 4-cm round density in the left lower lung field. Sputum cytology results were positive for malignancy.**

Human chorionic gonadotropin (hCG) level was three times the upper limit of normal. Which of the following lung cancer types would be most commonly associated with hCG hormone secretion?

a) Squamous cell
b) Anaplastic large-cell
c) Anaplastic small-cell
d) Adenosquamous cell
e) Adenocarcinoma

Question 3.28. **All of the following are true regarding treatment of gallbladder cancer EXCEPT:**

a) Lesions limited to the submucosa can be managed with cholecystectomy alone.
b) Extended cholecystectomy improves survival in Stage II (tumor invades perimuscular connective tissue) gallbladder cancer.
c) A prospective randomized study reported that more extensive surgery improves the survival of patients whose tumors involve the liver.
d) A second-look operation is warranted for Stage III (T3 tumors invade serosa, one adjacent organ, or extends into liver less than 2 (cm, or both)) gallbladder cancer, and further liver resection is needed.
e) The prevalence of laparoscopic cholecystectomy has increased the rate of recurrence at the trocar site.

Question 3.29. **Which of the following is true with regard to the diagnosis of gallbladder cancer:**

a) The use of ultrasound has greatly increased the rate of preoperative diagnosis of gallbladder cancer.
b) A large majority of gallbladder cancers are diagnosed preoperatively.
c) The majority of gallbladder cancers are diagnosed at an early stage.
d) The use of MRI has aided the rate of preoperative diagnosis of gallbladder cancer.
e) At the time of diagnosis, the majority of gallbladder cancers are technically resectable.

Question 3.30. **Which of the following is true regarding the treatment of gallbladder cancer?**

a) Because of the high sensitivity of this cancer to chemotherapy, the initial response to chemotherapy is very good.
b) Intraoperative radiotherapy improves the survival rate associated with surgery alone.
c) Papillary cancer has the same prognosis as tubular cancer.
d) Most treatment failures after complete surgical resection are caused by liver metastasis.
e) Radiotherapy is best for palliating obstructive jaundice caused by gallbladder cancer.

Question 3.31. **A patient is found to have a dilated biliary tract as revealed by ultrasound; CT scan demonstrates a 4-cm mass in the head of the pan-**

creas just lateral to the superior mesenteric vein and artery. There is no evidence of nodal or liver metastases. Endoscopic retrograde cholangiopancreatography (ERCP) demonstrates a distal dilation of the pancreatic duct, with a stricture of the duct near the head of the pancreas. Brush cytology is nondiagnostic. The next step in the management of this patient is:

a) CT scan–directed percutaneous biopsy of the pancreatic head mass
b) Mesenteric angiogram to determine the resectability of the mass
c) Obtain serum tumor markers CEA and CA 19–9 serum levels
d) Abdominal exploration with transduodenal biopsies of the pancreatic mass and pancreaticoduodenectomy only if the biospies demonstrate malignancy
e) Pancreatoduodectomy and resection of the superior mesenteric vein or portal vein if it is encased by tumor

Question 3.32.   A 32-year-old male homosexual who is human immunodeficiency virus (HIV)-negative has a long history of anal warts, but has recently experienced bright red blood with defecation. Physical examination reveals a small nonfixed nodule (1 cm) in the left anterolateral wall of the anal canal. Biopsy reveals cloacogenic carcinoma. There is no inguinal adenopathy. Therapy offered to this patient should be:

a) Abdominoperineal resection
b) Multimodality therapy (chemotherapy with 5-fluorouracil [5-FU], mitomycin C, plus irradiation), followed by wide local excision
c) Local excision plus bilateral inguinal node biopsy
d) Local excision alone
e) Interstitial and external irradiation

Question 3.33.   A 56-year-old woman who has been in excellent health was diagnosed with a locally advanced (T3) anal canal tumor, with bilateral inguinal adenopathy and a negative metastatic work-up. Histology of the primary tumor and nodes was poorly differentiated epidermoid carcinoma.

The patient was treated with concomitant irradiation and chemotherapy (5-fluorouracil and mitomycin C). With 3000 cGy to the pelvis, the inguinal adenopathy had completely regressed, but even at 4600 cGy, there was still a residual nodularity noted in the anal canal, which measured 1.0 cm. She completed the dose of 4600 cGy yesterday. The next step would be:

a) Biopsy of the residual nodule
b) Wide excision of the nodule
c) Abdominoperineal resection
d) Repeat the staging work-up
e) Follow-up only

Question 3.34.   A 40-year-old woman in otherwise good health was just diagnosed with an anal melanoma, just inside the anal verge. The tumor was 1 mm in depth, and there was no other evidence of disease. For the best chance of a possible cure, this patient should be offered:

a) A pelvic exenteration
b) An abdominoperineal resection (APR)

c) Wide local excision
d) Radiotherapy to the pelvis
e) Immunotherapy

Question 3.35.   Which of the following modalities is NOT used in the treatment of vulvar intraepithelial neoplasia (VIN)?

a) Wide local excision
b) CO_2 laser vaporization
c) 5-flourouracil cream
d) All of the aforementioned

Question 3.36.   Which part of the vulva has the ability to spread directly to the deep pelvic nodes, bypassing the inguinal-femoral nodes?

a) Mons pubis
b) Labia majora
c) Labia minora
d) Clitoris
e) Fourchette

Question 3.37.   Patients with locally advanced vulvar carcinomas who require more extensive surgery than radical vulvectomy may avoid the need for urinary or fecal diversion with which of the following approaches?

a) Anterior exenteration
b) Radical radiotherapy alone
c) Preoperative radiotherapy
d) Neoadjuvant chemotherapy

Question 3.38.   What is the optimal approach to a patient with a localized squamous cell carcinoma of the vagina that measures less than 0.5 cm in thickness who is treated with radiotherapy alone?

a) External beam radiotherapy alone
b) External beam and interstitial radiotherapy
c) Intracavitary radiotherapy alone
d) External beam and intracavitary radiotherapy

Question 3.39.   The Federation Internale Gynecology Oncology (FIGO) rules for the staging of cervical carcinoma permit all of the following examinations EXCEPT:

a) Cystoscopy
b) Intravenous pyelography
c) Lymphangiography
d) Skeletal radiographs
e) Hysteroscopy

Question 3.40.   Which of the following statements most accurately describes the behavior of breast cancer in the United States?

a) Breast cancer has the highest mortality of any tumor in US women.
b) The risk of developing breast cancer for women of any age is 1 in 8.

c)   The percentage of women who die from their breast cancer has increased by
     5% during the past 10 years.
d)   Thirty percent of women who have breast cancer ultimately die from their
     disease.
e)   The percent of patients who are initially seen with invasive ductal carcinoma
     has increased because of the influence of mammography.

Question 3.41. **The following statements concerning ductal carcinoma in
situ (DCIS) are correct EXCEPT:**

a)   The frequency of this diagnosis has been increasing with wider use of
     mammograms for screening purposes.
b)   Of the many subtypes, the comedocarcinoma DCIS has the worst prognosis
     and least favorable histologic pattern.
c)   Her-2neu protein overexpression, a poor prognostic indicator, has not been
     observed in the papillary and cribriform subtypes of DCIS.
d)   A high labeling index has been observed in the case of comedocarcinoma DCIS.
e)   Evaluation of estrogen receptor (ER) and progesterone receptor (PR) status is
     an important prognostic indicator for DCIS.

Question 3.42. **A well-educated 45-year-old woman has been diagnosed with
breast cancer and is being evaluated for surgical treatment. She is aware of
the importance of lymph node status as a prognostic indicator. Which of the
following statements is correct?**

a)   Even after excising the first six lymph nodes, the more lymph nodes that are
     removed, the easier it becomes to assess prognosis.
b)   Nodal metastasis is no longer believed to be the most significant prognostic
     factor in determining risk of relapse after 5 and 10 years because of the
     description of factors such as p53 tumor suppressor gene content, BRCA-1/
     BRCA-2 mutations, and Her-2neu protein overexpression.
c)   The presence of sinus histiocytosis in the lymph nodes always a poor
     prognostic indicator.
d)   The relapse rate at 5 years but not at 10 years is significantly greater for
     patients with $\geq$ 4 nodes with metastases as compared with patients who have
     1 to 3 nodes.
e)   The NSABP-04 trial demonstrated that after mastectomy, histologic grade and
     tumor size are helpful in further determining prognosis at 5 and 10 years in
     patients who have $\geq$ 4 nodes with metastases.

Question 3.43. **A 57-year-old American woman began menstruating at
age 12, went into menopause at age 52, and had her first child at age 34. She
currently uses estrogen replacement therapy. She has 1 glass of wine with
dinner every night and has a 50 pack-year history of smoking. Which of the
following statements regarding her risk of developing breast cancer is true?**

a)   The administration of even low doses of estrogen increases the risk of
     developing breast cancer at least fourfold in postmenopausal women. This
     effect is less prominent in premenopausal women.
b)   Alcoholic beverages may have a protective effect regarding breast cancer,
     provided the drinking is not excessive.

c)   Cigarette smoking, especially with a greater than 40 pack-per-year exposure, has been demonstrated to increase the likelihood of breast cancer.
d)   Menarche at age 12 confers twice the risk of breast cancer as does menarche at age 13.
e)   Women who have children in their 30s may still have less risk of developing breast cancer than women who remain nulliparous. This is believed to be related to the fact that nulliparous women will have more ovulatory cycles.

Question 3.44. **Studies of the biology of breast cancer have led to the discovery of various growth factors and hormones, as well as several oncogenes, which might play a role in the behavior of the malignant cells that define this disease. All of the following statements regarding the preceding are true EXCEPT:**

a)   In experimental systems, ER–negative cells are more sensitive to the effects of the inhibitory factor tumor growth factor beta (TGF-B) than are ER–positive cells.
b)   Autostimulation of breast cancer cells by autocrine and paracrine modulation of estrogen-induced growth factors may favor tumor growth.
c)   Antiestrogens have a cytocidal effect because of their ability to arrest cells in S phase.
d)   Families who have mutations in the tumor suppresser gene *p53* are prone to breast cancer as well as other tumors.
e)   Transgenic mice that express the oncogenes *myc, ras,* and HER-2neu in a tissue-specific pattern have an increased incidence of both benign and malignant breast pathology.

Question 3.45. **A 50-year-old man is initially seen with a new black nevus on the anterior chest just beneath the right nipple. Excisional biopsy demonstrates a Clark Level III, 1.5-mm thick nodular melanoma. The margins of excision for this lesion should be:**

a)   The margins should be the same as for any other malignant melanoma, and they should be guided by the anatomic site of the lesion.
b)   2-cm margins, given the thickness of the primary lesion
c)   1 cm
d)   The margins of excision are not relevant, but the excision should include pectoralis muscle fascia, because the lymphatics from the primary lesion drain via these channels.
e)   No further excision is necessary

Question 3.46. **Which of the following agents is used in the medical management of patients who have pituitary prolactinoma?**

a)   Octreotide
b)   Bromocriptine
c)   Somatostatin
d)   Prolactin
e)   None of the aforementioned

Question 3.47. **A 58-year-old man underwent a total thyroidectomy for follicular carcinoma. On permanent section review of the specimen, a portion of the tumor is found to extend beyond the thyroid capsule posteriorly. Postoperative care should include all of the following EXCEPT:**

a)   Thyroid stimulating hormone (TSH) should be suppressed between 0.1 to 0.4 mIU/mL.

b)   Reoperation with partial laryngeal resection
c)   Postoperative total body radioactive iodine (RAI) scan at 4 to 6 weeks
d)   Elevations of serum thyroglobulin levels should be treated with 100 to 250 mCi of RAI.
e)   Close follow-up every 6 months with neck examination for recurrence

Question 3.48. **Exposure to asbestos can lead to the following pleural manifestations EXCEPT:**

a)   Pleural calcifications
b)   Benign pleural plaques
c)   Benign effusion
d)   Malignant mesothelioma
e)   Benign mesothelioma

Question 3.49. **Besides asbestos exposure, other factors incriminated in the etiology of malignant mesothelioma in man include all of the following EXCEPT:**

a)   Exposure to zeolite fibers (erionite type)
b)   Prior history of radiotherapy
c)   Cigarette smoking
d)   A family history of malignant mesothelioma

Question 3.50. **The incidence of hepatocellular carcinoma (HCC) worldwide can be described as:**

a)   Equal (1:1) for men and women in both low- and high-incidence regions.
b)   Asians living in Asia are at similar risk for HCC as are Asians born in Asia but who move to the United States.
c)   Highest in China and Thailand, with 45 % of the entire world's cases occurring in China.
d)   Related to long-term exposure to alcohol and other carcinogens, including steroids, aflatoxins, vinyl chloride, and hepatic iron stores. These factors are the most significant in the etiology of HCC.

Question 3.51. **Treatment options for a 2-cm HCC can be described as follows:**

a)   Total hepatic radiation has a local control rate of 65% but is generally reserved for patients who have poor hepatic reserve.
b)   Intravenous 5-fluorouracil and doxorubin have been found to be the most effective combination for palliation of HCC symptoms.
c)   Surgical resection is limited to patients who have little hepatic dysfunction, whereas transplantation is typically reserved for patients with end-stage liver function and incidental HCC.
d)   Cryosurgical ablation of HCC has become the standard surgical approach for this carcinoma.

Question 3.52. **All of the following statements regarding the pathogenesis of gallbladder cancer are true EXCEPT:**

a)   Pyogenic biliary disease is a risk factor for gallbladder cancer.
b)   Chronic inflammation of the gallbladder has been implicated in gallbladder cancer.
c)   There is a definite association of gallstone disease with gallbladder cancer.

d) The incidence of gallbladder cancer in the "porcelain" gallbladder group is 12 to 61%.

e) There is no identified premalignant lesion in gallbladder cancer.

***Question 3.53.*   Recent molecular biology studies suggest an association of HCC with:**

a) Mutations of the *p16* tumor suppressor gene

b) Increased expression of cyclin D

c) Variable expression of the *BRCA-1* and *BRCA-2* genes

d) Mutations on chromosome 4 and in exon 7 on the *p53* gene

e) Rearranged *c-abl* proto-oncogene

***Question 3.54.*   Which of the following is true with regard to the diagnosis of gallbladder cancer:**

a) The use of ultrasound has greatly increased the preoperative diagnosis rate of gallbladder cancer.

b) A large majority of gallbladder cancers are diagnosed preoperatively.

c) The majority of gallbladder cancers are diagnosed at an early stage.

d) The use of MRI has aided the preoperative diagnosis rate of gallbladder cancer.

e) At the time of diagnosis, the majority of gallbladder cancers are technically resectable.

***Question 3.55.*   The risk of pancreatic cancer is increased in patients who:**

a) Have a history of exposure to nitrosamines and benzidine

b) Have a long history of tobacco and alcohol abuse

c) Have no family history of pancreatic cancer

d) Are found to have *k-ras* proto-oncogene expression in their blood

e) Have expression of the *MTS-1 gene (multiple tumor suppressor gene) on chromosome 9p21*

***Question 3.56.*   A 15-year-old boy is initially seen with pain and swelling in the right midthigh. The patient also has had intermittent fevers during the past few weeks and feels poorly. Radiograph of the right femur reveals a periosteal deficit with a soft-tissue extension yielding an onion-skin appearance. Bone biopsy reveals uniform sheets of small round cells with indistinct cytoplasmic borders and small round nuclei with nucleolar prominences. Immunoperoxidase stains performed reveal absence of the leukocyte antigen, factor VII, and myoglobin. Which of the following genes is most likely to be rearranged or mutated in the affected tissue?**

a) Retinoblastoma

b) *bcl-2*

c) *bcr*

d) *fli-1*

e) Dihydrofolate reductase

***Question 3.57.*   A 60-year-old woman is seen by her internist with a history of weight loss, anorexia, jaundice, and abdominal fullness. The initial step in her diagnostic work-up is:**

a) Non-contrast MRI of the upper abdomen

b) Upper abdominal ultrasonography, followed by CT scan

c) Transhepatic cholangiogram (THC)
d) Endoscopic retrograde cholangiopancreatography (ERCP), followed by immediate abdominal exploration
e) Whole body positron emission tomogram (PET) scan

Question 3.58. **The optimal management of a patient with a 3-cm squamous cell carcinoma of the anus who does not have distant metastasis involves:**

a) APR
b) Preoperative radiotherapy, followed by APR
c) Radiotherapy and single-agent chemotherapy (5-FU)
d) Radiotherapy and combination chemotherapy (5-FU and mitomycin C)
e) None of the aforementioned

Question 3.59. **A 47-year-old woman who has smoked two packs of cigarettes per day for 30 years has experienced a sensation of a mass in the anorectal area for the last month. She also notes that she has a couple of "lumps" in the right groin, but they do not bother her. On physical examination, there is a 3-cm mass beginning at the dentate line on the right anorectal wall, and also two firm 1.5-cm lymph nodes in the right groin. Biopsies of the anorectal mass and excisional biopsy of one of the lymph nodes demonstrate moderately well-differentiated epidermoid carcinoma in both sites.**
Further work-up should include all of the following EXCEPT:

a) Chest radiograph
b) Liver function tests
c) Tumor-associated antigens
d) Endoscopy
e) CT scans of abdomen and pelvis

Question 3.60. **Radiotherapy is the treatment of choice for patients who have squamous cell carcinoma of all of the following sites EXCEPT:**

a) Eyelids
b) Pinna of the ear
c) Nasolabial fold and alar nasi
d) Lip commissure
e) All of the aforementioned

Question 3.61. **Erythroplasia of Queyrat refers to squamous cell carcinoma in situ of the:**

a) Glans penis
b) Nasolabial fold
c) Vocal cord
d) Pinna of the ear
e) None of the aforementioned

Question 3.62. **Leukoplakia of which of the following sites is associated with the lowest risk of malignancy?**

a) Buccal mucosa
b) Floor of mouth
c) Tonsillar region

d)   Anterior one third of the tongue
e)   Base of tongue

Question 3.63.   Which of the following central nervous system tumors is found in patients who have neurofibromatosis type 2?

a)   Pituitary adenoma
b)   Craniopharyngioma
c)   Bilateral acoustic neuromas
d)   Medulloblastoma
e)   Unilateral acoustic neuromas

Question 3.64.   A 19-year-old male is seen by his primary care physician because of pain and swelling in his right lower extremity. The patient's examination discloses a 3-cm nodular tibial lesion approximately 6 cm inferior to the knee. A radiograph of the tibia reveals a sclerotic lesion with a lucent nidus.

The patient is referred to an orthopedic surgeon who performs an incisional biopsy and notes a circumspect red lesion. Pathology reveals reactive bone surrounding a vascular tumor without mitotic figures. The tumor has ample blood vessels and nerve fibers coursing throughout.

Appropriate additional therapy would include:

a)   Observation
b)   Radiotherapy
c)   Chemotherapy with high-dose methotrexate
d)   Radiotherapy plus chemotherapy with high-dose methotrexate
e)   Re-excision followed by radiotherapy

Question 3.65.   A 20-year-old man with a biopsy-proven osteogenic sarcoma of the mid-tibial shaft is seen for evaluation. Work-up reveals no evidence of distant metastases. The most appropriate therapeutic management at this point would be:

a)   Chemotherapy
b)   Chemotherapy followed by surgical removal of the lesion
c)   Chemotherapy followed by amputation
d)   Amputation at the proximal tibia
e)   Removal of the lesion followed by radiotherapy

Question 3.66.   Which of the following has the weakest epidemiologic association with the development of osteogenic sarcoma?

a)   Retinoblastoma gene expression
b)   *p53* tumor suppressor gene mutations
c)   Adolescence
d)   Trauma
e)   Paget's disease

Question 3.67.   A 35-year-old man who has osteogenic sarcoma is receiving high-dose methotrexate. All of the following are appropriate strategies for reducing toxicity EXCEPT:

a)   Administration of sodium bicarbonate intravenously
b)   Administration of leukovorin

c) Intravenous hydration
d) Administration of mesna
e) Monitoring of methotrexate levels

Question 3.68. **A 25-year-old man is initially seen with pain and swelling in the right knee. Radiographs show a well-demarcated lesion in the distal femur. The cortex is intact, and there is no extraosseous soft-tissue mass. Bone biopsy reveals a background of a benign spindle cell stroma with numerous multinucleated giant cells. CT scan of the chest is negative, and the CT scan of the distal femur and knee discloses no additional lesions. The most appropriate therapy at this point is:**

a) Aggressive local removal of the lesion
b) Amputation of the leg by hip disarticulation
c) Amputation of the leg at the mid-femur
d) Radiotherapy
e) Chemotherapy followed by surgical removal

Question 3.69. **All of the following have been associated with development of human soft- tissue sarcoma EXCEPT:**

a) Mutation of the *p53* gene
b) Rous sarcoma virus infection
c) Polyvinyl chloride exposure
d) Radiation exposure
e) Immunosuppression

Question 3.70. **What is the most common presenting symptom in patients who have mycosis fungoides?**

a) Lymphadenopathy
b) Fever
c) Pruritis
d) Weight loss
e) Night sweats

Question 3.71. **A 60-year-old man is initially seen with generalized erythroderma involving most of the skin surface. His symptoms developed suddenly and include intense pruritus. Physical examination demonstrates generalized erythroderma and areas of skin thickening. In addition, there are signs of excoriation and skin ulceration. Laboratory examination reveals high levels of circulating malignant atypical mononuclear cells. The presumptive diagnosis is a cutaneous T-cell lymphoma (mycosis fungoides). This patient has:**

a) Mycotic syndrome
b) Sézary syndrome
c) Lymphometroid syndrome
d) Fungoid phase

Question 3.72. **Which part of the body is routinely shielded in patients undergoing total skin electron beam therapy for mycosis fungoides?**

a) Perineum
b) Breasts

c)   Soles of the feet
d)   Eyes
e)   All of the aforementioned are shielded

Question 3.73.   Scoliotic changes associated with the use of radiotherapy in the pediatric patient can be avoided by:

a)   The use of twice daily (hyperfractionated) radiotherapy
b)   Including the entire epiphyses
c)   Use of large fractions ($\geq$300 cGy) given once weekly
d)   Use of concomitant chemotherapy
e)   None of the aforementioned

Question 3.74.   In the treatment of pediatric malignancies, the addition of combination chemotherapy has allowed significant reductions In the dose of radiotherapy required in all of the following diseases EXCEPT:

a)   Hodgkin's disease
b)   Wilms' tumor
c)   Ewing's sarcoma
d)   Rhabdomyosarcoma
e)   Both (a) and (b)

Question 3.75.   Which of the following tumors is the most common tumor to occur in the first year of life?

a)   Acute lymphoblastic leukemia (ALL)
b)   Neuroblastoma
c)   Wilms' tumor
d)   Brain-stem glioma
e)   Acute myeloid leukemia (AML)

Question 3.76.   All of the following statements regarding the association between genetic syndromes and pediatric central nervous system tumors are correct EXCEPT:

a)   The majority of pediatric brain tumors are not associated with an identifiable genetic sydrome.
b)   Neurofibromatosis is the genetic syndrome most frequently associated with pediatric brain neoplasms.
c)   Cerebellar hemangioblastomas are associated with von Hippel-Lindau disease.
d)   Turcot syndrome is associated with tumors of the posterior fossa.
e)   Tuberous sclerosis patients develop periventricular tumors.

Question 3.77.   All of the following statements comparing adult and pediatric brain tumors are true EXCEPT:

a)   Unlike low-grade tumors in adults, pediatric low-grade glial tumors rarely mutate into more malignant forms.
b)   Clinical studies suggest that pediatric high-grade glial tumors are less responsive to treatment than are those arising in older patients.
c)   Pediatric glial malignant tumors do not demonstrate the same cytogenetic and molecular genetic changes seen in adult high-grade gliomas.

d) High-grade glial tumor of the supratentorium is the most common brain tumor seen in adults.
e) Brain-stem gliomas are more common in children than adults.

Question 3.78.   Which of the following statements is FALSE regarding the use of hyperfractionated radiotherapy (HFRT) in patients who have pediatric brain tumors?

a) HFRT involves the use of more than one fraction of treatment per day, with larger than conventional doses per fraction.
b) HFRT is used to reduce the potential of late effects such as necrosis and subclinical damage.
c) HFRT allows the use of higher than conventional total doses.
d) Ongoing national randomized trials are testing the role of HFRT schedules in patients who have brain-stem gliomas and medulloblastoma.
e) All of the aforementioned are true.

Question 3.79.   Which of the following pediatric brain tumors carries the worst prognosis?

a) Craniopharyngioma
b) Cerebellar pilocytic astrocytoma
c) Brain-stem glioma in the medulla
d) Brain-stem glioma in the pons
e) Medulloblastoma

Question 3.80.   Which is the most frequent site of origin for an ependymoma arising in childhood?

a) Frontal lobe
b) Temporal lobe
c) Parietal lobe
d) Posterior fossa
e) Spinal cord

Question 3.81.   Which of the following pediatric brain tumors is the most common suprasellar tumor of childhood?

a) Germinoma
b) Craniopharyngioma
c) Meningioma
d) Embryonal cell carcinoma
e) Ependymoma

Question 3.82.   Which of the following malignant pediatric brain tumors is the most likely to be cured with surgery alone?

a) Glioblastoma multiforme
b) Embryonal carcinoma
c) Choroid plexus carcinoma
d) High-grade ependymoma
e) None of the aforementioned

Question 3.83. **The optimal approach to a child who has a Wilms' tumor with evidence of extension into and partial obstruction of the inferior vena cava involves:**

a) Surgical resection followed by postoperative radiotherapy
b) Preoperative chemotherapy followed by surgery
c) Surgical resection followed by postoperative chemotherapy
d) Surgical resection alone
e) None of the aforementioned

Question 3.84. **A 43-year-old woman with hypertension underwent a nonenhanced CT scan because of complaints of persistent abdominal fullness and fatigue. The scan showed an 8-cm left suprarenal mass with irregular borders. You are consulted to evaluate this patient before surgery, and you obtain a history of depressive symptoms, insomnia, and proximal muscle weakness. Her last menstrual period was 6 months ago. On physical examination, her skin is thin, and the supraclavicular and dorsocervical fat pads are enlarged. There are a few course terminal hairs on her face, areolae, and abdomen, but no temporal balding or clitoromegaly. Her routine laboratory evaluation, including electrolytes, is normal. The most efficient laboratory evaluation at this time would be:**

a) Serum androgens (testosterone, dihydroepiandrosterone (DHEAS), and androstanedione)
b) 24-hour urine free cortisol
c) Serum aldosterone
d) 24-hour urine for 17-hydroxycorticosteroids
e) 24-hour urine metanephrine

Question 3.85. **A 54-year-old man who has metastatic adrenal cancer was found to have some increase in the size of multiple liver metastases as revealed by a CT scan done 1 month ago. His mitotane dosage has been gradually increased since that time from 1 g bid to 2 g bid. He is admitted to the emergency room this evening complaining of severe dizziness and prostration. He states that he has a feeling of "not being in touch with reality." He is being hydrated with IV fluids. The best course of management now would be:**

a) Check a serum cortisol level to rule out adrenal insufficiency
b) Stop the mitotane and check the drug's serum level
c) Stop the mitotane and draw an 8 AM cortisol the next day
d) Give 100 mg hydrocortisone IV push now; stop the mitotane and draw a mitotane serum level
e) Give fludrocortisone acetate 0.1 mg daily; stop the mitotane and draw a serum level of the drug

Question 3.86. **Which of the following histologic subtypes of invasive breast cancer is associated with the worst prognosis?**

a) Infiltrating ductal carcinoma
b) Medullary carcinoma
c) Tubular carcinoma
d) Colloid carcinoma
e) Papillary carcinoma

Question 3.87. **A 67-year-old woman who has invasive ductal carcinoma of the right breast is found to have 2 of 10 lymph nodes that contain cancer at the time of her axillary lymph node dissection. The metastatic work-up is negative. Which of the following statements concerning this patient's therapeutic course is accurate?**

a) The benefit of tamoxifen therapy beyond 6 months is unclear.
b) If tamoxifen is used as the only therapy, the patient's chances for long-term survival will not be increased.
c) Toxicities (cumulative) limit the long-term use of tamoxifen.
d) Tamoxifen will increase the risk of atherosclerotic heart disease by raising the circulating levels of cholesterol.
e) Use of tamoxifen is associated with a slight increase in the risk of uterine cancer.

Question 3.88. **A 32-year-old man undergoing evaluation for a suspected pheochromocytoma is found to have bilateral renal and pancreatic cysts as revealed by computed tomography. Ophthalmologic evaluation discloses a retinal hemangioma.**

Which of the following statements regarding this patient's condition or syndrome is correct?

a) The patient has a high lifetime risk for renal cell carcinoma.
b) The patient has a high lifetime risk for angiosarcoma.
c) A renal cyst, if aspirated, would almost certainly contain benign renal epithelial cells.
d) This syndrome is caused by overexpression of a growth promoting gene.
e) Tumors arising in patients who have this syndrome frequently have an extra copy of chromosome 7.

Question 3.89. **A 65-year-old man who has a history of adenocarcinoma of the colon with hepatic metastases was treated with 5-FU in combination with leucovorin for six cycles. After an initial response, computed tomography disclosed enlarging metastases. Which of the following approaches is most reasonable at this time, given a desire on the part of the patient to have further antineoplastic treatment?**

a) Administration of oral hydroxyurea in combination with 5-FU
b) Administration of methotrexate in combination with 5-FU
c) Administration of cisplatin
d) Administration of irinotecan
e) Supportive care only, given the lack of potential benefit with any available agent

Question 3.90. **A 67-year-old otherwise healthy woman is seen with a rectal mass which, at the time of surgical resection, proves to be a rectal adenocarcinoma invading into the serosa. Two of ten resected lymph nodes contain tumor cells. Which of the following represents the most appropriate treatment for this patient after recovery from surgery?**

a) Administration of 5-FU in combination with leucovorin
b) Administration of 5-FU alone
c) Administration of 5-FU, methyl-lomustine (CCNU), and vincristine in combination with radiotherapy

d)   5-FU in combination with radiotherapy

e)   Radiotherapy alone

Question 3.91.   A 65-year-old woman is seen with a large fungating chest wall mass and metastatic bone lesions. She is diagnosed with Stage IV breast cancer. As her oncologist, you know that in this situation all of the following statements are correct EXCEPT:

a)   The fact that her tumor was ER–positive on review of the pathologic specimen and that her CALGB performance score was 0 (highest) predicts that she will have a good response to a combination chemotherapy regimen that includes doxorubicin.

b)   Although complete remission rates are approximately 10 to 20%, patients who receive combination chemotherapy have a median survival of 2 years.

c)   The cyclophosphamide, Adriamycin, 5-fluorouracil (CAF) combination may actually be slightly more effective than cyclophosphamide, methotrexate, and 5-fluorouracil (CMF); however, the toxicity is greater as well.

d)   If the initial therapy does not yield a response, the total response rate to salvage regimens, even when these consist of combinations of drugs is approximately 20 to 30%.

e)   In metastatic disease, a strategy of stopping chemotherapy after six to eight cycles is no better than continuing chemotherapy constantly until the disease progresses.

Question 3.92.   A 63-year-old woman was diagnosed with Stage IV breast cancer 2 years ago and was found to have an estrogen receptor– and progesterone receptor–positive tumor. Tamoxifen therapy was started and caused a partial response associated with a minimal tumor burden and no progression. The patient returns to your office for routine follow-up and asks you whether it is time to start her on chemotherapy in addition to her tamoxifen. How would you answer this question?

a)   The majority of studies addressing this question show no advantage of combination endocrine/chemotherapy treatment.

b)   You recommend chemotherapy because the patient has only had a partial response. The addition of chemotherapy to her treatment will thus enhance her chances of a more prolonged survival.

c)   Hormonal agents are contraindicated in patients receiving chemotherapy because these agents induce a quiescent chemoresistant state in the cancer cells.

d)   You recommend the administration of estrogen to prime the cancerous cells. This can result in an increase in the S-phase fraction, during which the cells are more chemosensitive, and therefore a greater cell kill ensues when cytotoxic drugs are administered.

e)   Postmenopausal women may paradoxically have a recrudescence of their tumors when chemotherapy is added to a successful hormonal chemotherapy.

Question 3.93.   On performing a routine breast examination, it is possible to encounter a number of findings that must be interpreted with caution. Which of the following interpretations of different physical signs is true?

a)   The presence of a bloody discharge almost always means that there is an underlying breast cancer, and therefore this finding warrants further investigation.

b) Regarding palpation of axillary lymph nodes, clinical judgment is inaccurate, with 75% false-negative findings and 50% false-positive findings.
c) The presence of pain is most common in the diagnosis of breast cancer. Therefore, a pathologic specimen needs to be obtained from the painful tissue to exclude the presence of neoplastic cells.
d) On palpation, fibrocystic disease seems to blend into the surrounding tissue, whereas cancerous lumps usually have well-defined borders and are fairly fixed into the rest of the glandular structure.
e) Cyclic breast pain is uncommon in premenstrual women. This symptom usually is due to perimenopausal hormonal surges and is commonly associated with an underlying carcinoma that flares with the endocrine stimulus.

Question 3.94. **Many studies have been carried out analyzing the indications for mammography as a screening tool for breast cancer. These studies have been plagued by different weaknesses and criticisms, and their meaning is still debated today. Other trials are still ongoing in the attempt to clarify this complex issue. Which of the following statements are correct?**

a) Studies that report survival rates or average survival time are likely to be particularly accurate, because they avoid biases that commonly occur when studying breast cancer incidence and mortality in response to mammography screening.
b) Lead time bias refers to the fact that the date of death of a woman from breast cancer will be delayed with the influence of mammography, therefore causing a bias in the interpretation of the results.
c) Length bias refers to bias incurred due to the discovery of more slow-growing tumors in the screened group, whereas patients who have more rapidly growing tumor will be diagnosed at other times. Thus, the screened group will seem to be doing better because of the less biologically malignant nature of their disease.
d) Counting the number of deaths from breast cancer in both group studies (screening and not screened) is prone to lead time and length time bias and should be avoided.
e) Length time bias refers to bias incurred due to the fact that screened women are diagnosed with larger or more progressed tumors that have been growing longer. This makes the issue of improved survival from screening efforts difficult to interpret.

Question 3.95. **All of these statements regarding the proper use of screening procedures for early detection of breast cancers are correct EXCEPT:**

a) Women over the age of 50 and under the age of 74 should have yearly mammographic examinations, because this has been shown to reduce their risk of dying from breast cancer by 70%.
b) Although it has not been conclusively demonstrated that women between the ages of 40 to 49 should have yearly mammograms, this issue should be decided between a patient and her physician in view of the particularities of her case.
c) The role for self breast examination (SBE) is not entirely clear, because there are no data to show that this practice definitely prolongs survival, even though it has been shown to lead to earlier detection. In spite of this, SBE is recommended routinely.

d) The interpretation of data regarding the efficacy of mammography screening in women 40 to 49 years old requires a longer follow-up (at least 8 years) to begin to detect different survival times between screened and non-screened groups.

e) Women who have a positive history of a first-degree relative with breast cancer should have their first mammography between 30 and 35 years of age.

Question 3.96.   An 88-year-old practicing lawyer has an annual physical examination. He is in excellent health except for a rectal examination that reveals a 2+ enlarged moderately firm prostate. The prostate specific antigen level was 8 μg/L. An ultrasound revealed a 1-cm hypoechogenic defect in the left lobe. A biopsy revealed a Grade II (of 10) carcinoma of the prostate. The bone scan results were normal, and abdominal CT scan results were negative. The most reasonable management would be one of the following:

a) Radical prostatectomy
b) Radiotherapy to the prostate and retroperitoneal nodes
c) Leuprolide
d) Flutamide combined with luteinizing hormone releasing hormone analogue
e) Observation at 4-month intervals

Question 3.97.   A 48-year-old woman had a Stage II (lymph node positive) breast cancer treated by lumpectomy and radiotherapy, followed by adjuvant chemotherapy with CAF. The cancer was strongly estrogen receptor– and progesterone receptor–positive. Following the chemotherapy, she started receiving tamoxifen therapy. During the chemotherapy, her menstrual periods ceased, and she developed severe hot flashes before the onset of tamoxifen therapy. The hot flashes became debilitating. Which of the following would you recommend?

a) Replacement estrogen therapy
b) A barbiturate
c) A progestational agent
d) Reassurance
e) Synthroid

Question 3.98.   A 64-year-old man is found to have multiple bilateral pulmonary nodules as revealed by chest radiograph 4 years after a right radical mastectomy for breast cancer. Results of a bone scan are negative, and search for other primary sources of cancer is not productive. This patient's second marriage occurred 6 months ago. The preferred method of management would be:

a) Stilbestrol, non–enteric coated, 5 mg tid
b) Medroxyprogesterone
c) CAF chemotherapy
d) Bilateral orchiectomy
e) Luteinizing hormone releasing hormone analogues

Question 3.99.   A 23-year-old man is seen with a testicular mass, retroperitoneal lymphadenopathy (7 cm), and a left supraclavicular lymph node. Chest CT scan and head CT scan results are normal. Preoperative levels of AFP,

1236 ng/mL, and beta hCG, 1826 mIU/mL. Radical orchiectomy reveals embryonal cell carcinoma, teratoma and yolk sac element. The patient receives three cycles of cisplatin, etoposide, and bleomycin. His serum markers normalize. Repeat CT scan of the chest demonstrates multiple bilateral pleural-based nodules in the lower lobes. Abdominal CT scan reveals that his abdominal mass is unchanged. Therapeutic options are :

a)   Salvage chemotherapy with vinblastine, ifosfamide, and cisplatin
b)   Biopsy of new lung nodules
c)   Retroperitoneal lymph node dissection and neck dissection
d)   High-dose chemotherapy with peripheral stem cell rescue
e)   Close observation

Question 3.100.   **Which of the following is not a typical presentation for a patient who has cancer of the pancreaticobiliary tree?**

a)   A 63-year-old man who has no family history of diabetes has experienced weight loss and nausea and has been found to be diabetic within the past 4½ months.
b)   After cholecystectomy 6 months ago (which failed to significantly relieve symptoms), a 58-year-old man has become severely jaundiced and complains of nausea and vomiting.
c)   A 67-year-old woman who has complained of back pain for almost 2 years notes that, although she has stopped losing weight, she is very weak, and her dresses have become very tight in the waist.
d)   A 61-year-old woman who has a history of episodic right subcostal and scapular pain for many years has become jaundiced after a severe attack associated with nausea and a single episode of vomiting.
e)   A 72-year-old man, with epigastric discomfort and upper back pain and nausea that has been progressive over 3 months, has become jaundiced.

Question 3.101.   **In which of these pancreaticobiliary cancers has multimodality therapy been tested in a randomized trial and shown to be of some benefit?**

a)   Gallbladder
b)   Klatskin's syndrome cancer of the proximal biliary ducts
c)   Bile duct cancer
d)   Pancreatic cancer
e)   Cancer of the ampulla of Vater

Question 3.102.   **Which of the following provides the optimal diagnostic evaluation regimen for a patient who has clinical obstructive jaundice?**

a)   Gastrointestinal contrast study, MRI of the pancreas, and ERCP with insertion of the biliary stent
b)   CT scan, ERCP with insertion of biliary stent, biopsy
c)   MRI, percutaneous transhepatic insertion of biliary stent, laparoscopy with biopsy
d)   Gastrointestinal contrast study, CT scan, selective hepatic and celiac arteriography, surgical biliary drainage
e)   CT scan, percutaneous transhepatic biliary drainage, gastric emptying study, biopsy

Question 3.103. **In the presence of advanced metastatic cancer of the pancreas to the liver, patients have been offered a variety of treatment options. Assuming that all patients also receive optimal pain and nausea control, these options might include:**

1) 5-Fluorouracil
2) Gemcitabine
3) Phases I or II trials of drugs or drug combinations
4) Radiotherapy
5) Supportive care only

Which of the following is most appropriate?

a) 1 or 2
b) 5
c) 1, 2, or 3
d) 1 and 4
e) 1, 2, 3, or 5

Question 3.104. **A 42-year-old man is seen with a testicular mass and retroperitoneal lymphadenopathy (8 cm in greatest diameter). Results of chest CT scan and physical examination are both negative. Radical inguinal orchiectomy reveals pure seminoma and serum AFP, 56 ng/mL, and beta hCG, 10 IU/mL. The patient is treated with three cycles of cisplatin, etoposide, and bleomycin. His markers normalize, and his CT scan of the abdomen reveals a residual 3-cm mass. Options for further management are:**

a) Radiotherapy to the residual mass
b) Cisplatin-ifosfamide–based salvage chemotherapy
c) Fine needle aspirate of the residual mass
d) Retroperitoneal lymph node dissection
e) Close observation

Question 3.105. **A 10-year-old child born with café au lait spots and numerous spongy palpable cutaneous lesions develops a grand mal seizure. CT scan reveals a large lesion in the right frontal lobe. Which of the following statements about the situation is correct?**

a) The lesion is most likely a metastasis.
b) Other family members are likely to be afflicted with soft-tissue sarcomas and breast cancer.
c) Each of the patient's siblings has a 25% chance of being afflicted with a similar syndrome.
d) The gene responsible for this syndrome codes for a protein with homology to guanosine triphosphate–activated proteins.
e) Skin lesions called adenoma sebaceum are common in this disorder.

Question 3.106. **A 65-year-old man is seen with progressive severe headaches, nausea, and vomiting. Neurologic examination is remarkable for an inability to write or do simple mathematic calculations. Visual field testing**

reveals inferior quadrantanopsia. Computed tomography demonstrates an intracranial lesion. The lesion is most likely located in the:

a) Cerebellum
b) Frontal lobe
c) Parietal lobe
d) Thalamus
e) Temporal lobe

Question 3.107. A patient who has severe headaches is referred for an MRI that shows a large gadolinium-enhancing infiltrative lesion of the right frontal lobe that crosses the midline. The radiologic impression is that of a probable glioblastoma multiforme or a high-grade astrocytoma. Which of the following represents the most appropriate therapeutic strategy?

a) Maximal resection followed by radiotherapy
b) Biopsy followed by chemotherapy
c) Biopsy followed by external bean radiotherapy
d) Biopsy followed by brachytherapy
e) Biopsy followed by chemotherapy and external bean radiotherapy

Question 3.108. A 35-year-old man is seen with incontinence and lower extremity weakness. MRI shows a heterogeneously gadolinium-enhancing lesion in the inferior spinal cord. The patient is referred for a surgical resection, which appears to be complete. Pathology reveals anaplastic astrocytoma. The natural history of this disease would most likely be:

a) Long disease-free survival without additional treatment
b) Long disease-free survival after postoperative radiotherapy
c) Long disease-free survival after postoperative radiotherapy and adjuvant nitrosourea chemotherapy
d) Long-term survival after postoperative radiotherapy, nitrosourea-based chemotherapy regimen, and re-resection after eventual recurrence
e) Death due to intra-axial spread despite radiotherapy, chemotherapy, and re-resection

Question 3.109. A 30-year-old man who has known HIV infection is seen with confusion, memory loss, and generalized seizure. Contrast-enhanced computed tomography reveals multiple enhancing lesions of the basal ganglia, thalami, and frontal lobes. The patient's toxoplasmosis titers are negative. Stereotactic biopsy of one of the accessible lesions is likely to reveal:

a) Small-cleaved malignant B lymphocytes
b) Large-cell immunoblastic lymphoma
c) Metastatic adenocarcinoma
d) Toxoplasmosis
e) Large-cell malignant T-lymphocytes

Question 3.110. A 3-year-old child underwent complete surgical removal of a posterior fossa medulloblastoma. Which of the following is the most appropriate therapy:

a) No further therapy

b)   Whole brain radiotherapy
c)   Craniospinal irradiation
d)   Administration of lomustine, vincristine, and prednisone
e)   Whole brain radiotherapy, followed by administration of lomustine, vincristine, and prednisone

Question 3.111.   **A 59-year-old heavy smoker is seen with a lung mass of 4 cm in diameter. Needle biopsy reveals adenocarcinoma. Mediastinoscopy reveals positive hilar nodes. The patient received right upper lobectomy and postoperative radiotherapy followed by chemotherapy. He remained disease free for 12 months, when he developed seizures. He was found to have a single 6-cm right frontal lobe enhancing lesion as revealed by computed tomography and was stabilized with antiseizure medicines and corticosteroids. The most effective therapy in this situation would probably be:**

a)   Readministration of the same chemotherapy given after lung surgery
b)   Resection of the lesion
c)   Resection of the lesion plus radiotherapy
d)   Whole brain radiotherapy
e)   Brachytherapy

Question 3.112.   **Which of the following is the symptom complex most closely associated with adenocarcinoma of the right colon?**

a)   Pain, constipation
b)   Weakness, pain
c)   Melena, constipation, diarrhea
d)   Bright red blood coating the stool
e)   Nausea and vomiting due to obstruction

Question 3.113.   **A 55-year-old man is seen with enlargement of the left testicle. Examination reveals a normal size, shape, and consistency of the left testicle, but there is an enlarged apparently fluid-filled structure inferior to the testicle. Ultrasonography discloses a normal testes, with a varicocele. Which of the following tumors would most likely give rise to this clinical finding?**

a)   Penile carcinoma
b)   Non-Hodgkin's lymphoma
c)   Renal cell carcinoma
d)   Bladder carcinoma
e)   Testicular carcinoma

Question 3.114.   **Which of the following statements concerning the histologic grading of adenocarcinoma of the prostate are correct?**

a)   The histologic grade correlates with the stage of the lesion, but has no independent influence on prognosis.
b)   The number of mitoses per 10 high power fields is the most important feature of the histologic grading system.
c)   Higher grade lesions are more common in older individuals.
d)   The grading system is based on dominant morphology in addition to the next most common pattern of differentiation.

e)   The histologic staging system is based on review of prostate pathology based on large autopsy series.

Question 3.115.   **The American Cancer Society recommends that healthy men over age 50 be screened for prostate cancer. What tests are recommended?**

a)   Annual digital rectal examination
b)   Annual prostate specific antigen (PSA) determination
c)   Annual digital rectal examination and annual PSA determination
d)   Annual digital rectal examination, PSA determination, and transrectal ultrasonographic examination
e)   Annual digital rectal examination, annual PSA determination, and transrectal ultrasound examination every 5 years

Question 3.116.   **Which statement is false regarding an extrafascial hysterectomy?**

a)   The uterine vessels are skeletonized.
b)   The pubovesicocervical fascia is separated from the cervix.
c)   The plane for bladder separation from the cervix is created by sharp instead of blunt dissection.
d)   The uterosacral ligaments are transected separately near their insertion.
e)   All of the aforementioned are true.

Question 3.117.   A 64-year-old woman is seen with a 3-month history of vague abdominal pain and increasing abdominal girth. Physical examination of the abdomen and pelvis reveals evidence of a fluid wave and a right-sided ovarian mass. Ultrasonography confirms the presence of ascites and a right-sided ovarian mass. The mass is complex in nature. The next most appropriate step in management would be:

a)   Referral for laparotomy
b)   Paracentesis to confirm the diagnosis, followed by whole abdominal radiotherapy
c)   Paracentesis to confirm the diagnosis, followed by platinum-based therapy
d)   MRI scanning and determination of serum tumor marker CA-125 level
e)   Colonoscopy to confirm the diagnosis, followed by 5-FU–based chemotherapy

Question 3.118.   **Which of the following statements concerning the surgical treatment of renal cell carcinoma is correct?**

a)   Patients who require a partial nephrectomy due to cancer in an anatomically or functionally solitary kidney have a 50% likelihood of local recurrence.
b)   Invasion of the renal vein by the primary tumor is a contraindication to radical nephrectomy.
c)   Local recurrence is the most common reason for relapse after radical nephrectomy.
d)   Stage for stage, regional nodal involvement confers a significantly worse prognosis after radical nephrectomy.
e)   Radical nephrectomy should be performed in those who have widely metastatic cancer because of the possibility of spontaneous tumor regression if the primary tumor is removed.

Question 3.119. **A 69-year-old woman with known chronic myelogenous leukemia who has been followed up in the stable phase for the past 6 years presents with sweats, fevers, increasing splenomegaly, and a white blood cell count of 40,000, with 35% blasts. Bone marrow examination reveals that 62% of nucleated cells are leukemic blasts. Cytochemical stains are negative. The most important additional piece of information that will aid in designing an immediate therapeutic strategy is:**

a)   HLA typing of the patient and her siblings
b)   Radionuclide ventriculogram
c)   Pulmonary function tests
d)   Immunophenotypic analysis of aspirated bone marrow cells
e)   Cytogenetic analysis of aspirated bone marrow cells

Question 3.120. **At least 70% of children who have acute lymphoblastic leukemia are likely to be cured; however, only approximately one third of adults who are seen with the same disease will have such a favorable outcome. Which of the following is the most important reason for this discrepancy?**

a)   Adults are more likely to have lymphoblasts harboring a t(9;22) abnormality.
b)   Adults who have ALL are more likely to have lymphoblasts that harbor a t(8;14) abnormality.
c)   Adults are more likely to have central nervous system disease.
d)   Adults have higher white blood cell counts than do children.
e)   It is more difficult to administer full-dose chemotherapy to adults.

Question 3.121. **A 68-year-old woman is seen with fatigue. Her physical examination reveals several 2-cm lymph nodes in the anterior cervical chain bilaterally. She has no splenomegaly. CBC discloses a hematocrit of 24%, platelet count of 220,000/μL, and a WBC of 98,000/μL, with 24% neutrophils and 76% mature appearing lymphocytes. Flow cytometry performed on peripheral blood mononuclear cells reveals a large population of CD20, CD5, and CD23 positive cells. Surface immunoglobulin is weakly positive.**

Which of the following studies is most critical in deciding on the appropriate therapeutic intervention at this time?

a)   Bone marrow aspirate and biopsy
b)   Cytogenetic studies on peripheral blood mononuclear cells
c)   Liver function tests and reticulocyte count
d)   CT scans of the chest, abdomen, and pelvis
e)   Gallium scan

Question 3.122. **A 42-year-old man notes the onset of subcutaneous nodules on his right leg and left arm. In addition to the aforementioned nodules, his physician notes the presence of bilateral groin and right axillary adenopathy, with lymph nodes measuring up to 3 cm in diameter. Biopsy of one of the subcutaneous nodules reveals infiltration with poorly differentiated large cells, which appear to be lymphoid in origin. Mitoses are frequent. Immunoperoxidase studies reveal that most of the cells have a T-cell origin and most coexpress the Ki-1 antigen (CD30). Cytogenetic studies performed on**

biopsy material reveal a t(2;5) abnormality. Computed tomography of the chest, abdomen, and pelvis reveals significant retroperitoneal adenopathy, but no mediastinal adenopathy. Bilateral bone marrow examination results are negative for tumor. The most appropriate therapy is:

a) Radiotherapy to the skin nodules and inguinal nodes
b) Chlorambucil and prednisone
c) Fludarabine
d) High-dose cyclophosphamide, doxorubicin, vincristine, prednisone, cranial prophylactic radiotherapy, and intrathecal methotrexate
e) Cyclophosphamide, vincristine, prednisone, doxorubicin chemotherapy

Question 3.123. **A 23-year-old man is seen with progressive chest pain and shortness of breath of 3 months' duration. Chest radiograph reveals a large anterior mediastinal mass. Further work-up includes chest, abdominal, and pelvic computed tomography that reveals a 12-cm anterior mediastinal mass, but no other adenopathy. The gallium scan results are positive only in the anterior mediastinum. Serum chemistry results are normal, except for a lactate dehydrogenase (LDH) level that is elevated. Pathologic examination of tissue obtained during mediastinoscopy reveals infiltration with neoplastic-appearing lymphoid cells, with frequent mitoses. Immunoperoxidase studies reveal the neoplastic lymphocytes to be of T-cell origin. Which of the following is the most appropriate therapy?**

a) Combination chemotherapy with cyclophosphamide, vincristine, doxorubicin, and prednisone (CHOP)
b) CHOP chemotherapy, followed by mediastinal radiotherapy
c) Mediastinal radiotherapy alone
d) CHOP chemotherapy, followed by prophylactic therapy (intrathecal chemotherapy and cranial irradiation) to the central nervous system
e) CHOP chemotherapy and prophylactic therapy (intrathecal chemotherapy plus cranial irradiation) to the CNS, followed by mediastinal irradiation

Question 3.124. **A 75-year-old man who is seen for evaluation of indigestion is found to have normal CBC and chemistry panel test results, except for a slightly elevated serum total protein. Serum protein electrophoresis reveals an M-spike of 2.5 g/dL. Immunoelectrophoresis reveals an IgG kappa monoclonal protein. The patient is then referred to an oncologist who performs the following studies: skeletal survey, normal; bone marrow aspirate and biopsy, normal cellular marrow without infiltration of unusual elements and only scattered plasma cells present; urine protein electrophoresis, normal; and β_2-microglobulin, normal. The next most appropriate therapeutic or diagnostic maneuver would be:**

a) Observation
b) Bone scan
c) Initiation of phenylalanine mustard therapy
d) Initiation of therapy with continuous infusion of vincristine, doxorubicin, and dexamethasone
e) Immunoglobulin gene rearrangement studies on peripheral blood cells

Question 3.125. **A 2-year-old previously healthy male child is seen with pruritis. Examination reveals crops of reddish brown lesions diffusely located over his skin. The remainder of his physical and laboratory examinations is unremarkable. Biopsy of one of the lesions reveals infiltration with normal-appearing mast cells. You tell the parents that:**

a)   This is a benign self-limited condition with no long-term sequelae.
b)   The patient is likely to develop acute leukemia within 3 years.
c)   This is a manifestation of extramedullary mast leukemia and should be treated with chemotherapy and possible bone marrow transplantation.
d)   Aggressive search for allergens is indicated.
e)   Serology for hepatitis A, B, and C is indicated.

Question 3.126. **A 51-year-old man undergoes upper gastrointestinal endoscopy because of severe heartburn that is partially responsive to antacids. In addition to areas of active gastritis, the endoscopist notes a 0.5-cm polypoid lesion in the gastric antrum. Pathologic examination of the endoscopically biopsied lesion reveals a hyperplastic polyp with normal underlying mucosa. The most appropriate strategy at this time is:**

a)   Repeat endoscopy in 6 months
b)   Partial gastrectomy
c)   Subtotal gastrectomy
d)   Colonoscopy
e)   Symptomatic treatment only

Question 3.127. **A 72-year-old man is found to have a PSA value of 12 ng/mL as revealed by routine screening. Transrectal ultrasound reveals a nodule in the right lobe of the prostate gland. Prostate biopsy reveals a Gleason Grade 5 adenocarcinoma of the prostate. Bone scan is negative, except for an area of increased uptake in the right humerus. Plain radiograph of this area is unremarkable. The most accurate conclusion that can be drawn from the available information is:**

a)   The patient probably has metastatic prostate cancer.
b)   The patient should have a computed tomogram of the humerus.
c)   The patient should have an MRI scan of the right humerus.
d)   The patient is likely to have tumor grossly confined to the prostate gland.
e)   Hormonal ablation therapy is indicated at this time.

Question 3.128. **A 63-year-old man is found to have a PSA of 18 ng/mL as revealed by routine screening. Physical examination and ultrasonography confirm the presence of a nodule confined to the right lobe of the prostate. Transrectal biopsy reveals Gleason Grade 5 adenocarcinoma of the prostate. The patient undergoes radical prostatectomy. Pathologic examination reveals extension of the tumor through the prostate capsule. Postoperatively, the patient's PSA level drops to the undetectable range; however, approximately 14 months after the operation, his PSA level is 2 ng/mL. MRI of the pelvis is unremarkable. PSA level repeated in 1 month's time is 3 ng/mL. The most appropriate strategy would be:**

a)   Repeat PSA in 6 months
b)   Reassure the patients that PSA elevations at this time are typical, due to regrowth of normal prostate tissue

c)   Supplemental irradiation treatment, approximately 6000 cGy
d)   Repeat operation to remove residual prostate cancer
e)   Leuprolide and flutamide

Question 3.129.   A 65-year-old business executive is found to have adeno-carcinoma of the prostate, Gleason Grade 6, which is clinically confined to the gland. The treatment options of either radical prostatectomy or definitive radiotherapy have been offered. Which of the following statements regarding these treatment options are correct?

a)   The likelihood of an undetectable PSA level at 5 years after either surgery or radiotherapy is virtually the same.
b)   Incontinence is more likely after radiotherapy.
c)   The risk of eventual impotence is very low (less than 10%) after radiotherapy.
d)   Diarrhea is more likely after radiotherapy.
e)   Patients can usually go back to work within approximately a week of radical prostatectomy.

Question 3.130.   A 75-year-old man is seen with symptomatic metastatic prostate cancer. Bone scan reveals areas of uptake throughout the skeleton. The patient has no significant past medical history. The best approach at this time would be:

a)   Leuprolide plus ketoconazole
b)   Radiotherapy to all symptomatic sites
c)   Diethylstilbestrol 1 mg daily
d)   DES 3 mg/d
e)   Leuprolide plus flutamide

Question 3.131.   All of the following statements concerning the epidemiology of bladder cancer are correct EXCEPT:

a)   Higher rates of bladder cancer are noted in black men compared with black women, white women, or white men.
b)   Cigarette smoking accounts for approximately 50% of bladder cancers in the United States.
c)   Occupational risk for bladder cancer occurs in the leather, rubber, and paint industries.
d)   Chronic cyclophosphamide use is associated with an increased risk of bladder cancer.
e)   Infections with *Schistosoma haematobium* are associated with both squamous cell and transitional cell carcinoma of the bladder.

Question 1.32.   A 58-year-old man is seen with gross hematuria. Intavenous pyelography is negative for upper urinary tract lesions. Urine cytology reveals cells that raise a high suspicion of transitional cell carcinoma. Cystoscopy reveals a 1-cm papillary lesion in the dome of the bladder. Pathologic examination reveals a histologic Grade II tumor that invades into the lamina propria but not into the muscularis. Random biopsies reveal moderate dysplasia in distant sites. No vascular invasion is noted on the pathologic specimen. Which of the following is the most appropriate strategy at this time?

a)   Metastatic work-up
b)   Intravesical mitomycin-C therapy

c) Radical cystectomy
d) Preoperative radiotherapy followed by radical cystectomy
e) Partial cystectomy

Question 3.133. **A 65-year-old woman develops vaginal bleeding. The patient undergoes a dilation and curettage of the uterus, with sampling of both the endometrial cavity and endocervical canal. Pathology reveals adenocarcinoma. The patient undergoes a total abdominal hysterectomy, bilateral salpingo-oophorectomy, pelvic washings, and lymph node sampling. Pathology reveals adenocarcinoma of the uterus; tumor invades over one half the depth of the myometrium but not into the following structures: the cervix, beyond the uterus, into parametrial structures, and into the vagina; also, the tumor did not invade the bladder, bowel, or metastasize to pelvic or periaortic lymph nodes. All of the following factors would make recurrence more likely EXCEPT:**

a) Clear cell cancer (compared with adenocarcinoma)
b) Poorly differentiated tumors
c) Increased depth of myometrial penetration
d) Positive peritoneal cytology
e) Prior history of oral contraceptive use

Question 3.134. **A 30-year-old man is seen with anemia, thrombocytopenia, and leukocytosis. A large percentage of the peripheral blood cells appear to be blasts. Which of the following findings on bone marrow examination would be associated with the best prognosis?**

a) Infiltration is characterized by nondescript blasts that are cytochemically negative, but myeloid antigen positive.
b) Erythroid hyperplasia is present (greater than 50% of the cells are erythroblasts); 20% of the total nucleated cells are blasts.
c) Infiltration is present, with monocytoid appearing blasts. Special stains are only positive for the nonspecific esterase.
d) Thirty percent of the nucleated cells are blasts; some of the megakaryocyte have simplified nuclei, and there are bilobed mature neutrophils.
e) Most of the nucleated cells are myelomonoblasts; there is an associated population of eosinophil-like cells that also have basophilic granules.

Question 3.135. **A 52-year-old man is seen with fevers, sweats, and bilateral cervical adenopathy. Biopsy of one of his cervical nodes reveals effacement of normal architecture, with infiltration by a monoclonal population of large B lymphocytes. Further staging studies reveal diffuse adenopathy in the anterior cervical chain, anterior mediastinum, and periaortic area nodes. Gallium scan is positive in each of these areas. Bilateral bone marrow examinations reveal no evidence of bone marrow infiltration. Serum chemistry test results are normal, except for a lactate dehydrogenase level that is elevated approximately two times the upper limit of normal. The most appropriate therapeutic strategy at this time would include:**

a) Combination therapy with methotrexate, bleomycin, cyclophosphamide, doxorubicin, dexamethasone, and vincristine

b) Combination therapy with cyclophosphamide, doxorubicin, vincristine, and prednisone
c) Combination therapy with doxorubicin, bleomycin, vinblastine, and dacarbazine
d) Total nodal lymphoid irradiation
e) Combination chemotherapy with cyclophosphamide, vincristine, prednisone, doxorubicin, intrathecal methotrexate, and prophylactic cranial radiotherapy

Question 3.136. **Each of the following represents a therapeutic advance in the treatment of children who have acute lymphoblastic leukemia EXCEPT:**

a) The administration of prophylactic intrathecal chemotherapy and/or cranial radiotherapy.
b) The addition of anthracyclines to the induction chemotherapy regimen.
c) The recognition that different chemotherapeutic strategies should be applied to patients on the basis of clinically assessable risk factors.
d) High-dose cytarabine is used as part of the post-remission management strategy.
e) Maintenance chemotherapy is used.

Question 3.137. **The most common malignant solid tumor arising in neonatal patients is:**

a) Astrocytoma
b) Germ cell tumor
c) Hepatoblastoma
d) Neuroblastoma
e) Wilms' tumor

Question 3.138. **Complete surgical excision of the primary tumor is virtually always necessary for long-term survival in which of the following childhood malignancies:**

a) Hepatoblastoma
b) "Infantile" fibrosarcoma
c) Lymphoma
d) Neuroblastoma
e) Retinoblastoma

Question 3.139. **A 52-year-old man is seen 1 year after resection of a Duke's B2 colon carcinoma. He is being seen at 3-month intervals, and a CEA rise from 3 to 10 ng/mL has been noted. The patient is asymptomatic, and recent chest radiographic findings were negative. The next plan of action should be:**

a) Observe and repeat CEA level determination in several months in order to determine the significance of the rise in CEA.
b) Obtain a CT scan of the abdomen and pelvis and, if negative, perform a radio-immunoguided diagnostic procedure using an anti-CEA monoclonal antibody.
c) Evaluate the patient for other causes of elevated CEA level, including peptic ulcer disease, jaundice, cirrhosis, or recent use of tobacco.
d) Obtain a whole body PET scan to look for disease outside of the abdomen.
e) Perform an exploratory laparotomy.

Question 3.140.   All of the following colorectal polyps are considered precancerous EXCEPT:

a)   Villous adenoma
b)   Tubular adenoma
c)   Hyperplastic polyps
d)   Tubulovillous adenomas
e)   4-cm adenoma

Question 3.141.   A 54-year-old man is seen with right lower quadrant abdominal pain and fever. Examination is suggestive of local peritonitis at the right lower quadrant of the abdomen. The admitting diagnosis in the emergency department is acute appendicitis. The patient is taken to the operating room, where he is noted to have an inflamed appendix, the tip of which has a fleshy appearing mass approximately 2 cm in size. Frozen section of the excised specimens demonstrates a 2-cm carcinoid tumor. The appropriate therapy is:

a)   Completion of the appendectomy, with restaging of the patient postoperatively and 5-FU– based chemotherapy
b)   Completion of the appendectomy, follow-up radiographic studies, and systemic therapy only if the patient develops a recurrence
c)   Close incision, administer octreotide analogue postoperatively
d)   Right hemicolectomy
e)   Evaluation for sites of other carcinoid tumors

Question 3.142.   A 75-year-old gentlemen is seen with new onset of rectal bleeding (most commonly noted following bowel movement). The patient is found to have an external hemorrhoid and a firm posterior rectal mass 6 cm above the dentate line as revealed by sigmoidoscopy. Biopsy demonstrates an invasive adenocarcinoma, although computed tomography of the abdomen does not demonstrate evidence of liver metastases, rectal wall invasion, or nodal metastases. The most appropriate therapy at this time is:

a)   Transanal excision in order to gain adequate local control
b)   Abdominoperineal resection
c)   Low anterior resection
d)   Preoperative radiotherapy followed by a limited resection of the rectum
e)   Low anterior resection followed by postoperative radiotherapy and infusional 5-FU–based chemotherapy

Question 3.143.   An 84-year-old man is seen with progressive weight loss, bloody diarrhea, and on examination is noted to have a markedly distended abdomen with ascites and a mass 4 cm above the anal verge. Endoscopic biopsy demonstrates a highly undifferentiated adenocarcinoma that involves two thirds of the rectal wall circumference. The best therapy in this situation is:

a)   Preoperative chemotherapy, radiotherapy, and abdominoperineal resection
b)   Abdominoperineal resection
c)   5-FU and levamisole alone

d)   Local treatment (laser photoablation) alone or in combination with diverting colostomy

e)   Intraoperative radiotherapy at the time of abdominoperineal resection

Question 3.144.   A 26-year-old man is seen with a long history of painful defecation and occasional pruritus. Examination of the anal region demonstrates a benign-appearing external hemorrhoid, and a 4-cm erythematous, slightly elevated skin lesion is noted in the anal canal. The patient has a history of condyloma acuminatum in the genital region. Biopsy of the anal lesion demonstrates a squamous cell carcinoma. The risk factors for the development of this disease are:

a)   Tobacco exposure

b)   Constant irritation of the perianal skin from anal pruritus and poor anal hygiene

c)   The papillomavirus in association with condyloma acuminatum

d)   Excessive UV light exposure that results in a mutation of the *p53* tumor suppressor gene

e)   Exposure to carcinogens such as benzene and fluorohydrocarbons

Question 3.145.   Metastatic work-up of a patient who has a 4-cm squamous cell carcinoma of the anus demonstrates a 2-cm left inguinal lymph node. Biopsy of the node reveals metastatic squamous cell carcinoma. The most appropriate therapy at this point would be:

a)   Abdominoperineal resection with left inguinal node dissection

b)   External beam radiotherapy with 3000 Gy to the perineal region, local excision of the anal tumor, and left inguinal node dissection

c)   Preoperative administration of 5-FU and mitomycin, with external beam radiotherapy and limited resection of the perianal region and left inguinal node dissection

d)   Concurrent therapy consisting of preoperative radiotherapy and 5-FU and mitomycin, followed by limited resection of the anal primary lesion and left inguinal node dissection

e)   External beam radiotherapy to the perineal and inguinal region

Question 3.146.   A 46-year-old woman is seen with perianal discomfort and rectal bleeding. On examination she is noted to have a 1-cm anal amelanotic skin lesion at the dentate line. Biopsy demonstrates malignant melanoma. The approach to treatment should be:

a)   Review of the pathology to determine if this amelanotic skin lesion is melanoma

b)   Preoperative radiotherapy and dacarbazine chemotherapy followed by limited resection

c)   Abdominoperineal resection

d)   Limited resection to control the local disease

e)   Limited resection followed by inguinal node dissection

Question 3.147.   A 25-year-old Latin man is seen with an exophytic skin lesion on the glans penis. Biopsy demonstrates an invasive squamous cell carcinoma. The management of this disease:

a)   Depends on the histologic grade of the primary lesion

b)   Requires metastatic work-up before management of the primary lesion

c)   Is limited resection or external beam radiotherapy, depending on the size and thickness of the lesion
d)   Is excision of the primary lesion and, depending on the tumor's size, thickness, and histologic aggressiveness, prophylactic lymph node dissection using cutaneous lymphoscintigraphy as a guide to demonstrate the nodal basin at risk
e)   Is preoperative chemotherapy and radiotherapy followed by limited resection

Question 3.148.   Patients with invasive carcinoma of the bladder who are seen with a suprapubic mass and bilateral lower extremity lymphedema are best treated:

a)   By intravesical therapy with mitomycin, doxorubicin, or bacille Calmette-Guérin (BCG)
b)   By partial cystectomy
c)   By radical cystectomy
d)   By radiotherapy
e)   By intravenous chemotherapy (methotrexate, vinblastine, doxorubicin, cisplatin)

Question 3.149.   External-beam radiotherapy may play a role in the management of which of the following types of gastric disease:

a)   Ménétrier's disease
b)   Gastric lymphoma
c)   Leiomyosarcoma
d)   Gastric ulcers secondary to *Helicobacter pylori*
e)   Adenomatous polyps of the stomach

Question 3.150.   A 46-year-old gentleman is seen with dyspepsia and epigastric pain. Upper GI endoscopy suggests a submucosal greater curvature mass, but the biopsy is nondiagnostic, and a CT scan of the abdomen demonstrates a 6-cm mass along the curvature without evidence of perigastric lymph nodes or hepatic disease. The patient undergoes exploratory laparotomy, and biopsy demonstrates a gastric leiomyosarcoma. The patient should:

a)   Receive chemotherapy and radiotherapy followed by a total gastrectomy
b)   Undergo a total gastrectomy regardless of the size of the tumor, because multifocal disease is unlikely
c)   Undergo limited resection in order to obtain clear surgical margins
d)   Undergo limited resection followed by postoperative radiotherapy
e)   Undergo palliative bypass because occult hepatic metastases are probable and are unlikely to be cured

Question 3.151.   All of the following predispose patients to gastric carcinoma EXCEPT:

a)   gastric adenomatous polyps
b)   previous gastric irradiation
c)   previous gastric operation
d)   presence of *H. pylori*
e)   atrophic gastritis

Question 3.152. **The standard surgical management of gastric carcinomas of the distal antrum should include:**

a) Extensive regional lymph node dissection (R1 and R2), as described in the Japanese literature
b) Total gastrectomy
c) Subtotal gastrectomy, including resection of the perigastric lymph nodes along the gastric arteries and omentectomy
d) Total gastrectomy with random lymph node biopsies and peritoneal washings
e) Esophagogastrectomy

Question 3.153. **Carcinoma of the breast in men:**

a) Generally has a better prognosis than similar stage disease in women
b) Is typically treated in a similar fashion as in women
c) Can be predicted by the presence of BRCA-1 and BRCA-2 gene mutations
d) Is clinically evident by unilateral gynecomastia in most men
e) Accounts for 5% of malignancies in men

Question 3.154. **A true statement regarding cystosarcoma phylloides is:**

a) It is a variant of lobular carcinoma in situ.
b) Most lesions are malignant and tend to spread rapidly to the regional lymph nodes.
c) It has a high grade of multifocality and is often bilateral.
d) Wide local excision or simple mastectomy is usually sufficient for therapy.
e) Preoperative chemotherapy is typically indicated for large primary lesions, followed by salvage mastectomy.

Question 3.155. **Which of the following statements regarding ductal carcinoma in situ (DCIS) and lobular carcinoma in situ (LCIS) of the breast are true?**

a) They are derived from similar cell types of the breast.
b) They have an equal risk of subsequent invasive malignancy.
c) They have an equal incidence of bilateral occurrence.
d) DCIS is typically associated with subsequent development of invasive disease. Patients with LCIS typically have occult invasion at the time of presentation.
e) The risk of synchronous invasive cancer is higher in patients with DCIS, and patients with LCIS may have bilateral disease.

Question 3.156. **A 46-year-old woman is seen with a 2.5-cm right upper outer quadrant breast mass and is noted on mammogram to have diffuse microcalcifications throughout the same breast. Needle directed biopsy demonstrates DCIS. The management of this lesion should be:**

a) Segmental resection, with evaluation of the surgical margins in order to determine if segmental resection alone is proper therapy
b) Lumpectomy followed by postoperative external beam radiotherapy to the remaining breast
c) Segmental resection with follow-up mammogram in order to determine the change in the calcification overtime

d) Total mastectomy
e) Lumpectomy and axillary lymph node dissection

Question 3.157.   The management of DCIS of the breast is controversial. Several new molecular markers have been developed in order to determine which patients have a worse prognosis. These include all but:

a) Her-2/neu protein overexpression
b) Flow cytometry in order to determine S-phase fraction of the tumor
c) Sialyl-Tn expression
d) Chromosome I aneusomy
e) p53 Tumor suppressor gene overexpression of the primary tumor

Question 3.158.   A 52-year-old woman is seen with a 2-cm right upper quadrant breast mass. Screening mammogram demonstrates no other lesions, and the axillary node basin appears clinically negative. Segmental mastectomy, radiotherapy, and total mastectomy have been shown to be equivalent therapy for the treatment of this primary lesion. What is the role of axillary lymph node dissection in a patient with a 2-cm breast cancer mass?

a) There is no role for axillary lymph node dissection, because this patient is likely to receive cytotoxic therapy following surgical resection of her breast cancer.
b) The patient should have lymph node sampling in order to reduce the morbidity associated with a complete axillary node dissection.
c) The patient should undergo complete axillary node dissection in order to adequately stage her disease.
d) She should begin tamoxifen regardless of the axillary node status.
e) The patient should receive high-dose chemotherapy regardless of the status of axillary nodes.

Question 3.159.   A 52-year-old woman is seen with an ill-defined right breast mass and dimpling of the skin. Biopsy of the skin demonstrates lymphatic invasion with adenocarcinoma. Results of a metastatic work-up with chest radiograph, CT scan of the abdomen, and bone scan were negative. The therapy at this point should be:

a) Modified radical mastectomy with postoperative cyclophosphamide, methotrexate, and 5-FU
b) Preoperative external beam radiotherapy and lumpectomy followed by postoperative cyclophosphamide, methotrexate, 5-fluorouracil treatment (CMF)
c) Combination chemotherapy with CAF (cyclophosphamide, doxorubicin, and 5-FU), followed by modified radical mastectomy if the patient responds to initial therapy, followed by postoperative radiotherapy
d) Four cycles of preoperative chemotherapy, and if there is a response, bone marrow transplantation with high-dose chemotherapy.
e) High-dose chemotherapy with stem cell transplantation, followed by salvage mastectomy

Question 3.160.   A patient with a history of breast cancer who was treated with lumpectomy and axillary node dissection followed by postoperative ra-

diotherapy 5 years earlier develops a recurrence in the ipsilateral breast. At this point, the patient should be treated by:

a) Lumpectomy with additional postoperative radiotherapy
b) Systemic chemotherapy
c) Total mastectomy
d) Tamoxifen alone
e) Additional radiotherapy isolated to the recurrence

Question 3.161. **A 46-year-old gentleman is seen with abdominal fullness and a palpable 6-cm lower abdominal mass. Work-up demonstrates a low-density mass in the retroperitoneum, and biopsy suggests a low-grade liposarcoma. The most appropriate therapy is:**

a) Preoperative chemotherapy followed by resection and postoperative external beam radiotherapy
b) Preoperative chemotherapy followed by resection
c) Complete surgical resection, if possible
d) Preoperative chemotherapy based on chemosensitivity of the primary lesion, complete surgical resection, followed by postoperative radiotherapy
e) Partial resection for palliation of symptoms followed by postoperative external beam radiotherapy

Question 3.162. **A patient with a retroperitoneal sarcoma has been followed up with routine CT scans of the abdomen after having complete surgical resection 2 years previously. The CT scan reveals a mass in the retroperitoneum adjacent to the left kidney. The patient is asymptomatic, and treatment should be:**

a) Surgical resection in order to reduce the tumor burden and hopefully to prevent further recurrences
b) Preoperative external beam radiotherapy combined with intraoperative radiotherapy and resection
c) High-dose external beam radiotherapy alone in order to preserve the kidney
d) Observation and resection only if the patient is symptomatic from disease
e) High-dose methotrexate

Question 3.163. **The treatment of cystic neoplasms of the pancreas include:**

a) External or internal drainage or biopsy
b) Postoperative intravenous 5-fluorouracil and external beam radiotherapy following surgical resection
c) Complete surgical resection
d) Palliative resection, including gastric and biliary bypass, if necessary
e) External beam radiotherapy alone

Question 3.164. **Splenectomy may be performed as part of the staging for Hodgkin's disease. Patients at highest risk for post-splenectomy sepsis are:**

a) Those patients who have splenectomy as a result of trauma, idiopathic thrombocytopenic purpura, or hereditary spherocytosis
b) Those patients who have splenectomy for metastatic non-hematopoietic disease

c)   Those patients with Hodgkin's disease and other diseases of the reticuloendothelial system

d)   Those who have coexisting bowel problems

e)   Those patients receiving chronic antibiotic prophylactic therapy

Question 3.165.   **In general, for a given cancer, the younger the patient the better the prognosis. All of the following statements regarding this issue are correct EXCEPT:**

a)   There are two age peaks for the incidence of acute lymphocytic leukemia (ALL): childhood and age over 50.

b)   Current protocols for ALL produce cure rates of 60 to 70% in children and 15 to 40% in adults.

c)   The greater curability of younger patients is due primarily to their better tolerance of chemotherapy.

d)   Cytogenetic, immunophenotyping, and molecular biology studies indicate that ALL is heterogenous.

e)   Hyperdiploidy occurs more commonly in pediatric ALL than in adult ALL.

Question 3.166.   **All of the following statements regarding the acute lympho-cytic leukemias or acute myeloid leukemias (AML) are correct EXCEPT:**

a)   Balanced translocations occur more commonly in adults with ALL and are associated with a worse prognosis.

b)   The 9:22 translocation (BCR/ABL) in ALL is an indication for allogeneic bone marrow transplantation in first remission.

c)   *p53* tumor suppressor gene mutations occur more commonly in pediatric leukemias.

d)   Blasts from older patients with de novo untreated AML more commonly display multidrug resistance gene (MDR) expression as compared to those obtained from younger patients.

e)   Older patients with AML commonly exhibit subtle degrees of hypocellularity and trilineage dysplastic changes in the marrow.

Question 3.167.   **All of the following statements concerning the epidemiology of Hodgkin's disease are correct EXCEPT:**

a)   Non-Hodgkin's lymphoma is increasing in incidence and is now more common than Hodgkin's disease.

b)   Hodgkin's disease in patients over 40 is more likely to be lymphocyte predominant or of mixed cellularity.

c)   Patients with Hodgkin's disease who are less than 16 years old are likely to be males with lymphocyte predominant histology.

d)   Like non-Hodgkin's lymphoma, Hodgkin's disease occurs in increasing incidence in immunosuppressed patients, including patients undergoing transplantation.

e)   In developing countries, Hodgkin's disease tends to frequently occur in young patients.

Question 3.168.   **All of the following statements regarding Hodgkin's disease are correct EXCEPT:**

a)   Lymphocyte predominant Hodgkin's disease is more often seen in males either under 15 years of age or over 40, is often localized to a single node, and is indolent in nature.

b)   Patients with mixed cellularity more often have constitutional symptoms and more often have stages III and IV disease compared to patients who have the lymphocyte predominant or nodular sclerosing types.
c)   Nodular sclerosis represents 70% of Hodgkin's disease cases in economically developed countries but is less common in developing countries.
d)   Granulomatous lesions in a lymph node increase the risk that Hodgkin's disease will be found elsewhere.
e)   Granulomatous lesions in an involved node are an adverse prognostic factor for patients with Hodgkin's disease.

Question 3.169.   All of the following statements concerning Hodgkin's disease are correct EXCEPT:

a)   Part or all of the EBV genome is found in the Reed-Sternberg (RS) cells of up to 50% of patients who have Hodgkin's disease.
b)   There is a direct correlation between the abundance of lymphocytes in the lymph nodes of patients with Hodgkin's disease and a slow rate of progression of the disease.
c)   The Reed-Sternberg cells of lymphocyte-predominant Hodgkin's disease are CD15 positive, whereas the Reed-Sternberg cells of the mixed cellularity and nodular sclerosis types are CD15 negative.
d)   Although the lymphoid infiltrate in a Hodgkin's lymph node may be polymorphous, cytogenetic and molecular studies indicate clonality of the Reed-Sternberg cells.
e)   Patients with the lymphocytic depleted subtype have a relatively poor prognosis.

Question 3.170.   All of the following regarding the RS cell are correct EXCEPT:

a)   Both B- and T-cell antigens have been demonstrated on the RS cell.
b)   The RS cell may express immunoglobulin and/or T-cell receptor gene rearrangements.
c)   Hodgkin's disease is characterized by the t(14;18) translocation that results in amplification of *bcl-2* oncogene products.
d)   The CD15 antigen can rarely be demonstrated on RS cells.
e)   RS cells frequently express activation antigens such as interleukin-2 receptors.

Question 3.171.   All of the following regarding the immune response in Hodgkin's disease are correct EXCEPT:

a)   The immune defect is present at the time of diagnosis and presumably precedes the onset of the disease.
b)   Cellular immunologic deficits persist even in patients who achieve long-term remissions with radiotherapy and/or chemotherapy.
c)   Herpes zoster appears most commonly within the first year after treatment.
d)   Systemic infection with encapsulated organisms such as pneumococci and *Haemophilus influenzae* appear predominantly in splenectomized patients.
e)   Pneumococcal vaccine should be given following splenectomy.

Question 3.172.   All of the following statements regarding Hodgkin's disease are correct EXCEPT:

a)   It tends to involve central rather than peripheral lymph nodes.
b)   The disease spreads by contiguity to adjacent lymph nodes.

c)   Hematogenous spread may account for stage IV disease.
d)   Relapse at pretreatment sites of tumor after complete remission is more likely
     in patients who have Hodgkin's disease compared with those who have non-
     Hodgkin's lymphoma.
e)   The liver is generally involved in the presence of splenic involvement.

Question 3.173. **All of the following statements regarding nitrogen mustard,
vincristine, procarbazine, prednisone (MOPP) or daunorubicin, bleomycin,
vinblastine, dacarbazine (ABVD) therapy for Hodgkin's disease are correct
EXCEPT:**

a)   Patients who relapse after combination chemotherapy with MOPP or ABVD
     have a much lower response to retreatment with the original combination
     treatment compared with the alternative combination.
b)   ABVD is superior to MOPP in that infertility and secondary tumors are less
     frequent.
c)   In comparative studies, downward dose modification with MOPP occurs more
     commonly than with ABVD.
d)   Hybrid regimens derived from MOPP and ABVD as well as alternating
     MOPP–ABVD therapy have proved superior to MOPP or ABVD with regard to
     disease-free and overall survival.
e)   In comparative studies, ABVD is equivalent to MOPP in terms of disease-free
     survival.

Question 3.174. **All of the following statements regarding mycosis fungoides
are correct EXCEPT:**

a)   The earliest and most prominent symptom is pruritis.
b)   The earliest manifestations are slightly scaly erythematous lesions that wax
     and wane.
c)   The neoplastic cell is a CD4 helper T cell.
d)   T-cell gene rearrangements are relatively constant in biopsies from different
     sites within a given patient.
e)   As the disease progresses, ulceration and infection may occur, which leads to
     Pautrier's abscesses in the skin.

Question 3.175. **All of the following statements regarding mycosis fungoides
are correct EXCEPT:**

a)   Early skin lesions respond to topical corticosteroids.
b)   Repetitive treatment with psoralen followed by UV light produces a 40 to 80%
     remission rate, depending on the number and size of the plaquelike lesions.
c)   Remissions produced with tar and UV light are often of long duration.
d)   Depth of UV penetration must be adjusted to the depth of the lesions. Short
     wavelength (UVC) penetrates more deeply and is therefore better for deep
     lesions.
e)   The overall response to electron beam therapy is almost 100%.

Question 3.176. **Which of the following statements regarding the treatment
of mycosis fungoides is correct?**

a)   Repetitive application of topical nitrogen mustard will produce tumor
     regression by cytotoxic effect.

b)   Myelosuppression is a significant toxicity of topical nitrogen mustard.
c)   *Cis*-retinoic acid is inactive.
d)   Diffuse erythroderma is associated with circulating cells that have a different genetic and immunology profile than those from skin lesions.
e)   The Sézary syndrome responds to extracorporeal photopheresis.

Question 3.177.   A 50-year-old farmer is seen with a 2-month history of chronic hoarseness. Examination reveals a lesion of the right true vocal cord, with horseshoe extension onto the contralateral anterior third of the left true vocal cord. The lesion appears to be superficial and does not appear to have significant supraglottic, subglottic, or paraglottic extension. The vocal cord has normal mobility. Biopsy of this lesion is consistent with an invasive squamous carcinoma. The best possible management regarding survival and quality of life is:

a)   Interstitial radiotherapy implants
b)   Laryngeal preservation with chemotherapy and radiotherapy
c)   Surgical excision with frontal lateral laryngectomy
d)   Laser surgical excision followed by radiotherapy
e)   External beam radiotherapy

Question 3.178.   A 55-year-old housewife with a T1N0M0 squamous cell carcinoma of the soft palate was treated by definitive radiotherapy and has minimal complaints of xerostomia. She discontinued her 1.5 pack per day smoking habit when she received the diagnosis. The patient's greatest risk for mortality is due to:

a)   Myocardial infarction caused by coronary artery disease
b)   Radiation-induced sarcoma
c)   Second primary malignancy of the lung or upper aerodigestive tract
d)   Squamous cell carcinoma of the cervix
e)   Radiation-induced chronic interstitial fibrosis

Question 3.179.   A 38-year-old woman is seen with a left parotid mass that has rapidly developed over the past 6 weeks. The mass is located primarily in the tail of the gland and is mobile from underlying structures; its greatest dimension is 2.5 cm, and there is no palpable lymphadenopathy within the neck. Facial nerve function is bilaterally symmetric. The patient undergoes superficial parotidectomy, with anatomic preservation of the facial nerve. Complete surgical excision of the neoplasm with tumor-free margins surrounding the gland is performed. Final pathologic review is consistent with a low-grade mucoepidermoid carcinoma. Seven accompanying lymph nodes are positive. Further management of this patient requires:

a)   Postoperative radiotherapy
b)   Additional surgery with complete parotidectomy and resection of the facial nerve, followed by postoperative radiotherapy
c)   Magnetic resonance imaging to evaluate for a contralateral salivary gland simultaneous primary tumor
d)   Observation only
e)   Postoperative radiotherapy with adjuvant chemotherapy to manage microscopic disseminated systemic disease

Question 3.180. A 49-year-old African American man recently developed urinary frequency and nocturia attributed to benign prostatic hypertrophy (based on physical examination) or to chronic prostatitis following gonococcal infection 25 years ago. His PSA level was found to be 14 ng/mL. Six transrectal prostatic biopsies disclosed prostatic carcinoma in two specimens. Risk factors for prostate cancer in this patient include:

a) Age
b) Prior history of sexually transmitted disease
c) Race
d) Benign prostatic hypertrophy
e) Chronic prostatitis

Question 3.181. Which of the following statements regarding the pathology of prostate cancer is correct?

a) Most cancers are poorly differentiated.
b) Prostate cancers occur equally distributed throughout the prostate gland.
c) Prostate intra-epithelial neoplasia (PIN) is a well-recognized "precursor" of prostate cancer.
d) Gleason grade 8 prostate cancers are a favorable prognostic group of tumors.
e) Prostate cancer never occurs before age 45.

Question 3.182. A 62-year-old asymptomatic carpenter is found to have prostatic enlargement on digital rectal examination, and his PSA level is 7 ng/mL. Transrectal biopsy discloses carcinoma from all sites in the right lobe, and none in the left lobe. Before considering a radical prostatectomy, metastasis should be excluded. Which of the following is the most sensible?

a) Laparotomy with retroperitoneal node dissection
b) Biopsy of the bone marrow
c) Laparoscopy with pelvic node biopsies
d) Measurement of PSA level after a 2-month course of leuprolide
e) Radiology skeletal survey

Question 3.183. A 48-year-old man is seen with headaches and increasing shoe size. Pictures taken 5 years ago compared with his current appearance suggest a marked change, with increasing prominence of the frontal bone. After an appropriate work-up is done to document the likely clinical cause of these changes, the most appropriate therapy would be:

a) Octreotide
b) Streptozocin and 5-fluorouracil
c) Doxorubicin, streptozocin, and 5-fluorouracil
d) Cranial irradiation
e) Trans-sphenoidal hypophysectomy

Question 3.184. The most appropriate postoperative therapy for patients with properly staged epithelial ovarian cancer, stage Ia, grade 1, is:

a) Observation
b) Single-agent chemotherapy
c) Combination chemotherapy

d) Pelvic irradiation
e) Combination chemotherapy and pelvic irradiation

Question 3.185. **Of the following, which is the essential initial step in the therapeutic strategy for ovarian malignancies:**

a) Computed tomography
b) Bone marrow harvest
c) Paracentesis
d) Exploratory laparotomy
e) Induction chemotherapy

Question 3.186. **Other than prophylactic oophorectomy, the only known documented means of reducing the probability of developing invasive epithelial ovarian cancer is the following:**

a) Serial measurements of the serum tumor marker CA-125
b) Transvaginal ultrasonography (TVUS)
c) Low-fat diet
d) Oral contraceptives
e) Aerobic exercise

Question 3.187. **A 59-year-old man had a pedunculated polypoid mass of 1.5 cm colonoscopically removed from his descending colon 17 months ago after a bout of hematochezia. The pathologic specimen was lost. He has just returned from a vacation to a tropical country and complains of 3 weeks of lower abdominal crampy pain. His hemoglobin level is 10.7 mg/dL; WBC, 9000/μL; neutrophils, 62%; lymphocytes, 29%; monocytes, 4%; and eosinophils, 5%. Stool culture revealed no enteric pathogens, and one stool sample for ova and parasites was negative. The next diagnostic step should be:**

a) A therapeutic trial of loperamide
b) Colonoscopy
c) Barium enema
d) Gastroscopy
e) Two more stool cultures for ova and parasites

Question 3.188. **The proclivity for a primary tumor to form distant metastases is:**

a) A random event that typically occurs when only a few malignant cells are dispersed from the primary tumor.
b) Dependent only on hematogeneous routes of spread
c) A multistep process involving an orderly sequence of events at the molecular level
d) Supported solely by Paget's "seed and soil" hypothesis
e) Preferential to certain organ systems, depending on mechanical factors only

Question 3.189. **All of the following are important prognostic factors for survival of patients with metastatic pulmonary disease EXCEPT:**

a) Short disease-free interval
b) Long (>40 days) tumor doubling time

c) Less than four metastatic lesions
d) Control of the primary tumor
e) Lung as the sole site of metastatic disease

Question 3.190. **The surgical technique of resection for metastatic pulmonary disease includes all of the following EXCEPT:**

a) Staged bilateral thoracotomy
b) Median sternotomy
c) Exploration of the lung in both inflated and deflated condition
d) Abandoning pulmonary resection if pneumonectomy or chest wall resection is required for complete surgical eradication of disease
e) Examination of mediastinal lymph nodes by frozen specimen

Question 3.191. **A 35-year-old man is seen with a large (8- x 10-cm) mass on the proximal thigh. Which of the following is true regarding biopsy of this lesion?**

a) Because the patient has not noticed a change in the lesion in 6 months, a follow-up visit should be scheduled in 6 months to determine if a biopsy is indicated for this stable lesion.
b) An experienced pathologist can diagnose malignant sarcomas by fine-needle biopsy.
c) Excisional biopsy of this large lesion is indicated because it is probably malignant, and an incisional biopsy would only disseminate disease.
d) A transverse biopsy excision is preferred for incisional biopsies of extremity soft-tissue sarcoma.
e) Frozen-section analysis is not justified if at least a 1-cm specimen is sent for permanent section review.

Question 3.192. **Which statement best reflects our understanding of soft-tissue sarcomas?**

a) The AICC classification of soft-tissue sarcomas reflects the universal organization of sarcomas based on anatomic site of the primary.
b) The AICC staging system for soft-tissue sarcomas is based on TNM status, with tumor size the only important prognostic factor.
c) There is no universally accepted classification system for soft-tissue sarcomas.
d) The AICC clinicopathologic staging system for soft-tissue sarcoma depends primarily on tumor size and lymph node status.
e) Histogenetic classification of sarcomas has been accepted because sarcomas have one cell type and are easily distinguishable.

Question 3.193. **All of the following statements regarding the treatment for extremity soft-tissue sarcomas are correct EXCEPT:**

a) Internal hemipelvectomy can be performed for attempted limb salvage even if sarcoma is invading the ilium.
b) Brachytherapy is most effective for low-grade tumors because it improves local control by 65% when compared with surgery alone.
c) Adjuvant chemotherapy is well established for osteosarcoma and Ewing's sarcoma.

d) Advances in multimodality therapy and improved operative techniques have allowed limb salvage for more than 90% of extremity soft-tissue sarcomas.

e) The role of preoperative radiotherapy limb salvage is more pronounced for those with large tumors.

Question 3.194.   All of the following statements concerning soft-tissue tumors are correct EXCEPT:

a) Liposarcoma is one of the most common soft-tissue tumors.

b) Desmoid tumors are treated with local excision and brachytherapy.

c) The potential for metastasis of malignant fibrous histiocytoma (MFH) is directly related to the size and the grade of the primary tumor.

d) Alveolar rhabdomyosarcoma carries an extremely poor prognosis.

e) Patients who have classic Kaposi's sarcoma have a higher incidence of secondary malignancies such as lymphoma.

Question 3.195.   A 5-year-old boy was seen with a prolonged history of anemia, thrombocytopenia, fevers, and joint pains. He had been followed by a pediatric rheumatologist with the diagnosis of juvenile rheumatoid arthritis when his blood counts began to deteriorate. Soon thereafter, blasts were seen on the peripheral smear, and a diagnosis of acute lymphoblastic leukemia was made. Which one of the following statements is true about this child's course?

a) The child's age places him in a good prognostic group, although this may be influenced by other factors such as ploidy, chromosome translocation, or the intitial white blood cell count.

b) The prolonged course of follow-up with the diagnosis of juvenile rheumatoid arthritis before the diagnosis of ALL, along with a prolonged course of nonsteroidal medications, compromised the child's care.

c) Males tend to do worse than females with childhood ALL, and this appears to be principally related to testicular disease.

d) If this 5 year old does not have a complex translocation, transplantation might be indicated in first remission.

e) One of the major advances in the treatment of childhood ALL was the development of CNS preventative therapy. For this 5 year old, standard CNS preventative therapy would most likely include daily intrathecal medication.

Question 3.196.   An 11-year-old boy is seen with a diagnosis of acute lymphoblastic leukemia. At the time of presentation, he has a t(9;22); an initial white blood cell count of 466,000/μL; hemoglobin, 11.3 mg/dL; platelet count, 52,000/μL; no evidence of CNS disease at diagnosis; and no evidence of a bulky mass. Which would be the best approach for this child, assuming that he attains a remission within a 4-week period of time?

a) This child should receive conventional therapy, including cranial irradiation to prevent CNS disease in the future.

b) If this child has an overall good response to therapy, as measured by rapid clearance of blasts on a Day 7 bone marrow aspiration, he will do well with conventional therapy.

c)   If a matched sibling donor is available, transplantation in first remission will yield the best possible cure rate for this child.

d)   Because of the initial high white blood cell count, the therapeutic approach should include prophylactic testicular irradiation to prevent the testes from serving as a reservoir for leukemia cells.

e)   The duration of therapy for this child has not been adequately determined, and 5 years of treatment would be considered the standard length of therapy for such a patient with high-risk features.

Question 3.197.   For adults with acute myeloid leukemia who are under the age of 60 years, given access to appropriate antibiotics, blood bank support, and clinical expertise, the best results occur when intensive induction therapy is followed by:

a)   Continuous maintenance treatment
b)   Standard-dose intensification
c)   High-dose intensification
d)   Immunotherapy
e)   No treatment

Question 3.198.   The prognosis of acute myeloid leukemia depends on many features. Given an attentive staff in a hospital with adequate resources, the chief determinant of outcome is:

a)   Age
b)   FAB cytologic type
c)   Karyotype
d)   Chemotherapeutic regimen
e)   Bone marrow transplantation in first remission

Question 3.199.   A 60-year-old man with a heavy smoking history has an episode of painless gross hematuria. His physician refers him to a urologist. He undergoes cystoscopy and is found to have a 2-cm pedunculated tumor on the left wall of the bladder. The lesion is completely resected, and pathology reveals that it is a grade I or grade III papillary transitional cell carcinoma confined to the epithelium (Ta). The correct management for this patient is:

a)   Observation
b)   Installation of BCG for 6 weeks
c)   Installation of BCG for 6 weeks followed by maintenance BCG
d)   Intravesical mitomycin C
e)   Cystectomy

Question 3.200.   A 65-year-old man with a several-year history of recurrent multifocal superficial bladder cancer with associated carcinoma in situ (CIS) has received several types of intravesical therapy. On follow-up examination he was found to have a high-grade (III of III) recurrence with muscular invasion ($\geq$T2). Results of a metastatic work-up are negative. The most appropriate treatment for this patient at the present time is:

a)   Observation
b)   Radiotherapy

c) Cystectomy
d) Neoadjuvant chemotherapy followed by cystectomy
e) Neoadjuvant chemotherapy followed by radiotherapy

Question 3.201. A 67-year-old man is 2 years status post cystectomy for a T3a N0 M0 transitional cell carcinoma of the bladder. He received no adjuvant chemotherapy or radiotherapy. He now is seen with a 2-cm lesion in the right lower lobe of the lung. The rest of the findings from his metastatic work-up are negative. The most appropriate management for this patient at this time is:

a) Repeat chest radiograph in 3 months
b) Resection of pulmonary lesion
c) Four to six cycles of MVAC chemotherapy
d) Four to six cycles of MVAC chemotherapy followed by resection of residual mass
e) Irradiation to pulmonary lesion

Question 3.202. A 50-year-old man goes to his doctor because of a nonproductive cough that he has had for 2 weeks. Physical examination of the chest is unremarkable. However, a spleen edge is palpable 2 cm below the left costal margin. Chest radiographic findings are negative. Blood studies show the following:

		Differential distribution (percent)	
Hct	45%		
Hgb	15.0 gm%	**Neutrophil**	68
Platelet	420,000/mm^3	**Band form**	15
WBC	30,000/mm^3	**Myelocyte**	10
		Monocyte	2
		Lymphocyte	5

The hematology resident who is on call submits a good specimen of bone marrow to the laboratory, the results of which, within 48 hours, report the absence of the Philadelphia chromosome. The next course of action should be:

a) Treat vigorously with antibiotics, because this is a mild leukemoid reaction.
b) Await the determination of serum vitamin B12 and B12 binding levels.
c) Await results of *bcr/abl* gene rearrangement studies.
d) Repeat cytogenetic studies.
e) Determine the leukocyte alkaline phosphatase level.

Question 3.203. A 65-year-old man is found on physical examination to have an enlarged spleen that is palpable 9 cm below the left costal margin. His liver is palpable 1 cm below the right costal margin. Peripheral blood studies show:

		Differential distribution (percent)	
Hct	10.5 gm%		
Hgb	30.0%	**Neutrophil**	58
Platelet	28,500/mm^3	**Band form**	15
WBC	192,000/mm^3	**Myelocyte**	10
		Metamyelocyte	10
		Promyelocyte	4
		Myeloblast	3

Examination of the peripheral blood discloses tear drop forms and nucleated erythroid cells. A bone marrow biopsy shows intervening islands of fibrosis alternating with granulocytic and megakaryocytic hyperplasia. The **LEAST** likely diagnosis is:

a)   Agnogenic myeloid metaplasia
b)   Chronic myeloid leukemia
c)   Polycythemia vera
d)   Essential thrombocytosis
e)   Myelodysplastic syndrome

Question 3.204.   When a patient has a nonmetastatic gestational trophoblastic tumor and desires to preserve fertility, initial therapy should entail:

a)   Local uterine resection
b)   Combination chemotherapy
c)   Repeat uterine curettage
d)   Single-agent chemotherapy with either paclitaxel or cisplatin
e)   Single-agent chemotherapy with either actinomycin-D or methotrexate

Question 3.205.   Following remission with chemotherapy for a gestational trophoblastic tumor, patients should be counseled that in future conceptions:

a)   They have a higher risk of spontaneous abortion.
b)   They may anticipate a normal reproductive outcome.
c)   They have a higher risk of requiring cesarean section.
d)   They have a higher incidence of congenital anomalies.
e)   They have a higher risk of tubal pregnancies.

Question 3.206.   Ameloblastoma of the mandible is commonly treated with which of the following:

a)   Radiotherapy
b)   Block resection, leaving the lower border of the mandible intact
c)   Hemimandibulectomy and rib graft
d)   Cisplatin
e)   Curettage followed by radiotherapy

Question 3.207.   A 59-year-old architect under treatment for metastatic prostatic carcinoma 3 years following radical prostatectomy is receiving leuprolide and flutamide. After 11 months, he complains of intermittent dull sacral pain. Bone scan demonstrates an increased uptake that cannot be distinguished from osteoarthritic changes. His PSA level has risen from 0.7 to 3.9 ng/mL. The proper course of action is:

a)   Prescribe nonsteroidal anti-inflammatory drugs and reassess in 3 months
b)   Discontinue flutamide and prescribe nonsteroidal anti-inflammatory drugs
c)   Double the dose of flutamide
d)   Continue flutamide and discontinue the leuprolide
e)   Discontinue leuprolide and flutamide, and prepare for castration

Question 3.208.   A 76-year-old teacher found to have osseous metastatic disease with adenocarcinoma cells in his marrow and an enlarged prostate

underwent orchiectomy 8 years ago. A supraclavicular lymph node was
found when he visited his doctor with complaints of cough and shortness
of breath. On biopsy, metastatic small-cell carcinoma was found. Chest
radiograph showed increased bronchovascular markings and a moderately
enlarged heart. The patient underwent diuresis with furosemide, with improvement in his dyspnea but not his cough. The next diagnostic study
should be:

a) Bronchoscopy
b) Prostatic biopsy
c) Mediastinoscopy
d) CT scan of the neck
e) CT scan of the lung

Question 3.209.   **A 60-year-old salesman who has metastatic carcinoma of
the prostate to vertebral bodies and the pelvis complains of excruciating pain
that is unrelieved by 120 mg of sustained-released morphine every 8 hours.
He has relapsed from total androgen deprivation, and states that the pain is
usually in his back, but sometimes in his shoulders. Pain often radiates
through the femoral or sciatic nerve distribution.**
    **The patient admits to prior use of crack cocaine and heavy alcohol intake.
The proper approach to treating his pain is:**

a) High-dose chemotherapy with autologous stem-cell re-infusion
b) Increase in morphine dose, including intravenous administration in a hospice
   setting
c) Intravenous pamidronate
d) Strontium 89
e) External beam radiotherapy

Question 3.210.   **Which statement regarding the management of localized
prostate cancer is TRUE:**

a) Radical prostatectomy is an operation that has fallen into disfavor and is
   uncommonly done.
b) All men who are younger than 70 years of age should undergo irradiation or
   prostatectomy for localized prostate cancer.
c) Eighty percent of men with localized (T1,2N0M0) disease who undergo
   prostatectomy are free of any evidence of disease at 5 years.
d) Irradiation is effective as a palliative treatment for (T1,2N0M0) prostate cancer,
   but is not a useful approach if long-term disease control is sought.
e) After prostate irradiation, monthly administration of intramuscular testosterone
   enanthate is safe and effective in maintaining potency.

Question 3.211.   **A 60-year-old woman develops abdominal discomfort and
increasing abdominal girth. She denies having nausea, constipation, or
weight loss. Previous history includes cholecystectomy, appendectomy,
and total abdominal hysterectomy and biteral salpingo-oophorectomy.
Physical examination reveals ascites; CT scan of the abdomen and pelvis
confirms the presence of ascites with several 2- to 3-cm peritoneal masses.
Paracentesis yields exudative fluid; cytology shows adenocarcinoma. The**

patient's blood chemistry profile is normal; radiographic findings are normal; Tumor markers CA-125 and CEA are 350 and 6.0, respectively. The next step should be:

a) Repeat paracentesis for immunoperoxidase studies and electron microscopy
b) Laparoscopy with biopsy
c) Laparotomy with maximal surgical cytoreduction
d) Upper GI endoscopy with ERCP
e) Chemotherapy with paclitaxel and cisplatin

Question 3.212. A 25-year-old man develops rapidly worsening substernal chest pain as well as swelling of his arms and face. On physical examination, he has superior vena cava syndrome, with no other abnormalities. Chest radiograph reveals a large anterior mediastinal mass, with three nodules in the right lung. CT scans of the chest/abdomen reveal no additional abnormalities. Routine laboratory evaluation is normal, except for an LDH level of 650. Tumor marker levels are as follows: hCG, normal; alpha-fetoprotein, 40,000. The appropriate management is:

a) Begin radiotherapy immediately to relieve superior vena cava syndrome.
b) Biopsy the mediastinal mass using a parasternal approach
c) Perform a CT-directed needle biopsy of the mediastinal mass.
d) Initiate chemotherapy immediately with cisplatin, etoposide, and bleomycin (BEP).
e) Initiate chemotherapy immediately with cyclophosphamide, doxorubicin, vincristine, and prednisone (CHOP).

Question 3.213. A 45-year-old man develops a mass in the right side of his neck. He feels fatigued but is otherwise asymptomatic. Physical examination reveals a 2 × 3-cm right posterior cervical lymph node, and a 2 × 2-cm right axillary lymph node. CT scans of the chest and abdomen reveal multiple mediastinal and retroperitoneal lymph nodes ranging from 1 to 3 cm in diameter. Biopsy of the right cervical lymph node is interpreted as "anaplastic neoplasms, favor carcinoma". Results of immunoperoxidase staining are; cyto-keratin (−), S-100 protein (−), leukocyte common antigen (+), epithelial membrane antigen (+), chromogranin (−), vimentin (−). The most appropriate management is:

a) Chemotherapy with cisplatin and etoposide
b) Chemotherapy with cytosine arabinoside and idarubicin
c) Chemotherapy with cyclophosphamide, doxorubicin, vincristine, and prednisone
d) Rebiopsy of axillary lymph node for electron microscopy examination
e) Chemotherapy with 5-fluorouracil, doxorubicin, and mitomycin C

Question 3.214. A 60-year-old man is seen with symptoms of nausea, vomiting, and weight loss. Upper endoscopy is normal, but the upper GI series with bowel flowthrough reveals a partially obstructing mass in the distal duodenum/proximal jejunum. The next step in his work-up should be:

a) Consider radiotherapy.
b) Assess for operative risk factors, including malnutrition, then surgery.
c) Obtain a preoperative CT scan.

d)   Proceed immediately to Whipple procedure (pancreaticoduodenectomy).

e)   Inform the patient that palliative care is appropriate.

Question 3.215.   **A 90-year-old man is seen with a small bowel obstruction that fails to respond to nonoperative management. At exploration, he is found to have a midjejunal intussusception of 15 cm with vascular compromise of the distal most involved bowel. The operative surgeon should:**

a)   Reduce the intussusception and observe the bowel for vascular supply.

b)   Perform a resection of all involved segments and primarily re-anastomose the jejunal ends.

c)   Close the patient's wound after placing a distal jejunal feeding access.

d)   Perform an ileocolostomy.

e)   Irrigate the peritoneum.

Question 3.216.   **A 55-year-old woman is taken to the operating room for right lower quadrant pain and a presumptive diagnosis of appendicitis. At operation, a 2.5-cm carcinoid of the appendix is found and confirmed on frozen section. Which of the following is the best operation:**

a)   Simple appendectomy

b)   Right hemicolectomy

c)   Right hemicolectomy and exploration for metastatic lesions

d)   Closing of the patient's wound and administration of octreotide

e)   Closing of the patient's wound and administration of streptozocin and 5-fluorouracil

Question 3.217.   **A patient with a widely metastatic carcinoid who is experiencing intractable flushing could be treated with each of the following EXCEPT:**

a)   Surgical debulking

b)   Chemotherapy

c)   Calcium channel blockers

d)   Somatostatin analogues

e)   Intraperitoneal chemotherapy

Question 3.218.   **A 62-year-old woman is seen with a 6-month history of 1- to 2-cm bilateral axillary lymph nodes. She is otherwise asymptomatic. Biopsy shows follicular small-cleaved cell non-Hodgkin's lymphoma. Her staging studies demonstrate several 1-cm cervical nodes, but no other peripheral adenopathy. Chest radiographic findings are negative, and an abdominal/pelvic computed tomogram demonstrated several 2-cm retroperitoneal lymph nodes. Her Hct is 39%; WBC is 6.4/mm^3, with a normal differential; aspirate platelet count is 175,000/mm^3. A bone marrow shows several paratrabecular lymphoid infiltrates constituting less than 10% of the marrow space. The most appropriate therapeutic strategy at this time is:**

a)   Follow up the patient clinically with serial physical examination and periodic radiographic studies.

b)   Administer single-agent cyclophosphamide.

c)   Administer cyclophosphamide, vincristine, doxorubicin, and prednisone (CHOP) for six cycles.
d)   Administer CHOP followed by autologous transplantation.
e)   Administer six courses of fludarabine.

Question 3.219. **A 50-year-old man was diagnosed with stage III diffuse large-cell lymphoma 18 months ago. At diagnosis, he had a normal LDH level, and there was no extranodal involvement. His prognostic group, by the International Index, was low-intermediate risk. He received six cycles of CHOP at standard dose and had entered a complete remission by the end of three cycles. The patient now is seen with an abdominal mass of 5 cm, and a retroperitoneal lymph node of 2 to 3 cm. He is asymptomatic, otherwise healthy, and has no comorbid disease. What is the most appropriate therapy at this time?**

a)   Cyclophosphamide, doxorubicin, vincristine, and prednisone (CHOP) for four cycles to achieve a complete remission
b)   Involved-field radiotherapy
c)   A second-line combination chemotherapy regimen such as ESAP (etoposide, methylprednisone, cytarabine, and cisplatin)
d)   CHOP for four cycles and radiotherapy
e)   A second-line regimen such as dexamethasone, ara-C, and prednisone (DHAP), and if disease responsiveness is demonstrated, high-dose therapy with hematopoietic stem-cell support

Question 3.220. **In differentiating polycythemia vera from secondary polycythemia, the following feature favors secondary polycythemia:**

a)   An increased red blood cell mass
b)   An increased eythropoietin level
c)   An increased leukocyte alkaline phosphatase score
d)   A palpable spleen
e)   A leukocyte count of 11,500/mm^3

Question 3.221. **In the therapy of polycythemia vera with phlebotomy alone, one expects:**

a)   Similar incidence of subsequent acute leukemia relative to patients treated with alkylating agents or phosphorus 32
b)   An increased rate of thrombotic complications in patients over the age of 70
c)   Reduction in the patient's platelet count
d)   Reduction in the patient's leukocyte count
e)   A rise in the mean corpuscular volume of the patient's red blood cells

Question 3.222. **On routine gynecologic examination a 41-year-old married woman was found by palpation and sonography to have a mass in her left ovary. Work-up disclosed a carcinoma in the distal transverse colon, and at laparotomy she had bilateral ovarian metastases, and one implant on the omentum. All disease apparently was resected by an ileo-descending colostomy, total abdominal hysterectomy, and bilateral salpingo-oophorectomy and omentectomy. Twenty days postoperatively, the patient's CEA level was found to be 11. Your approach would be:**

a)   Administer fluorouracil and levamisole for 1 year
b)   Colonoscopy

c)   MRI of the liver
d)   CT scan of the lungs
e)   CEA level determination

Question 3.223.   **A patient is referred to you for assistance in managing his established diagnosis of Kaposi's sarcoma. His physician has elected not to recommend chemotherapy, because none of the numerous cutaneous and oral lesions are in highly visible areas. The patient has 223 CD4 cells per cubic millimeter. His HIV RNA titer is 150,000 copies per cubic millimeter. Medications include didanosine (ddl) monotherapy, which the patient has received for the past 6 months. The patient states that he is intermittently febrile and has a dry cough and dyspnea with moderate exertion. Physical examination reveals more than 50 cutaneous KS lesions and several obvious oral plaques. The pulmonary examination is unremarkable. The chest radiograph shows an indistinct multilobar infiltrate that the radiologist feels could be consistent with either *Pneumocystis carinii* pneumonia (PCP), tuberculosis (TB), or Kaposi's sarcoma (KS), although the infiltrate is not typical of any of these conditions. Which of the following is NOT an acceptable initial management approach at this time?**

a)   Empirical anti-tuberculous therapy
b)   Sputum induction for TB and PCP
c)   Bronchoscopy to evaluate the presence of endobronchial KS lesions
d)   Respiratory isolation until the diagnosis of TB can be excluded
e)   Reconsider changing to combination anti-retroviral therapy, including a protease inhibitor

Question 3.224.   **You are charged with developing guidelines for a large health maintenance organization regarding the early recognition of Kaposi's sarcoma to permit more expeditious management. You recognize that some patients are at a higher risk for this malignancy, probably induced by two viral infections, HIV and human herpesvirus type 8 (or the Kaposi's sarcoma herpesvirus). Which of the following patients would be considered to have the HIGHEST KS risk?**

a)   A woman who received HIV infection via vaginal intercourse with a bisexual partner
b)   A homosexual man who engaged primarily in receptive anal intercourse
c)   A child of an HIV infected mother who used drugs by injection
d)   A bisexual man whose homosexual activity was primarily oral
e)   A hemophiliac who has been infected with HIV for the past 12 years, with a history of recurring herpes labialis

ANSWERS

Answer 3.1.   **The answer is (e).**

Eighty percent of cases of medullary carcinoma of the thyroid occur sporadically. The remaining cases occur as either part of MEN (multiple endocrine neoplasia) syndrome or as part of a non–MEN familial pattern. Typically, familial cases are associated with multifocal tumors and bilateral C-cell (calcitonin-producing) hyperplasia. Total thyroidectomy with ipsilateral cervical node dissection is appropriate for management of gross disease for this locally invasive tumor. CEA and calcitonin may predict recurrence. Radiotherapy is useful for treatment of metastatic disease but not for residual thyroid tissue.

For Detailed Discussion: (1) Chapter 100, "Neoplasms of the Thyroid."

Answer 3.2.   **The answer is (a).**

The AMES staging system takes into account patient age, presence of metastases, and size and extent of the tumor. Men older than 40 (and women older than 50) are considered to be high risk, as are patients whose tumors either extend beyond the thyroid capsule or are greater than 5 cm in size. Lymph node metastases are not a poor prognostic indicator in papillary carcinoma.

For Detailed Discussion: (1) Chapter 100, "Neoplasms of the Thyroid."

Answer 3.3.   **The answer is (d).**

The incidence of occult papillary carcinoma in the remaining thyroid gland after less than total thyroidectomy ranges from 6 to 15%. For that reason, radioactive iodine therapy is seldom necessary. High-risk patients can be determined by using the AMES criteria. Anaplastic carcinomas may, albeit rarely, arise from residual papillary carcinomas.

For Detailed Discussion: (1) Chapter 100, "Neoplasms of the Thyroid."

Answer 3.4.   **The answer is (c).**

Even though passive smokers are exposed to much lower concentrations of carcinogens than are active smokers, environmental tobacco smoke has become the only agent ever classified by the Environmental Protection Agency as a human carcinogen for which an increased cancer risk has actually been observed at typical environmental levels of exposure.

For Detailed Discussion: (1) Chapter 107, "Cancer of the Lung." (2) American Cancer Society. Facts and Figures. Washington, DC: American Cancer Society, 1996.

Answer 3.5.   **The answer is (d).**

Lung cancer also occurs in association with occupational and environmental exposure to carcinogenic agents from sources other than tobacco smoke. Beryllium exposure occurs in electronic, aerospace, and nuclear reactor parts manufacturing plants; nickel exposure occurs at refineries; chromium exposure occurs at pigment manufacturing plants; and arsenic exposure occurs at smelteries and pesticide manufacturing plants.

For Detailed Discussion: (1) Chapter 107, "Cancer of the Lung." (2) American Cancer Society. Facts and Figures. Washington, DC: American Cancer Society, 1996. (3) Frank AL, Thoracic Oncology. Philadelphia: WB Saunders, 1989, p 8.

Answer 3.6.   **The answer is (e).**

Expression of *myc* family genes has been demonstrated in SCLC cell line and nude mouse xenograft studies using in situ hybridization techniques, but the significance of the increased expression of *myc* family genes remains uncertain.

For Detailed Discussion: (1) Chapter 107, "Cancer of the Lung." (2) American Cancer Society. Facts and Figures, 1995.

Answer 3.7. **The answer is (a).**

The *ras* genes code for a protein—p21—that is located on the inner surface of the plasma membrane. The p21 gene has GTPase activity that participates in signal transduction and cell cycle regulation. These oncogenes are activated by point nucleotide mutations that alter the amino acid sequence of p21.

For Detailed Discussion: (1) Chapter 107, "Cancer of the Lung." (2) American Cancer Society. Facts and Figures. Washington, DC: American Cancer Society, 1996.

Answer 3.8. **The answer is (a).**

Lung tumors can be induced in mice with tobacco nitrosamine and dimethylamine. Ninety percent of tumors contain the transforming gene *K-ras.* The most likely mechanism of action for this carcinogen is DNA methylation.

For Detailed Discussion: (1) Chapter 107, "Cancer of the Lung." (2) American Cancer Society. Facts and Figures, 1995. (3) Belinsky SA, et al. Relationship between the formation of promutagenic adducts and the activation of the K-ras protooncogene in lung tumors from A/J mice treated with nitrosamines. Cancer Res 1989;49:5305.

Answer 3.9. **The answer is (b).**

Tumor cells that produce a growth factor and express its receptor may show self-stimulatory or autocrine growth. Bombesin, a peptide identical to gastrin releasing peptide, is a potent stimulator of clonal growth for human NSCLC as well.

For Detailed Discussion: (1) Chapter 107, "Cancer of the Lung." (2) American Cancer Society: Facts and Figures, 1995. (3) Belinsky SA, et al. Relationship between the formation of promutagenic adducts and the activation of the K-ras protooncogene in lung tumors from A/J mice treated with nitrosamines. Cancer Res 1989;49:5305. (4) Cuttitta F, et al. Bombesin-like peptides can function as autocrine growth factors in human small-cell lung cancer. Nature 1985;316:823.

Answer 3.10. **The answer is (d).**

There is a definite increased risk of lung cancer in association with aerodigestive malignancies, laryngeal carcinoma in particular. The incidence of primary lung cancer following the treatment of laryngeal carcinoma ranges from 4 to 9%. Nonsquamous carcinomas are found as well and occur more frequently in women.

For Detailed Discussion: (1) Chapter 107, "Cancer of the Lung." (2) American Cancer Society. Facts and Figures, 1995. (3) Belinsky SA, et al. Relationship between the formation of promutagenic adducts and the activation of the K-ras protooncogene in lung tumors from A/J mice treated with nitrosamines. Cancer Res 1989;49:5305. (4) Yellin J. Bronchogenic carcinoma associated with upper aerodigestive cancers.Thorac Cardiovasc Surg 1986;91:674.

Answer 3.11. **The answer is (d).**

This patient had a pleural effusion of unknown etiology. An infectious cause such as tuberculosis is unlikely in the absence of fever. Lung cancer is a possibility in view of the smoking history, but the lack of a parenchymal lesion on chest CT scan and normal findings on bronchoscopy make this possibility unlikely, although a peripheral adenocarcinoma cannot entirely be ruled out. The most important information is the history of shipyard work in the distant past, which indicates occupational asbestos exposure. Malignant mesothelioma is a strong possibility (rather than benign asbestos effusion, which usually occurs earlier after asbestos exposure). The results of pleural fluid cytology and needle biopsy of the pleura are often negative in malignant pleural mesothelioma, which is today an important cause of "idiopathic" pleural effusion. The best approach is therefore a thoracoscopy, which allows the diagnosis of malignant mesothelioma in more than 80% of patients and rules out benign asbestos effusion as well as another carcinoma. It would be inappropriate to use a sclerosing agent or give a course of corticosteroids without an established diagnosis. Repeating a chest radiograph in 3 months is also inappropriate because the effusion can recur quickly in patients who have malignant mesothelioma. Thoracoscopy causes less morbidity than does thoracotomy. The diagnosis must be confirmed before contemplating treatment options.

For Detailed Discussion: (1) Chapter 108, "Malignant Mesothelioma."

Answer 3.12. **The answer is (d).**

This patient has classic features of acute promyelocytic leukemia. In contrast to other subtypes of AML, patients who have acute promyelocytic leukemia are frequently first seen with leukopenia. The other notable presenting feature is the tendency toward hemorrhage due to disseminated intravascular coagulopathy incited by the release of procoagulant granules inside the malignant promyelocytes. Elevations in this patient's prothrombin time and proximal thromboplastin time are consistent with the possibility of consumptive coagulopathy. The bone marrow aspirate shows sheets of dysplastic-appearing promyelocytes and myeloblasts. The peroxidase stain would be highly positive; many Auer bodies would also be seen.

Although standard antileukemic induction chemotherapy, such as 3 days of anthracycline plus 7 days of cytosine arabinoside, is reasonable therapy for patients presenting with acute promyelocytic leukemia, recent studies have demonstrated the remarkable ability of the vitamin A analogue, all-*trans* retinoic acid, to lead to a rapid resolution of the coagulopathy and gradual improvement in blood counts, such that approximately 85% of patients treated with this oral medicine alone achieve remission within 30 to 60 days. Studies performed in Europe and the United States have suggested that it is reasonable to begin with all-*trans* retinoic acid. However, a French study has demonstrated the advantage of adding chemotherapy should the patient experience a marked elevation in white blood count, which is an all-*trans* retinoic acid–related side effect.

For Detailed Discussion: (1) Chapter 142, "Acute Myeloid Leukemia in Adults." (2) Fenaux P, et al. Effect of all transretinoic acid in newly diagnosed acute promyelocytic leukemia: results of a multicenter randomized trial. Blood 1003;82:3241 3240.

Answer 3.13.   **The answer is (e).**

Following extensive brain irradiation, children, especially those less than 7 years of age, are at high risk of developing long-term intellectual and endocrinologic sequelae. It is appropriate to re-evaluate the child for evidence of tumor recurrence, but usually an MRI of the head and spine (occasionally supplemented by cerebrospinal fluid cytologic examination) will be sufficient. The majority of children who have received 2400 cGy or greater of craniospinal irradiation will have learning disabilities; many will have demonstrable declines in overall intelligence. These children should be referred for educational and intellectual assessment and placement in an appropriate school setting. In addition, those children receiving greater than 3000 cGy to the hypothalamic region are at significant risk for growth failure due to growth hormone insufficiency. Other hormonal abnormalities may appear over time. These children should be followed up by an endocrinologist, and hormonal replacement should be started if clinically indicated.

For Detailed Discussion: (1) Chapter 166, "Brain Tumors in Children."

Answer 3.14.   **The answer is (d).**

The tumor removed is most likely a medulloblastoma. Approximately 20 to 30% of children with medulloblastoma will have disseminated disease to other parts of the central nervous system at the time of diagnosis. Determination of such dissemination is important in treatment planning and long-term management of the patient. Patients with disseminated disease have a poorer prognosis, and treatment with craniospinal radiotherapy plus local boost radiotherapy alone is usually insufficient to control disease, and thus, the addition of chemotherapy is usually warranted. Small round cell tumors, such as medulloblastoma, are almost always primary central nervous system tumors, and extensive evaluations for an occult systemic primary tumor are not indicated.

For Detailed Discussion: (1) Chapter 166, "Brain Tumors in Children."

Answer 3.15.   **The answer is (c).**

The clinical presentation and MRI appearance are classical for a diffuse intrinsic brain-stem glioma. In such circumstances, surgical biopsy is often misleading due to sampling error and may cause increased neurologic morbidity. The presence of multiple cranial nerve deficits, the long tract findings, and balance difficulties suggest a poor prognosis, independent of whether the tumor is low- or high-grade on biopsy. Although the majority of patients will die within 18 months of diagnosis, patients will usually, at least transiently, respond to local radiotherapy. Other variants of childhood brain-stem gliomas, such as tectal tumors or exophytic cervicomedullary tumors (which may be more amenable to surgical resections), carry a more favorable prognosis.

For Detailed Discussion: (1) Chapter 166, "Brain Tumors in Children."

Answer 3.16.   **The answer is (c).**

Retinoblastoma is one of the very few malignancies in pediatric oncology that is diagnosed clinically, without pathologic confirmation. Needle biopsies are rarely, if ever, indicated for retinoblastoma. More than 50 years ago, it was demonstrated that planned or unplanned puncturing of the eye allowed tumor cells to seep out of the eye, causing orbital invasion and death. Ophthalmologic examination under anesthesia is important to exclude small foci of disease that may be present in the other eye. MRI imaging of the head and orbit is often used to exclude orbital or central nervous system spread of the tumor. Enucleation of the afflicted eye is often indicated in unilateral disease because of the extent of the tumor at presentation, and as discussed previously, should be done without prior pathologic confirmation of a clinical diagnosis made by an ophthalmologist familiar with this entity. Radiotherapy may be consider as a treatment option to salvage the eye.

For Detailed Discussion: (1) Chapter 98, "Neoplasms of the Eye."

Answer 3.17.   **The answer is (a).**

Recurrent retinoblastoma typically occurs within months or even up to a few years after diagnosis. Recurrent disease more than 10 years after initial diagnosis, as in this case, would be extremely unlikely. Both osteosarcoma and glioblastoma multiforme must be considered because of the high risk of second malignancies in patients with a history of bilateral retinoblastomas, especially those who received radiotherapy for their primary disease. If warranted after careful clinical examination, a head CT or MRI could be obtained to exclude a mass lesion. Migraine headaches or sinusitis are important considerations, because common illnesses also occur more commonly in patients who have a history of a malignancy.

For Detailed Discussion: (1) Chapter 98, "Neoplasms of the Eye."

Answer 3.18.   **The answer is (c).**

This patient has shown a good response to tamoxifen in all sites except the choroid region, which is part of the central nervous system. Changing to aggressive chemotherapy would not be in the patient's best interest at this time. Biopsy of these lesions is inappropriate; this diagnosis is made based on clinical and ultrasound findings. Initiation of radiotherapy to both eyes would be the treatment of choice, but should be proceeded by an imaging study of the brain to ensure that other central nervous system lesions that may also benefit from treatment are not present before designing a field. Cryotherapy is not a treatment for this type of eye cancer.

For Detailed Discussion: (1) Chapter 98, "Neoplasms of the Eye."

Answer 3.19.   **The answer is (b).**

The use of radiotherapy in a child who has the retinoblastoma gene has been associated in large and long-term studies with an increase in relative risk for a second malignancy, either in or outside of the radiation treatment field. With bilateral disease, this child has a genetic mutation whether or not she has a family history. With laterally directed radiation fields, no loss of eyelashes or eyebrows would be encountered; dry eyes and cognitive impairment would not be anticipated. Pronounced temporal bone hypoplasia would also not be encountered because a 2½-year-old child has already had significant increase in head circumference from infancy. Most likely, temporal bone hypoplasia, if it occurred at all, would be quite mild.

For Detailed Discussion: Chapter 98, "Neoplasms of the Eye."

Answer 3.20. **The answer is (c).**

The proportion of squamous cell cancers appears to be decreasing as the proportion of adenocarcinoma increases. Adenocarcinoma now appears to be the most frequent histologic type in the United States and Japan, but squamous cell carcinoma continues to be the predominant type in Europe.

For Detailed Discussion: (1) Chapter 107, "Cancer of the Lung."

Answer 3.21. **The answer is (c).**

Adenocarcinoma usually originates in the periphery of the lung and more commonly occurs in women. It tends to metastasize early to regional lymph nodes and distant sites, particularly the brain. Patients may have a history of associated chronic interstitial lung disease, that is, scleroderma, sarcoidosis, and so on.

For Detailed Discussion: (1) Chapter 107, "Cancer of the Lung."

Answer 3.22. **The answer is (e).**

Both typical and atypical carcinoid tumors are characterized by an organoid growth pattern. Histologic patterns may include spindle cell, palisading, rosette-like, or papillary patterns. Typical carcinoid tumors often have cytologic pleomorphism, but necrosis is absent, and mitotic figures are rare.

For Detailed Discussion: (1) Chapter 107, "Cancer of the Lung." (2) Arrigoni MG. Atypical carcinoid tumors of the lung. Thorac Cardiovasc Surg 1972;64: 413.

Answer 3.23. **The answer is (a).**

SCLC has a very aggressive clinical course and is therefore considered a distinct pathologic entity. SCLC usually is not amenable to surgery, so it is essential to distinguish this form histologically from NSCLC. Immunohistochemistry for keratin can be very helpful in difficult diagnostic circumstances.

For Detailed Discussion: (1) Chapter 107, "Cancer of the Lung."

Answer 3.24. **The answer is (d).**

Pleural involvement occurs at initial presentation in approximately 15% of patients who have lung cancer, and 50% of patients with disseminated lung cancer develop pulmonary effusion during the course of their illness. A number of pathogenic mechanisms have been implicated, but positive cytology does not significantly influence survival.

For Detailed Discussion: (1) Chapter 107, "Cancer of the Lung." (2) Mounthin CF. Prognostic implications of the International staging system for lung cancer. Semin Oncol 1988; 3:236. (3) Light RW. Pleural Effusion. Philadelphia: Lea & Febiger, 1983.

Answer 3.25. **The answer is (a).**

Pericardial involvement arises either from direct extension of the tumor or because of retrograde spread through mediastinal and epicardial lymphatics. Lung cancer is the most common neoplasm that produces pericardial metastasis, accounting for 37% of the reported cases. In many cases, the diagnosis is not made ante mortem. Breast cancer also often causes pericardial effusion, but not as a presenting complaint.

For Detailed Discussion: (1) Chapter 107, Cancer of the Lung." (2) Press O, et al. Management of malignant pericardial effusion and tamponade. JAMA 1988;257:1088.

Answer 3.26. **The answer is (c).**

SIADH results from secretion of arginine vasopressin, which is almost exclusively as-sociated with SCLC, with an overall reported frequency of 5 to 10%. Subclinical SIADH is much higher, around 35 to 40%. Besides the listed causes, renal failure, central nervous system trauma or space occupying lesion, and hypothyroidism need to be ruled out. Hyponatremia resulting from the secretion of atrial natriuretic factor also can occur in some patients.

For Detailed Discussion: (1) Chapter 107, "Cancer of the Lung." (2) Bliss DP. Ex-pression of the atrial natriuretic factor gene in small cell lung cancer tumors and tu-mor cell lines. JNCI 1990;82:305.

Answer 3.27. **The answer is (b).**

Human chorionic gonadotropin levels have been reported to be elevated in different series in 13 to 41% of patients who have lung cancer. This marker is more commonly associated with large-cell carcinoma. The only potential clinical manifestation is gy-necomastia in men. Gynecomastia is a rare finding in lung cancer patients.

For Detailed Discussion: (1) Chapter 107, "Cancer of the Lung." (2) Broder LE. Lung Cancer. New York: Grune & Stratton, 1983.

Answer 3.28. **The answer is (c).**

For gallbladder cancer limited to the submucosa, cholecystectomy is sufficient. However, for a Stage II lesion, many authors recommended cholecystectomy plus lymph node dissection at the porta hepatis (extended cholecystectomy). For gall-bladder cancer found at subsequent review of pathology, a second-look operation is indicated for Stage III cancer. The prevalence of laparoscopic cholecystectomy for treatment of symptomatic cholelithiasis has increased the number of trocar site recurrences. Because of the rarity of this disease, there have been no prospective randomized trials to direct its treatment.

For Detailed Discussion: (1) Chapter 116, "Neoplasms of the Gallbladder."

Answer 3.29. **The answer is (a).**

The recent use of ultrasound in the diagnosis of biliary pathology has increased the preoperative diagnosis rate of gallbladder cancer; approximately 50% of gallbladder cancers are diagnosed preoperatively by various modalities. However, gallbladder cancers are usually diagnosed at a later stage. Only 30% of gallbladder cancers are considered technically resectable.

For Detailed Discussion: (1) Chapter 116, "Neoplasms of the Gallbladder."

Answer 3.30. **The answer is (b).**

The papillary form of gallbladder cancer has the best prognosis. However, regardless of the subtype of this tumor, chemotherapy is uniformly ineffective. Intraoperative radiotherapy has been shown to be beneficial in comparison to surgery alone. However, when treatment failure occurs, it usually takes the form of local recurrence. Radiotherapy has not been helpful in relieving obstructive jaundice.

For Detailed Discussion: (1) Chapter 116, "Neoplasms of the Gallbladder."

Answer 3.31. **The answer is (e).**

The CT scan and ERCP suggest the presence of a periampullary malignancy, most likely adenocarcinoma of the pancreatic duct. Only 40% of patients who have adenocarcinoma of the pancreas will have tumors localized to the gland, and only 50% of these tumors will ultimately be resectable. Mesenteric angiography is useful for defining the vascular anatomy around the pancreas and in particular for identifying aberrant origins of the hepatic artery. Angiography may also identify large vessel encasement of tumor that is suspected as a result of CT scanning. This procedure should only be used in selected patients. Neither CEA or CA 19–9 serum levels are useful markers for pancreatic cancer screening but may be useful for postoperative surveillance and judging response to treatment. Both tests can be misleading because of false-negative results. Abdominal exploration is appropriate management for patients who have potentially resectable disease, although only 50% of patients will be found to be candidates for pancreatoduodectomy. In view of the findings from the ERCP, transduodenal biopsy is unnecessary, because the index for suspicion of malignancy is high. The diagnosis of pancreatic cancer may be difficult by frozen section analysis and can be confused with chronic pancreatitis. Performing a biopsy in this situation may only delay continuation of the procedure. Cancer localized to the head of the pancreas should be treated by pancreatoduodectomy, with resection and reconstruction of the superior mesenteric or portal veins. Both veins can be resected without an excessive rate of complications. Patients undergoing complete resection of their tumors have the best chance of survival, although 5-year survivors are rare. The median survival after complete resection is only approximately 14 months.

For Detailed Discussion: (1) Chapter 119, "Neoplasms of the Exocrine Pancreas." (2) Conlon KC, et al. Long-term survival after curative resection for pancreatic ductal adenocarcinoma. Ann Surg 1996;223:273.

Answer 3.32. **The answer is (d).**

Small anal lesions (T1) without sphincter invasion may be locally excised and result in an excellent patient survival, as high as 90%. Although multimodality therapy is an option, one would definitely not want to do a wide local excision after therapy. It is unnecessary, and healing may be difficult.

For Detailed Discussion: (1) Chapter 122, "Neoplasms of the Anus." (2) Greenall MJ. Epidermoid cancer of the anal margin: pathologic features, treatment and clinical results. Am J Surg 1985;149:95.

Answer 3.33. **The answer is (a).**

Additional chemotherapy, possibly *cis*–platinum–based, along with an additional small increment of irradiation to the primary site (to 54–60 Gy) may be useful in achieving cure in patients who have biopsy-proven persistent disease, so a biopsy in the next 2 to 3 weeks may be useful in determining whether the patient should have additional treatment. If the biopsy is negative, the nodularity may be merely residual scar tissue, and the patient should be followed up closely.

For Detailed Discussion: (1) Chapter 122, "Neoplasms of the Anus." (2) Flam MS, et al. Definitive combined modality therapy of carcinoma of the anus. A report of 30 cases including results of salvage therapy in patients with residual disease. Dis Colon Rectum 1987;30:495.

Answer 3.34. **The answer is (b).**

In a series of 85 anorectal melanoma patients from Memorial Sloan-Kettering Cancer Center, there was a subset of patients who did very well, namely, women who had an APR. Of the 10 long-term survivors, all were women, and nine had undergone an APR. Three of these patients had tumors that were less than 2 mm in depth.

For Detailed Discussion: (1) Chapter 122, "Neoplasms of the Anus." (2) Brady MS, et al. Anorectal melanoma: A 64 year experience at Memorial Sloan-Kettering Cancer Center. Dis Colon Rectum 1995; 38:146.

Answer 3.35. **The answer is (d).**

Vulvar intraepithelial neoplasia can be treated by a variety of methods. Wide local excision is often used; however, due to the multifocal nature of the disease, negative margins are often difficult to obtain. Carbon dioxide laser vaporization to a depth of 3 mm has also been used. Current evidence suggests that laser therapy may be as effective as surgical excision. 5-FU cream is another alternative therapy used in patients who have VIN.

For Detailed Discussion: (1) Chapter 129, "Neoplasms of the Vulva and Vagina."

Answer 3.36. **The answer is (d).**

The majority of the vulva drains first to the inguinal-femoral lymph nodes and subsequently to the deep pelvic lymph nodes. Ipsilateral tumors drain initially to the ipsilateral inguinal-femoral nodes, whereas midline lesions can spread to either the right or left side. The one part of the vulva that is capable of direct spread to the pelvis is the clitoral-urethral region. However, current evidence suggests that this pattern of spread is quite rare.

For Detailed Discussion: (1) Chapter 129, "Neoplasms of the Vulva and Vagina."

***Answer 3.37.* The answer is (c).**

Large tumors of the vulva with encroachment or involvement of the anorectal area or urethra require more extensive surgery than radical vulvectomy. Patients who have these tumors usually require urinary or fecal diversion. Newer approaches have been reported that treat these patients with a combination of preoperative radiotherapy followed by radical vulvectomy. Because of the sensitivity of the vulva to radiation, radiotherapy alone is not recommended.

For Detailed Discussion: (1) Chapter 129, "Neoplasms of the Vulva and Vagina."

***Answer 3.38.* The answer is (c).**

The approach to patients who have vaginal carcinoma treated with radiotherapy depends on the size of the tumor. Small (0.5-cm) lesions have a high rate of control with intracavitary radiation alone. For larger lesions, because of the increased risk of positive pelvic nodes, external beam treatment to the pelvis is also included. In addition, most radiotherapists recommend interstitial radiation in conjuction with external beam treatment for lesions >0.5 cm in size.

For Detailed Discussion: (1) Chapter 129, "Neoplasms of the Vulva and Vagina."

***Answer 3.39.* The answer is (c).**

FIGO rules state that "for staging purposes" (in patients who have cervical carcinoma), the following examinations are permitted: cytoscopy, inspection, colposcopy, endocervical curettage, hysteroscopy, proctoscopy, intravenous pyelography, chest radiograph, and skeletal radiographs. Examinations such as lymphangiography, laparotomy, laparoscopy, computed tomography, and magnetic resonance imaging are not permitted and cannot be used for staging purposes, despite the fact that such examinations or procedures provide valuable information for planning therapy.

For Detailed Discussion: (1) Chapter 130, "Neoplasms of the Cervix."

***Answer 3.40.* The answer is (d).**

Lung cancer has surpassed breast cancer as the number one cause of cancer death in US women. A woman's lifetime risk of developing breast cancer is 1 in 8; however, as women grow older, the relative risk decreases. An average healthy 50-year-old woman has a 4.4% risk. The death rate from breast cancer has remained stable for the past half century and is now actually declining. The introduction of widespread screening mammography has actually increased the percent of women who are diagnosed with ductal carcinoma in situ.

For Detailed Discussion: (1) Chapter 136, "Neoplasms of the Breast."

***Answer 3.41.* The answer is (e).**

The frequency of this diagnosis has been increasing with the wider use of screening mammograms. Of the different histologic patterns observed in DCIS, the comedo carcinoma variety has the least favorable histology and the worst prognosis. These tumors have a high labeling index and S-phase fraction, as well. Papillary and cribriform varieties are less aggressive, and this seems to correlate with the absence of HER-2neu overexpression of these cells. The evaluation of ER and PR status in DCIS has not yet been clearly established as an important prognostic indicator.

For Detailed Discussion: Chapter 136, "Neoplasms of the Breast."

Answer 3.42. **The answer is (e).**

Removing more than six lymph nodes at surgery does not enhance the assessment of patients' prognoses. Nodal metastasis remains the most powerful prognostic indicator to date. Sinus histiocytois is a good prognostic indicator. Patients who have ≥4 nodes clearly have a worse prognosis at 5 and 10 years.

For Detailed Discussion: (1) Chapter 136, "Neoplasms of the Breast."

Answer 3.43. **The answer is (d).**

In underdeveloped countries, menarche may be delayed due to poor nutrition, and this may be one of the factors related to the lower incidence of breast cancer in those areas. Menopause after the age of 55 confers a twofold risk compared with a menopause age of 45. Cigarette smoking is unrelated to breast cancer. Alcohol has a dose-response relationship to breast cancer, with women who drink three glasses of wine having up to a 50% increase in the risk of developing breast cancer. Women who have children in their late 30s have a higher risk of developing breast cancer than those who have had children before the age of 20. Women who give birth in their 30s have a greater risk than women who remain nulliparous. Low-dose estrogen replacement may be associated with a less than twofold increased risk of breast cancer.

For Detailed Discussion: (1) Chapter 136, "Neoplasms of the Breast."

Answer 3.44. **The answer is (c).**

Tamoxifen has been shown to cause a G1 cell cycle phase block, behaving more like a cytostatic rather than a cytocidal factor. Families who have Li-Fraumeni syndrome have an increased incidence of several tumor types due to mutations in the *p53* gene.

For Detailed Discussion: (1) Chapter 136, "Neoplasms of the Breast."

Answer 3.45. **The answer is (b).**

There have been several multicenter randomized trials that examined the margins of excision for cutaneous melanoma. The first, conducted by Veronesi at the World Health Organization, demonstrated that patients who were treated with either 1-cm or 3-cm margins had similar long-term survivals if the primary tumor was less than 2-mm in thickness. However, the data suggest that the local recurrence rate is higher in those patients who have thin margins excised for primary lesions that are 1 to 2 mm in thickness. It is therefore recommended that patients who have primary tumors greater than 1 mm in thickness should undergo margin excision of at least 2 cm;

these margins should only be compromised in anatomic sites such as the head and neck region. A second multicenter randomized surgical trial by Balch and associates demonstrated no difference in long-term survival in those patients whose primary tumors ranged from 1 to 4 mm in thickness, whether the margin was either 2 or 4 cm. The results of these studies demonstrate that patients who have primary lesions less than 1 mm in thickness can be adequately treated with 1-cm margins. However, those patients with primary tumors are thicker than 1 mm should likely have surgical margins $\geq$2 cm.

For Detailed Discussion: (1) Chapter 138, "Malignant Melanoma." (2) Verones U, et al. Thin Stage I primary cutaneous malignant melanoma. N Engl J Med 1988; 318:1159. (3) Balch CM, et al. Efficacy of 2 cm surgical margins for intermediate-thickness melanomas (1 to 4 mm): Results of a multi-institutional randomized surgical trial. Ann Surg 1993;218:262.

Answer 3.46. The answer is (b).

The traditional modalities used in the treatment of pituitary adenomas have been surgery and radiotherapy. However, in a number of tumor types the use of medical management has become increasingly popular. The paradigm for this approach is the use of the dopamine agonist bromocriptine in patients who have pituitary prolactinomas. Although bromocriptine is associated with high rates of regression, patients need to take this medication for the remainder of their lives. Moreover, a significant portion of patients have unpleasant and often unacceptable side effects at the dose levels used. In addition, a few tumors are resistant to medical therapy as judged by insufficiently lowered prolactin levels and, in some patients, continued tumor growth. Octreotide is a long-acting somatostatin analogue that is used in patients who have acromegaly.

For Detailed Discussion: (1) Chapter 99, "Pituitary Neoplasms."

Answer 3.47. The answer is (b).

Although this a high-risk lesion given the patient's age and extent of extracapsular extension, reoperation with laryngeal resection is not appropriate. This patient needs close follow-up and thyroxine suppression. Patients who have elevations of thyroglobulin levels and positive total body scans should be treated with 100 to 250 mCi of radioactive iodine. Even direct involvement of the trachea with tumor should be treated with sharp dissection rather than tracheal resection.

For Detailed Discussion: (1) Chapter 100, "Neoplasms of the Thyroid."

Answer 3.48. The answer is (e).

So-called benign pleural mesotheliomas are fibrous tumors of the visceral or parietal pleura and are usually not related to asbestos exposure. The most common associated signs are clubbing and/or osteoarthropathy, but pleural effusion is exceptional. Surgical excision is curative.

For Detailed Discussion: (1) Chapter 108, "Malignant Mesothelioma."

Answer 3.49.   **The answer is (c).**

Cigarette smoking acts synergistically with asbestos exposure to produce lung cancer. According to Selikoff [Selikoff IJ and Hammond EC. Ashestos and smoking (editorial). JAMA 1979; 242:458], the death rates for lung cancer compared to individuals who neither smoked nor worked with asbestos were increased 5 times for men who work with asbestos, and 53 to 90 times for those with both exposure to cigarettes and asbestos. Smoking has not been shown to increase the risk of malignant mesothelioma, however.

For Detailed Discussion: (1) Chapter 108, "Malignant Mesothelioma."

Answer 3.50.   **The answer is (c).**

Worldwide, the incidence of HCC is highest in China and Thailand and lowest in Ireland and the United Kingdom. HCC is relatively rare in the United States and predominately occurs in Asians and African-Americans. Although most HCC is caused by hepatitis B exposure, usually many years after the initial infection, there are other etiologic agents for HCC. Steroids, in particular androgens, and elevated hepatic iron stores, as seen in hematochromatosis, have been demonstrated to increase the risk of HCC. Oral contraceptive use is associated with hepatic adenomas rather than HCC. Aflatoxins may increase the risk of HCC, but the data are inconclusive. Vinyl chloride has been shown to be an initiating event in hepatic angiosarcomas. Although the risk of developing hepatitis B has decreased with blood testing and increased public awareness, immunization for hepatitis B is important for prevention of chronic hepatitis and cirrhosis. Infants in high-risk areas should be immunized, because the chance of becoming a chronic carrier of hepatitis B is highest in the neonatal period.

For Detailed Discussion: (1) Chapter 114, "Primary Neoplasms of the Liver."

Answer 3.51.   **The answer is (c).**

Although the outcome from treatment of HCC is generally poor, in those patients who have small (<2cm) single tumors without vascular involvement, 5-year survivals of up to 85% have been reported. Patients who have small tumors and neither active hepatitis B infection or end-stage disease have been treated with hepatic transplantation. Most patients are initially seen with larger tumors, because the symptoms from HCC are not specific for this disease. Attempts at screening with α-fetoprotein have been largely unsuccessful, even in high-risk regions. External beam radiotherapy is useful as palliative therapy. Chemotherapy appears to be most effective when given through hepatic artery infusions rather than by intravenous routes. fluorodeoxyuridine (FUDR) and doxorubicin combinations are the most active agents.

For Detailed Discussion: (1) Chapter 114, "Primary Neoplasms of the Liver."

Answer 3.52.   **The answer is (c).**

There is no clear association between gallstone disease and gallbladder cancer. Gallbladder cancer has been associated with pyogenic or parasitic biliary disease in the Asian population. Chronic inflammation of the gallbladder also has been implicated in the etiology of gallbladder cancer. In the case of porcelain gallbladder, where calcification of the gallbladder is a result of inflammation, the risk of gallbladder cancer is especially high. There is no identifiable premalignant lesion in gallbladder cancer.

For Detailed Discussion: (1) Chapter 116, "Neoplasms of the Gallbladder."

Answer 3.53. **The answer is (d).**

Although hepatitis B infection has been associated with development of HCC, available data are scant regarding specific gene mutations. Mutations of the *p16* tumor suppressor gene have been found in several different gastrointestinal malignancies, although the incidence in HCC is unknown. Cyclin D overexpression has been found in breast cancer. The BRCA genes have been found to be expressed in a high percentage of particular families who have breast, ovarian, and colon malignancies. Recent studies of these malignancies have found individuals who have mutations on chromosome 4q. In addition, *p53* exon 7 mutations have been found in some patients who have HCC; however, expression of the abnormal p53 protein may relate to genetic instability of the tumor rather than an initiating event.

For Detailed Discussion: (1) Chapter 114, "Primary Neoplasms of the Liver."

Answer 3.54. **The answer is (a).**

The recent use of ultrasound in the diagnosis of biliary pathology has increased the preoperative diagnosis rate of gallbladder cancer; approximately 50% of gallbladder cancers are diagnosed preoperatively by various modalities. However, gallbladder cancers are usually diagnosed at a later stage. Only 30% of gallbladder cancers are considered technically resectable.

For Detailed Discussion: (1) Chapter 116, "Neoplasms of the Gallbladder."

Answer 3.55. **The answer is (b).**

Although *k-ras* proto-oncogene expression occurs in almost 90% of patients who have pancreatic cancers, there are no data to support the use of this molecular marker for early detection of pancreatic malignancies. The *k-ras* gene encodes for a protein that is an important mediator in the regulation of cell cycle progression. Although methyl nitrosourea can induce *k-ras* mutations, a relationship between this gene and other chemicals to the development of pancreatic cancer in humans is unknown. Patients who have pancreatic cancer are approximately 5 to 13 times more likely to have a family history than are controls. The multiple tumor suppressor (MTS) gene encodes for the p16 protein inhibitor of the cell cycle and regulates the cyclin D/Cdk complex. Allelic deletions of the MTS gene have been shown to occur in increased number in patients who have pancreatic cancer. Both tobacco and alcohol have been implicated as etiologic factors in the development of pancreatic cancer. Several studies also suggest that patients who have chronic pancreatitis are at increased risk for pancreatic cancer.

For Detailed Discussion: (1) Chapter 119, "Neoplasms of the Exocrine Pancreas."

Answer 3.56.   The answer is (d).

The patient was initially seen with the classic clinical radiographic and pathologic findings of Ewing's sarcoma of the bone. This tumor is a malignant small-cell sarcoma occurring in adolescents and children. Given the nonspecific appearance of this tumor on hematoxylin and eosin staining, it is important to rule out other small cell tumors that can affect the bone, such as lymphoma, neuroblastoma, or small-cell carcinoma of the lung. Immunoperoxidase stains can be performed to rule out non-Hodgkin's lymphoma (leukocyte common antigen), angiosarcoma of the bone (factor 8), and neuroblastoma (neuron-specific, although results could possibly also be positive in Ewing's sarcoma). A Ewing's tumor may harbor foci of infection, which could account for the high sedimentation rates and systemic symptoms that patients are often initially seen with. Moreover, the lesions tend to be permeative, which accounts for the onion-skin appearance seen radiographically on the periosteum. Ewing's sarcoma and primitive neuroectodermal tumors both have a characteristic t (11; 22) translocation, which results in a fusion transcript known as ews/fli-1. Molecular biology techniques such as polymerase chain reaction (PCR)–based detection of the presence of this chimeric transcript could also prove to be another sensitive way to confirm the diagnosis of Ewing's sarcoma.

The treatment of Ewing's sarcoma is multidisciplinary in nature. As such, therapy for a patient with a distal femoral Ewing's lesion would probably be neoadjuvant chemotherapy, surgical resection of the bone, and limb salvage, followed by radiotherapy and further chemotherapy. Active agents would include vincristine, actinomycin O, and cyclophosphamide. Surgery appears to be required for optimal local control.

For Detailed Discussion: Chapter 139, "Bone Tumors."

Answer 3.57.   The answer is (b).

These signs and symptoms are suggestive of malignant obstruction of the biliary tract. Right upper quadrant ultrasound is a useful first step because it is noninvasive and is essentially free of complications. The frequency of detecting malignancy is from 53 to 90%. The presence of ascites or bowel gas can limit the utility of ultrasonography. CT scanning provides more accurate evaluation of the biliary tract, head of the pancreas, and liver. Magnetic resonance imaging provides similar imaging qualities as CT scanning, but requires gadolinium contrast to delineate tumors. ERCP is particularly sensitive for the diagnosis of pancreatic cancer, because it is useful for defining the biliary and pancreatic ducts and obtaining brush biopsies of the ductal system. ERCP can be useful for placing biliary stents in jaundiced patients who are not candidates for abdominal exploration. Transhepatic cholangiogram is useful for identifying lesions in a totally obstructed biliary tree, but it can be technically difficult to pass a catheter through the common bile duct into the duodenum. Whole body PET scanning is a relatively new modality for evaluating for the presence of metastases but is not typically used as a first step in the diagnosis of pancreatic cancer.

For Detailed Discussion: (1) Chapter 119, "Neoplasms of the Exocrine Pancreas."

Answer 3.58.   The answer is (d).

The optimal management of a patient who has localized anal carcinoma is combined modality therapy consisting of chemotherapy and radiotherapy. Surgery is presently reserved for patients who have very early disease or patients who fail combined modality therapy. Combination chemotherapy consisting of 5-FU and mitomycin C has been shown to be superior to single-agent 5-FU.

For Detailed Discussion: (1) Chapter 122, "Neoplasms of the Anus."

Answer 3.59.   The answer is (c).

Tumor-associated antigens are investigative only, but all of the other tests are useful in assessing the extent of disease.

For Detailed Discussion: (1) Chapter 122, "Neoplasms of the Anus."

Answer 3.60.   The answer is (e).

Although early stage squamous cell carcinomas of the skin are easily cured with either surgical excision or radiotherapy, surgery remains the treatment of choice in the majority of lesions and patients. In selected sites, the cosmetic outcome and control rates of radiotherapy are superior to surgery. These sites include the eyelids, pinna of the ear, nasolabial fold, alar nasi, and the lips.

For Detailed Discussion: (1) Chapter 137, "Neoplasms of the Skin."

Answer 3.61.   The answer is (a).

Squamous cell carcinom in situ of the skin typically appears as a scaly, erthyematous plaque on sun-exposed areas. Bowen's disease is synonymous with carcinoma in situ. This term should be restricted to lesions present on non–sun-exposed areas. Bowen's disease that occurs on the glans penis is also known as erythroplasia of Queyrat.

For Detailed Discussion: (1) Chapter 137, "Neoplasms of the Skin."

Answer 3.62.   The answer is (a).

Early premalignant changes or in situ carcinomas of the oral mucosa occur either as red (erythroplasia) or white (leukoplakia) patches. These lesions are readily apparent on visual examination. The prognosis of leukoplakial lesions depends on the site of presentaton. The great majority (>90%) of leukoplakial lesions of the buccal mucosa are benign. In contrast, leukoplakial lesions of other sites, for example, the floor of the mouth, are benign in <30% of patients.

For Detailed Discussion: (1) Chapter 137, "Neoplasms of the Skin."

Answer 3.63.   The answer is (c).

Neurofibromatosis type 2, or bilateral acoustic neurofibromatosis, is characterized by bilateral acoustic neuromas, schwannomas, and meningiomas. Overall, the most common central nervous system tumors in neurofibromatosis are optic gliomas, acoustic neuromas, astrocytomas, neurilemmomas, meningiomas, and neurofibromas. Unilateral acoustic neuromas are rarely seen in neurofibromatosis type 2.

For Detailed Discussion: (1) Chapter 137, "Neoplasms of the Skin."

Answer 3.64. **The answer is (a).**

This patient displays a classic history of osteoid osteoma, a benign bone lesion usually occurring in young adults (male predominance), most commonly in the fibula or tibia. There is usually abrupt onset of pain, which may often awaken the patient at night. Pain is a prominent symptom because these benign tumors are highly enervated. Radiologic findings are characteristic and reveal an eccentrically placed sclerotic lesion in a long bone with a central clear nidus. The nidus is the actual tumor that often appears red to the surgeon because of its rich blood supply. The optimal therapy is complete excision. There is no need for re-excision unless reoccurrences develop, nor is there need for adjuvant chemo- or radiotherapy.

For Detailed Discussion: (1) Chapter 139, "Bone Tumors."

Answer 3.65. **The answer is (b).**

Preoperative chemotherapy is now the standard approach for patients who are initially seen with osteogenic sarcoma. The advantages of this strategy compared with adjuvant chemotherapy, in which chemotherapy would be delayed until surgical recovery, include early treatment of micrometastatic foci, facilitation of limb salvage, and identification of patients who have a very good prognosis based on excellent response to the chemotherapy. Moreover, some studies have shown that the duration of the postoperative chemotherapy treatment may be markedly diminished with the use of such neoadjuvant chemotherapy. In fact, the response to the "upfront" chemotherapy is the most important prognostic indicator for ultimate outcome. Postoperative radiotherapy may be considered for those sites where adequate margins are difficult to obtain, although it must be noted that osteosarcoma is a relatively radioresistant tumor.

For Detailed Discussion: (1) Chapter 139, "Bone Tumors."

Answer 3.66. **The answer is (d).**

Inherited mutations in the retinoblastoma gene that account for clinical retinoblastoma are also associated with the development of osteogenic sarcoma. Other tumor suppressor genes such as *p53* and *p16* also may lead to increased incidence of this bone tumor. Chronic bone injury in patients who have Paget's disease, radiotherapy, or orthopedic hardware leads to an increased frequency of the occurrence of osteosarcoma and malignant fibrous histiocytoma compared with age-matched individuals. Osteogenic sarcoma is believed to occur in adolescence because of rapid bone growth. Although the clinician frequently elicits a history of trauma, it is likely that the injury may call attention to a pre-existing lesion.

For Detailed Discussion: (1) Chapter 139, "Bone Tumors."

Answer 3.67. **The answer is (d).**

It has long been known that doses of methotrexate in the 8 to 12 g/m^2 range are well tolerated and effective therapy for patients who have osteogenic sarcoma. Leukovorin rescue, which supplies reduced folates preferentially to normal tissues, is generally begun 24 hours after the therapy and is continued every 6 hours for approximately 12 doses or until the serum methotrexate level falls to 0.1 micromolar or less. Methotrexate is excreted almost entirely by the kidney; high intratubular methotrexate concentrations can result in precipitation, which leads to renal impairment. It is therefore important to ensure that there is adequate hydration and that the acid-base balance favors the relatively more soluble ionized form of methotrexate (which is a weak acid). There is no role for the use of mesna, a reducing agent capable of limiting the oxidant-mediated bladder injury caused by cyclophosphamide or ifosfamide.

For Detailed Discussion: (1) Chapter 139, "Bone Tumors."

Answer 3.68.   **The answer is (a).**

This patient is initially seen with the typical clinical scenario, radiologic appearance, and pathologic findings for a benign giant cell tumor of the bone. The majority of these tumors involve the distal femur and proximal tibia and have a typical radiographic appearance of a solitary demarcated lytic lesion. Rarely is the cortex expanded, nor is there a break. Although this is a benign lesion, numerous multinucleated giant cells are usually found. Pathologic fractures and metastases may occur, but are rare. The most important clinical problem is local recurrence; therefore, an aggressive surgical approach is necessary (but almost never an amputation). Thorough evacuation of the cavity, sometimes with phenol injection followed by packing with polymethyl-methacrylate, can reduce the local recurrence rate. Radiotherapy seems to have little role as primary or adjuvant therapy for these tumors.

For Detailed Discussion: (1) Chapter 139, "Bone Tumors."

Answer 3.69.   **The answer is (b).**

The development of human soft-tissue sarcomas has been associated with various factors: (1) progression from a benign precursor, such as angiosarcoma developing from chronic lymphedema; (2) genetic mutation, such as von Recklinghausen disease, Li-Fraumeni syndrome, Werner syndrome, or Gardner's syndrome; (3) EBV virus infection in HIV-positive patients; (4) prior radiation exposure; (5) prior exposure to various chemicals; (6) trauma; and (7) immunosuppression in AIDS patients who have Kaposi's sarcoma. Rous sarcoma virus is a simian virus that induces soft-tissue sarcomas in chickens.

For Detailed Discussion: (1) Chapter 140, "Soft Tissue Sarcomas."

Answer 3.70.   **The answer is (c).**

Mycosis fungoides, or cutaneous T-cell lymphoma, is a low-grade non-Hodgkin's lymphoma. Patients typically have very indolent courses extending over many years. However, the majority of patients eventually die of their disease or from secondary infections. Most patients experience months to years of nonspecific cutaneous symptoms before the establishment of diagnosis. Pruritus is the most common symptom in the early phase of the disease and is the problem that most often prompts a visit to the dermatologist. Systemic symptoms (fever, weight loss) and lymphadenopathy are signs of more advanced disease.

For Detailed Discussion: (1) Chapter 151, "Mycosis Fungoides and the Sézary Syndrome."

Answer 3.71.   **The answer is (b).**

Mycosis fungoides (cutaneous T-cell lymphoma) has a variety of presentations. Many patients are seen following a long history of nonspecific cutaneous complaints (premycotic phase), followed by the development of skin plaques (mycotic phase), and finally the tumor (fungoid) phase. This patient has a common variant of mycosis fungoides known as the generalized erythroderma (l' homme rogue) variant. Symptoms may appear suddenly and include intense pruritus that may be confused with an allergic reaction. Physical examination often reveals areas of skin thickening or atrophy, excoriations, and ulceration. Patients with erythroderma who have >5% of circulating malignant convoluted mononuclear cells have the so-called Sézary syndrome. Sézary syndrome is associated with a poorer prognosis than other types of mycosis fungoides.

For Detailed Discussion: (1) Chapter 151, "Mycosis Fungoides and the Sézary Syndrome."

Answer 3.72.   **The answer is (d).**

Radiotherapy in the form of total skin electron beam therapy is useful in patients who have mycosis fungoides. Treatment is often administered four times a week to a total dose of 30 to 36 Gy. Only the eyes are shielded routinely (with internal or external lead eye shields). Supplemental boost treatments are required for the soles of the feet, perineum, and under the breasts.

For Detailed Discussion: (1) Chapter 151, "Mycosis Fungoides and the Sézary Syndrome."

Answer 3.73.   **The answer is (b).**

The use of radiotherapy in the pediatric population requires tremendous care, experience, and patience. A number of late effects can be avoided simply by careful adherence to radiotherapeutic principles. The scoliotic changes associated with radiotherapy can be minimized by ensuring dose uniformity across the epiphyses. Hyperfractional approaches, that is, the use of smaller fractions delivered over the same overall treatment time, is another technique for decreasing late effects without compromising tumor control. However, even with hyperfractionated treatment, scoliosis will result without uniform coverage of the epiphyses. Large fractions will lead to a higher rate of late effects, because late effects are a function of fraction size. Concomitant chemoradiotherapy does not decrease the risk of late effects. In fact. chemotherapy may serve as a radiosensitizer and increase the *risk* of late effects.

For Detailed Discussion: (1) Chapter 159, "Principles of Pediatric Radiation Oncology."

Answer 3.74.   **The answer is (e).**

Radiotherapy alone was for many years used as the sole and primary treatment of a number of pediatric malignancies. However, high doses were often necessary to control sites of gross disease, which resulted in significant late sequelae. The use of combination chemotherapy in conjunction with radiotherapy has allowed the reduction of the radiation dose in a number of pediatric malignancies—including Hodgkin's disease and Wilms' tumor—without compromising local control but with less late effects. On the other hand, attempts at radiation dose reductions in the treatment of other malignancies—including Ewing's sarcoma and rhabdomyosarcoma—have been associated with increased risk of local recurrence. In these two malignancies, alternative means of reducing hyperfractionation schedules to a twice-a-day treatment, should be attempted.

For Detailed Discussion: (1) Chapter 159, "Principles of Pediatric Radiation Oncology."

Answer 3.75.   **The answer is (b).**

Leukemia is the most common cancer in the first quinquennium of life. However, neuroblastoma is by far the most common tumor in the first year of life. The incidence of neuroblastoma declines progressively and eventually disappears by adolescence. The incidence of lymphoblastic leukemia also declines through adolescence and into adulthood. In contrast, the incidence of bone tumors, lymphoma, and AML steadily increase after the first quinquennium of life.

For Detailed Discussion: (1) Chapter 160, "The Character of Childhood Cancer: Incidence, Origins, and Diagnosis."

Answer 3.76.   **The answer is (d).**

The etiology of the majority of pediatric brain tumors is unknown. However, several tumors are associated with specific identifiable genetic syndromes. The most frequent association is seen between neurofibromatosis and visual pathway gliomas, other glial tumors, and meningiomas. Overall, 20% of children with neurofibromatosis harbor optic nerve gliomas or develop other central nervous system tumors. Other syndromes associated with pediatric brain tumors include von Hippel-Lindau syndrome, Turcot syndrome, and tuberous sclerosis. von Hipple-Lindau syndrome is associated with cerebellar hemangioblastomas. Turcot syndrome patients develop medulloblastomas in the posterior fossa. Tuberous sclerosis is associated with periventricular giant cell astrocytomas and, ocassionally, ependymomas above and below the tentorium.

For Detailed Discussion: (1) Chapter 166, "Brain Tumors in Children."

Answer 3.77.   **The answer is (b).**

Clinical studies have suggested a biologic difference exists between pediatric and adult high-grade tumors, the latter of which appear to be somewhat more responsive to treatment. Pediatric low-grade glial tumors rarely transform into more malignant forms during the childhood years, whereas malignant dedifferentiation is commonly seen in adult patients. The most common tumor types differ between the adult and pediatric population. Although glioblastoma multiforme is the most common adult brain tumor, the most common pediatric brain tumors are medulloblastoma and brain-stem glioma. In addition, preliminary evidence suggests that pediatric glial tumors do not demonstrate the same cytogenetic and molecular changes seen in adult high-grade gliomas and glioblastoma multiforme. Determination of the unique biologic and genetic properties of childhood glial tumors is crucial to the understanding of the molecular pathogenesis of these tumors.

For Detailed Discussion: (1) Chapter 166, "Brain Tumors in Children."

Answer 3.78. **The answer is (a).**

Conventional radiotherapy is delivered in once-daily fractions five times a week. There is currently considerable interest in the use of altered fractionation schedules (hyperfractionated radiotherapy and accelerated radiotherapy). Hyperfractionated radiotherapy (HFRT) involves the use of more than one fraction per day of radiation, with smaller than conventional doses per fraction. The rationale behind HFRT is that late effects such as necrosis and subclinical damage are more dependent on fraction size than total dose. Thus, HFRT schedules should result in less late effects. In addition, the use of HFRT also allows the use of higher than conventional doses of radiation. Several ongoing national randomized trials are testing the efficacy and toxicity of HFRT radiation schedules in pediatric patients who have brain-stem gliomas and medulloblastoma.

For Detailed Discussion: (1) Chapter 166, "Brain Tumors in Children."

Answer 3.79. **The anwer is (d).**

Brain-stem gliomas carry the most unfavorable prognosis of all pediatric brain tumors, with only 10 to 15% of patients remaining alive 3 years following treatment. Of the brain-stem gliomas, the more common pontine tumor, particularly when it is diffuse, is the most aggressive and associated with the poorest outcome compared with tumors arising in the medulla of the upper cervical spine.

For Detailed Discussion: Chapter 166, "Brain Tumors in Children."

Answer 3.80. **The answer is (d).**

The most common site of origin of a ependymoma arising in childhood is the posterior fossa. Unlike adult lesions, the majority of ependymomas, especially those arising in the posterior fossa, are histologically benign. Excluding cases of posterior fossa tumors with extension to the upper cervical spine, childhood spinal ependymomas are quite rare.

For Detailed Discussion: (1) Chapter 166, "Brain Tumors in Children."

Answer 3.81. **The answer is (b).**

Craniopharyngioma is the most common suprasellar tumor of childhood. The majority of pediatric germ cell tumors arise in the pineal section, although 20% have primary suprasellar origins. Ependymomas occur primarily in the posterior fossa. Meningiomas are exceedingly rare in childhood.

For Detailed Discussion: (1) Chapter 166, "Brain Tumors in Children."

Answer 3.82. **The answer is (c).**

Unlike any other form of malignant childhood brain tumor, choroid plexus carcinomas can be cured with surgery alone. Approximately 70% of children who have choroid plexus carcinomas are free of disease 5 years following total surgical excision, independent of whether radiotherapy or chemotherapy is given.

For Detailed Discussion: Chapter 166, "Brain Tumors in Children."

Answer 3.83. **The answer is (b).**

Wilms' tumor can grow into the renal vein and extend retrograde down the gonadal vein (in the case of left-sided tumors) or anterograde into the inferior vena cava and beyond. In patients who have advanced disease, the tumor can extend to the right atrium. There may be preoperative clinical or imaging signs of tumor extension in the renal vein that can obstruct the inferior vena cava wholly or in part. The optimal management involves preoperative cytoreduction with chemotherapy. Attempts at resection without prior cytoreduction are associated with increased surgical morbidity. Tumor shrinkage usually follows neoadjuvant chemotherapy, which makes the standard abdominal approach feasible, and thus avoids thoraco-abdominal incisions and cardiac bypass.

For Detailed Discussion: (1) Chapter 171, "Renal Tumors of Children."

Answer 3.84. **The answer is (b).**

This patient who has a large, irregular adrenal mass most likely has adrenal cancer. Over half of the patients with adrenal cancer have some evidence of adrenal hypersecretion, commonly Cushing's syndrome. The patient's symptoms of insomnia, depression, and amenorrhea, as well as her signs of epidermal thinning and supraclavicular and dorsocervical fat accumulation, are highly suggestive of this condition. It is critical to confirm the diagnosis of Cushing's syndrome to prepare for the likelihood of adrenal insufficiency following tumor removal and to monitor the patient for tumor recurrence. The most efficient way to confirm the diagnosis of Cushing's syndrome is by measurement of free cortisol with radioimmunoassay in a 24-hour urine specimen. In more than 90% of patients who have Cushing's syndrome, the urine free cortisol (UFC) is greater than 200 mcg/24 h, whereas 97% of normal individuals have UFC values less than 100 mcg/24 h. 17-hydroxycorticosteroids can also be measured in the same urine specimen, but there are more false-positives with this test due to obesity, depression, stress, alcoholism, and interference of other medications in the assay results. Although the patient has hirsutism, this can be seen with Cushing's syndrome alone. The lack of any other manifestation of virilization (temporal balding or clitoromegaly) makes it unlikely that the lesion is a purely virilizing tumor. Thus, measurement of serum androgens would not be the most efficient evaluation. Dehydroepiandrosterone sulfate can be helpful in distinguishing an adrenal adenoma from an adrenal carcinoma. Finally, aldosterone-secreting adrenal cancers are very rare and usually present with hypokalemia in addition to hypertension. Thus, measurement of serum aldosterone would not be the most efficient laboratory evaluation.

For Detailed Discussion: (1) Chapter 101, "Neoplasms of the Adrenal Cortex."

Answer 3.85. **The answer is (d).**

Patients who are receiving mitotane for metastatic adrenal cancer are always at risk for adrenal insufficiency (AI), which should be suspected if these patients develop symptoms such as dizziness, extreme fatigue, or prostration. Beginning mitotane therapy or increasing the dose, however, can be associated with extreme fatigue, anorexia, and even dizziness, independent of AI, particularly when the dose is increased rapidly. Finally, mitotane toxicity causes dizziness and other disturbing central nervous system symptoms, including a "disassociated" feeling. Random serum cortisol levels (particularly in the evening) are likely to be quite low in patients who are receiving mitotane, even without frank AI. Thus, drawing a cortisol sample at this time might be misleading. Stopping the mitotane and obtaining a mitotane level should be done, but such an action is not sufficient to address the problem of suspected adrenal insufficiency. Although obtaining an 8 AM cortisol level is an appropriate screening test for AI (a level > 18 mcg/dL rules out AI), this patient requires symptomatic relief and should be treated for presumed AI with hydrocortisone. A single dose of 100 mg hydrocortisone will not interfere with eventual diagnosis; a dramatic response to treatment is suggestive of AI. Because mitotane is fat-soluble, the mitotane level may take several weeks or months to fall. A firm diagnosis of AI requires an adrenocorticotropic hormone stimulation test (250 mcg cosyntropin IV push), with measurement of cortisone at baseline, 30, and 60 minutes. This can be done 48 to 72 hours after the hydrocortisone dose is given. If the baseline cortisone does not at least double, or if there is no cortisol value > 18 mcg/dL, then the patient should be considered to be adrenally insufficient. The treatment is hydrocortisone (12–15 mg/m^2) po daily.

For Detailed Discussion: (1) Chapter 101, "Neoplasms of the Adrenal Cortex."

Answer 3.86. The answer is (a).

The pathologist plays an increasingly important role in the management of patients who have carcinoma of the breast. Initial assessment must include determination of whether or not the tumor is in situ (no invasion through the basement membrane, confined either to a duct or a lobule) or if the tumor is actually invasive. Of the invasive carcinomas, those that grow in a papillary configuration are rare, but it is rare for these benign-behaving tumors to invade the surrounding stroma; therefore, there is a cure rate of 100% if the lesion is completely excised. Medullary carcinomas, constituting 5 to 10% of breast cancers, are circumscribed lesions that attain large dimensions but demonstrate low-grade, barely infiltrating properties. Tubular and colloid carcinoma have similarly favorable neutral histories.

For Detailed Discussion: (1) Chapter 136, "Neoplasms of the Breast."

Answer 3.87. The answer is (e).

Tamoxifen is a safe and effective drug both for patients with Stage II breast cancer who will be given the drug as adjuvant therapy and for patients who have advanced breast cancer. Tamoxifen is a partial estrogen agonist/antagonist. The weak estrogen-like properties account for a slight decrease in the level of cholesterol in postmenopausal women, some changes in the vaginal cytology, and a few excess cases of uterine cancer (generally low stage) that have been reported. Probably because most postmenopausal patients are estrogen receptor–positive, most will respond to tamoxifen. Those who have estrogen receptor–positive disease are much more likely to respond to tamoxifen therapy than are those whose tumors do not express the estrogen receptor (48 vs 15% response rate). Although the likelihood of response to one of the various available hormone therapies (tamoxifen, megestrol acetate, or progesterone) is approximately equal, tamoxifen is safer and better tolerated than other regimens.

When used for adjuvant therapy, it appears that prolonged tamoxifen administration is better than brief tamoxifen therapy. Tamoxifen actually confers a survival advantage of up to 4 years in postmenopausal women, and therefore should be given for at least 1 to 2 years after diagnosis of such patients. The estrogen-like effects of tamoxifen lower the circulating cholesterol in women taking this drug; therefore, even prolonged use is not likely to be associated with coronary disease.

For Detailed Discussion: (1) Chapter 136, "Neoplasms of the Breast."

Answer 3.88. **The answer is (a).**

The patient has von Hippel Lindau disease. von Hippel-Lindau disease is a familial disease in which patients may develop several types of neoplasms, most notably clear-cell renal cell carcinoma (which occurs in approximately 40% of patients with this syndrome) as well as renal cysts (frequently multiple, bilateral, and containing malignant cells); retinal hemangiomas; hemangioblastoma of the cerebellum and spinal cord; pheochromocytomas; and pancreatic carcinomas and cysts. von Hippel-Lindau disease is linked to the short arm of chromosome 3. The gene accounting for this familial syndrome has been cloned and encodes a protein that inhibits the elongation of RNA transcription. One allele of this gene is almost always absent or lost in sporadic clear-cell renal cell carcinomas. It is interesting that other clear-cell carcinomas also exhibit loss of chromosomal material on the short arm of chromosome 3 in a region distinct from the von Hippel-Lindau gene. Papillary renal carcinoma (also known as chromophilic carcinoma) frequently displays an extra copy of chromosomes 7 or 17, or loss of the Y chromosome. These latter tumors make up only approximately 10 to 15% of all types of renal cell carcinomas, whereas the clear-cell type accounts for approximately 80% of cases.

For Detailed Discussion: (1) Chapter 124, "Neoplasms of the Renal Pelvis and Ureter." (2) Motzer RJ, et al. Renal cell carcinoma. NEJM 1996;355:865.

Answer 3.89. **The answer is (d).**

Although 5-FU continues to have a central role in the treatment of patients who have metastatic colorectal carcinoma, this patient appears to have 5-FU refractory disease. The target enzyme of 5-FU (after its metabolism to fluorinated deoxyuracil monophosphate [FdUMP]) is the thymidylate synthase enzyme that converts dUMP to thymidine-5'-phosphate, using reduced folates as cofactors. Leucovorin promotes the binding of FdUMP to thymidylate synthase, which results in greater enzyme inhibition. Addition of leucovorin to 5-FU may produce higher rates of tumor regression than when 5-FU is used as a single agent. However, the toxicity, particularly diarrhea, is magnified when these two drugs are used in conjunction. Nonetheless, several trials have suggested that the combination approach can lead to a better quality of life, chiefly due to a long duration of response and survival. Alternative biochemical modulation of 5-FU with methotrexate, cisplatin, PALA (N-[phophonacetyl]-L-apartic acid), and hydroxyurea each have been or are under study; to date, none of these approaches have been shown to exhibit convincingly superior benefits to those obtained with either 5-FU alone or 5-FU and leucovorin. However, the camptothecin analogues, all topoisomerase 1 inhibitors (inhibit DNA repair by preventing religation of cleaved strands) have been shown to be effective in patients with 5-FU refractory disease. The best studied, and currently clinically available drug, irinotecan (CPT-11 Yakult Horisha, Tokyo), can be given every 3 weeks in 30- to 90-minute intravenous infusions. CPT-11 produces few hematologic abnormalities, but significant diarrhea can occur. An acute cholinergic syndrome, characterized by severe vomiting, cramps, and diarrhea, has also been noted.

For Detailed Discussion: (1) Chapter 121, "Adenocarcinoma of the Colon and Rectum."

Answer 3.90. **The answer is (d).**

Perhaps because rectal cancers are not movable due to the lack of an omental attachment to the bowel, radiotherapy has an important role in reducing local and systemic relapses after surgery for those patients who have lymph node and/or serosal involvement without evidence of metastatic cancer . Although one National Surgical Adjuvant Breast & Bowel Project rectal cancer trial did show a slight benefit to a combination of methyl-lomustine, vincristine, and 5-fluorouracil treatment without radiotherapy, there have been two large, well-performed randomized trials that have documented a benefit for a combination of postoperative chemotherapy and external beam radiotherapy for the improvement of overall survival in patients with locally advanced rectal adenocarcinoma. The combination diminishes regional recurrence when compared with radiotherapy alone, chemotherapy alone, or surgery alone. However, methyl-lomustine treatment is associated with an unacceptable risk of late secondary leukemias. Whether or not the combination chemotherapy used in the adjuvant therapy of rectal cancer should include leucovorin and/or levamisole in addition to 5-FU was the subject of a recently closed, large randomized trial.

For Detailed Discussion: (1) Chapter 121, "Adenocarcinoma of the Colon and Rectum." (2) O'Connell MJ, et al. Improved adjuvant therapy for rectal cancer by combining protracted-infusion fluorouracil with radiation therapy after curative surgery NEJM 1994;331:502.

Answer 3.91. **The answer is (a).**

There are no accurate predictive markers for response of a tumor to chemotherapy. Although performance status, tumor burden, and absence of prior exposure to chemotherapy increase the chance of a response, estrogen receptor status dose not actually predict response to chemotherapy; therefore, this statement is wrong. Initial response rate of patients who have Stage IV disease is approximately 40 to 70%; however, the complete remission rate is only 10 to 20%. In general, more aggressive and continuous chemotherapy confers a better quality of life, because the complications from the cancer itself seem to cause more discomfort than the drugs themselves. The most effective drug for the treatment of breast cancer appears to be doxorubicin. However, the CAF combination does not have a clear advantage over the regimen of cyclophosphamide, methotrexate, and 5-fluorouracil, even though some studies do show a small difference in favor of CAF. This is especially important considering that CAF is more toxic. Answers d and e are both correct statements.

For Detailed Discussion: (1) Chapter 136, "Neoplasms of the Breast."

Answer 3.92. **The answer is (a).**

At this time, combination treatment cannot be recommended for Stage IV disease, because there is no solid clinical evidence supporting this modality. The patient has experienced a partial remission and stable disease with tamoxifen therapy for 2 years. This represents successful hormonal therapy. There is no evidence that giving chemotherapy at this time will enhance the patient's survival. There are also no definitive data suggesting that hormonal therapy is contraindicated, although some experimental studies do show an increased resistance of cancer cells to chemotherapy after treatment with tamoxifen. Although some studies suggest a role for estrogen priming to increase the S-phase fraction, this has yet to be confirmed.

For Detailed Discussion: (1) Chapter 136, "Neoplasms of the Breast."

Answer 3.93. **The answer is (d).**

Cancerous breast masses usually have a well-defined margin as opposed to fibrocystic disease, which blends into the surrounding tissue. Adenomas are well-defined but are encapsulated and highly mobile when palpated. The most common cause of bloody nipple discharge is a benign papilloma, although the discharge must always be evaluated. Although palpation of axillary lymph nodes is notoriously inaccurate, the true figures from a large NSABP trial are less dismal, with 38% false-negatives and 25% false-positives. Pain is uncommon in the presentation of breast cancer and is usually due to benign disease, especially when cyclic pain is encountered during the perimenstrual period in young women.

For Detailed Discussion: (1) Chapter 136, "Neoplasms of the Breast."

Answer 3.94. **The answer is (c).**

Lead time bias refers to the fact that with screening, patients may be diagnosed earlier, even though their date of death will be the same. This would make it seem that these women have a longer survival time, which is false. The correct way to avoid lead and length bias is to count the deaths from breast cancer in both groups and avoid using indicators such as survival rates and average survival.

For Detailed Discussion: (1) Chapter 136, "Neoplasms of the Breast."

Answer 3.95. **The answer is (a).**

There is enough evidence that mammography reduces mortality in the group of women 50 to 74 years of age that its routine yearly use is recommended. However, the reduction in mortality is 30%, not 70%. The rest of the statements are all true.

For Detailed Discussion: (1) Chapter 136, "Neoplasms of the Breast."

Answer 3.96. **The answer is (e).**

Scant data are available to record the outcome of prostate cancer in men over 80 years. There is a high probability that this man will die of causes other than prostate cancer. Hence, in the absence of symptoms (eg, nocturia, difficulty urinating) observation is appropriate. Hormonal therapy could be administered in the future if progressive, symptomatic disease occurs. The low histologic grade portends a slow-growing cancer.

For Detailed Discussion: (1) Chapter 126, "Neoplasms of the Prostate."

Answer 3.97. **The answer is (c).**

A patient who has a receptor-positive breast cancer should not receive estrogen replacement therapy, because this treatment could stimulate existing cancer cells. Progestogens are employed (in large doses) for treating advanced breast cancer; there is no evidence that smaller doses stimulate breast cancer. Hence, use of progestogen (20–40 mg/d) in the treatment of disabling menopausal symptoms is appropriate and effective.

For Detailed Discussion: (1) Chapter 136, "Neoplasms of the Breast."

Answer 3.98. **The answer is (c).**

Bilateral orchiectomy or other anti-androgen hormonal agents would be effective methods of management. However, chemotherapy also can play a significant role in countering this disease. In view of the patient's recent marriage, and a possible desire to maintain sexual prowess, chemotherapy is an appropriate initial therapy. If no response occurs, or later after reactivation of the cancer occurs, orchiectomy or luteinizing hormone releasing hormones could be used.

For Detailed Discussion: (1) Chapter 136, "Neoplasms of the Breast."

Answer 3.99. **The correct answer is (c).**

This is a classic presentation for bleomycin pseudonodules. The paradoxical fall in tumor markers, with the development of new "disease" in previously normal areas is almost certainly related to bleomycin pseudonodules. These findings should not in any way deter the correct management of this clinical setting, which is complete resection of postchemotherapy residual abnormalities (abdomen plus neck).

For Detailed Discussion: (1) Chapter 128, "Neoplasms of the Testes."

Answer 3.100. **The answer is (d).**

One third of patients who have cancer of the tail of the pancreas are found to be diabetic within 6 months of the diagnosis of pancreatic cancer. A cholecystectomy that fails to relieve symptoms permanently should be a cause for concern, particularly after laparoscopic cholecystectomy, a procedure that is not conducive to thorough exploration of the pancreas. Peritoneal metastases and ascites are very common in pancreatic cancer patients. Although usually a late finding, liver metastases are often absent. Episodic pain and suprascapular or medial scapular pain, as well as "shoulder" pain, are typical of cholelithiasis. Jaundice and nausea suggest a common duct stone. Uncinate process cancers are notoriously difficult to diagnosis, with late jaundice occurring as the cancer invades into the pancreatic head.

For Detailed Discussion: (1) Chapter 119, "Neoplasms of the Exocrine Pancreas."

Answer 3.101. **The answer is (d).**

Only pancreatic cancer has been subjected to randomized controlled trials involving multidisciplinary therapy. The Gastrointestinal Tumor Study Group demonstrated a significant survival advantage for radiotherapy (40-Gy split course) in combination with 5-FU, 500 mg/m^2 IV, on each of the first 3 days of each course of radiation and then (following a 28-day delay) weekly for 18 to 24 months compared with observation after complete resection. Patients who have locally advanced pancreatic cancer with no distant metastases may also benefit from treatment with either 40-Gy split or 60-Gy, double-split course radiotherapy, with 5-FU given as in the adjuvant trial but with maintenance continuing until relapse.

For Detailed Discussion: (1) Chapter 119, "Neoplasms of the Exocrine Pancreas." (2) Douglass HO. Current approaches to the multimodality management of advanced pancreatic cancer. Hepato-Gastrointestinal 1992;40:433.

Answer 3.102. **The answer is (b).**

Staging and evaluation of pancreatic cancer should be directed at relief of jaundice and assessment of the patient for metastatic disease. If the patient has been jaundiced for only a short period of time (7–10 days) and is otherwise in good physical condition, evaluation for possible resection should take priority, because there is no evidence that preoperative biliary decompression offers any advantage over early (within 1 week) resection. Imaging by MRI is not currently superior to that of CT scanning, particularly spiral CT and intravascular contrast. If biliary decompression is desirable, ERCP routinely drains bile into the gastrointestinal tract, whereas percutaneous drainage results in inconvenience to the patient, continued acholic stools, pain at the insertion site, and occasional electrolyte problems until conversion to internal drainage is performed. Delayed gastric emptying is a problem in many pancreatic cancer patients, and, when associated with partial obstruction in the duodenum, is an indication for gastrojejunostomy. Thus, optimal work-up involves a quick study to rule out liver metastases and ascites (CT scan), followed by relief of jaundice if the tumor is unresectable (ERCP), and then percutaneous fine needle aspiration biopsy to confirm the diagnosis.

For Detailed Discussion: (1) Chapter 119, "Neoplasms of the Exocrine Pancreas."

Answer 3.103. **The answer is (e).**

Unfortunately, no treatment has been shown to have a significant impact on the survival of patients who have advanced metastatic pancreatic cancer. Untreated, the median survival in the presence of liver metastates is 90 days. Optimal supportive care may improve this slightly. 5-fluorouracil has been the standard of treatment for 30 years, with response rates well below 20%. Gemcitabine has a similar or slightly better rate of response but received FDA approval because quality of life was better for patients receiving gemcitabine than for those given 5-fluorouracil. Many authorities feel that there is no standard treatment for patients with pancreas cancer and that Phases I or II studies or supportive care alone are all appropriate treatments. In the presence of metastatic disease, radiotherapy has little to offer because of the short life expectancy of the patients.

For Detailed Discussion: (1) Chapter 119, "Neoplasms of the Exocrine Pancreas."

Answer 3.104. **The answer is (d).**

The presence of serum α-fetoprotein despite histopathologic evidence of pure seminoma mandates management as a non-seminomatous germ cell tumor. The presence of a significant residual mass after chemotherapy mandates post-chemotherapy retroperitoneal lymphadenectomy. This procedure may be curative if teratoma is detected. If active germ cell cancer is found, then, depending on the amounts of residual disease, additional chemotherapy may be indicated.

For Detailed Discussion: (1) Chapter 128, "Neoplasms of the Testes."

Answer 3.105.   **The answer is (d).**

This child has neurofibromatosis, which may be associated with several types of nervous system tumors. Glial tumors are the most common central nervous system neoplasm. Although most patients do not have any specific inherited syndrome, neurofibromatosis Types I and II are autosomal dominant diseases (approximately 50% of all children of an affected individual will have the disease), which is characterized by cutaneous neurofibroma (as opposed to the adenoma sebaceum lesions typical of a much more rare autosomal dominant disorder, tuberous sclerosis [usually associated with benign giant cell astrocytomas]); café au lait spots; bone abnormalities; and a variety of intracranial neoplasms. Approximately 1 of 6 patients with one of the neurofibromatosis syndromes will develop a brain tumor, usually anaplastic astrocytomas, although meningioma and/or schwannoma have been known to occur in patients with neurofibromatosis Type II (who also tend to develop bilateral acoustic neuroma tumors). The gene responsible for neurofibromatosis Type I is located on chromosome 17 and encodes a protein with homology to the catalytic domain of mammalian guanosine triphosphate–activating proteins. The normal function of the protein may be to inactivate the growth-promoting signal transduction activity of the *ras* proto-oncogene. Neurofibromatosis Type II is linked to chromosome 22. The high-grade tumor glioblastoma multiforme may harbor *p53* gene mutations, including those in patients with the Li-Fraumeni syndrome, which are associated with a high incidence of breast cancer and soft-tissue sarcoma.

For Detailed Discussion: (1) Chapter 97, "Neoplasms of the Central Nervous System." (2) Blatt J, et al. Neurofibromatosis and childhood tumors. Cancer 1986;57:155.

Answer 3.106.   **The answer is (c).**

Generalized signs of intracranial tumors, most usually of glial origin, may be headache, nausea, vomiting, or seizures, but may also be specifically related to the area of involvement. Generalized symptoms and signs of increased intracranial pressure include papilledema, diplopia, cranial nerve palsies, and changes in the level of consciousness. Focal symptoms due to tumor of the frontal lobe include changes in mental status, reduced attention span, poor judgment, labile behavior, and loss of social inhibition. Motor abnormalities and expressive aphasia may occur in tumors of the posterior frontal lobe. Temporal lobe tumors may cause auditory hallucinations or problems in receptive speech, impairment of recent memory, and inability to name objects. Tumors of the non-dominant temporal lobe may produce spatial disorientation and lack of taste perception, hearing, or vision. Parietal lobe lesions may produce neglect syndromes contralateral to the side of the lesion, abnormalities of sensation, or inability to localize parts of the body. Gerstmann's syndrome is a disorder of the dominant parietal lobe, which is associated with an inability to write, calculate, and to discriminate between right and left. Complex motor tasks may be impossible. Visual field testing may reveal an inferior quandrantanopsia or hemianopsia. Occipital lobe tumors cause visual defects. Thalamic tumors often produce either increases in intercranial pressure, pain syndromes, or hemisensory loss/hemiparesis. Cerebellar tumors cause ataxia, nystagmus, and a tendency to fall to the affected side.

For Detailed Discussion: (1) Chapter 97, "Neoplasms of the Central Nervous System."

Answer 3.107.   **The answer is (a).**

Even for high-grade unresectable glial tumors, surgery should be undertaken, unless there are compelling medical reasons that would make the procedure too risky. In addition to making a firm diagnosis, the surgeon should attempt to remove as much tumor as safely possible, despite the infiltrative character and general unresectability of these lesions. Although adjuvant chemotherapy may extend the patient's life beyond that would be expected with surgery alone, the extent of surgery achieved appears to have an important impact on overall survival. The greater the extent of residual tumor left after surgery, the shorter the survival. This relationship is true independent of age, performance status, and histology. Therefore, unless the lesion is completely surgically inaccessible, biopsy alone is not justified. Radiotherapy plus surgery has afforded a better chance of longer survival than with surgery alone or surgery plus chemotherapy. The standard radiotherapy is single daily fraction radiation to a total dose of 60 Gy plus adjuvant nitrosourea. The benefit of adjuvant chemotherapy is more pronounced in patients with anaplastic astrocytoma compared with patients who have higher grade glioblastoma multiforme.

For Detailed Discussion: (1) Chapter 97, "Neoplasms of the Central Nervous System." (2) Simpson, et al. Influence of location and extent of surgical resection on survival of patients with glioblastoma multiforme: Results of three consecutive Radiation Therapy Oncology Group (RTOG) clinical trials. Int J Radiat Oncol Biol Phys 1993;26:239.

Answer 3.108.   **The answer is (e).**

Once a spinal cord tumor is identified by MRI scanning, the goal of surgery is to remove as much of the tumor as possible (as well as to make a diagnosis). For ependymomas, meningiomas, and neurofibromas, total removal is clearly possible. For astrocytomas, especially the anaplastic variety, usually only partial removal can be accomplished, although the recent surgical literature suggests that a more aggressive approach with a goal of total removal may be feasible. Nonetheless, over two thirds of all patients with anaplastic astrocytomas of the spinal cord die of their disease due to intra-axial spread, despite postoperative radiotherapy that appears to be helpful for patients who have low-grade astrocytomas or ependymomas. Although some patients who have anaplastic astrocytomas will respond to chemotherapy, others will sustain growth despite chemotherapy, as well as growth after repeat surgery. Recurrence is the rule, with spread throughout the neural axis and eventual demise of the patient.

For Detailed Discussion: (1) Chapter 97, "Neoplasms of the Central Nervous System."

Answer 3.109. **The answer is (b).**

The recent increase in incidence of primary central nervous system lymphoma is explained only in part by the increasing number of immunosuppressed individuals due to the AIDS epidemic and because of an increased frequency of organ transplantation recipients who require profound immunosuppression to prevent rejection. The reason for the increased incidence of non-AIDS–related primary central nervous system lymphoma is not known. Patients who have AIDS–related central nervous system lymphoma usually are seen with confusion, memory loss, focal deficits, seizures, and lethargy. A patient with HIV infection who presents with multiple enhancing central nervous system lesions is likely to have toxoplasmosis or lymphoma. Patients who have negative toxoplasmosis titer results may bear a higher likelihood of having lymphoma. The non-Hodgkin's lymphomas that develop in the central nervous system of AIDS patients are most commonly immunoblastic (B-cell) lymphomas, but occasionally may be small-cleaved or large noncleaved B-cell tumors. T-cell tumors and metastatic solid tumors are much less common. Once an AIDS–related primary central nervous system lymphoma is diagnosed, the treatment of choice is whole-brain radiotherapy (usually 40 Gy over 3 weeks). Although chemotherapy has been used in only a small number of patients with AIDS–related primary central nervous system lymphoma, there are increasing data that support the use of high-dose systemic chemotherapy and intrathecal chemotherapy as an adjunct to radiotherapy in other cases of primary central nervous system lymphoma.

For Detailed Discussion: (1) Chapter 97, "Neoplasms of the Central Nervous System." (2) Formenti SC, et al. Primary central nervous system lymphoma in AIDS: Results of radiation therapy. Cancer 1989;63:1101.

Answer 3.110. **The answer is (c).**

Medulloblastoma is the most common brain tumor of children and generally occurs in the posterior fossa. Theses tumors usually are seen in children under age 5 and are manifested by symptoms related to hydrocephalus, including nausea, emesis, headache, and unsteadiness. Poor prognostic factors include cerebrospinal fluid involvement (evaluation done several weeks after surgery to prevent misleading results) and young age. The impact of tumor size is controversial. The most important therapy is complete surgical removal, if possible. Due to the possibility of disseminated disease, the introduction of craniospinal axis irradiation has made a major impact on the likelihood of cure. Survival rates of greater than 50% have been reported when a dose of 35 to 45 Gy to the brain and 30 to 36 Gy to the spine have been delivered. There is much interest in determining whether or not a lower dose of craniospinal radiation might be associated with an equally high survival while decreasing the risk of cognitive deficits. Chemotherapy has been beneficial only in those patients who have very large tumors and/or recurrent disease.

For Detailed Discussion: (1) Chapter 97, "Neoplasms of the Nervous System." (2) Deutch M. Medulloblastoma staging and treatment outcome. Int J Radiat Oncol Biol Phys 1988;14:1103.

Answer 3.111. **The answer is (c).**

A patient who has controlled primary lung cancer and no evidence of disease except for a single brain metastasis is clearly a candidate for surgical resection. There have been several retrospective series that have compared the benefit of surgery and radiotherapy versus radiotherapy alone for symptom relief and overall survival of such patients. For example, Patchell compared survival in patients who had metastatic brain tumors treated with radiotherapy alone versus patients undergoing surgery plus radiotherapy. Median survival was 10 months in the group receiving radiotherapy alone, but 19 months in the combined treatment group. Certainly for lesions that fail to respond symptomatically to irradiation (either so-called stereotactic radiation, whole-brain radiation, or interstitial brachytherapy), complete removal of a single lesion can provide the best form of local control. Chemotherapy would have little role in this situation, especially in the case of non–small-cell lung cancer, which is relatively chemoresistant.

For Detailed Discussion: (1) Chapter 97, "Neoplasms of the Central Nervous System." (2) Patchell RA, et al. Randomized trial of surgery in the treatment of single brain metastasis. NEJM 1990;322:494.

Answer 3.112.   The answer is (b).

Due to the larger lumen caliber in the right colon, obstruction is rare. Stool consistency in the right colon is liquid, which also minimizes the chance for obstruction. Lesions can grow to relatively large size before a symptom such as pain occurs. Occult bleeding in this setting can lead to significant anemia (with microcystic red blood cell indices) and weakness on that basis. Melena is much more common in left colonic or rectal/rectosigmoid lesions. Tenesmus and diarrhea would be unusual presenting symptoms in patients who have right colonic lesions, but are not uncommon in individuals with a distal sigmoid or rectal lesion. Patients who have left colonic lesions often describe colicky pain and frequently have obstruction; blood may be mixed with the stool. Patients with rectal lesions often describe steady, gnawing pain, and frequently have obstruction, but commonly have bright red blood coating the stool. Although rectal sigmoid and left colon–sided cancers traditionally have accounted for most colon cancers, right-sided lesions are becoming increasingly common.

For Detailed Discussion: (1) Chapter 121, "Adenocarcinoma of the Colon and Rectum."

Answer 3.113.   The answer is (c).

Varicocele, caused by retrograde blood flow into the internal spermatic vein, results in palpable dilation of the plexus of veins adjacent to the testicles and occurs in approximately 10 to15% of men. It is a common cause of male infertility, perhaps because of increased testicular temperature. However, approximately 2% of all male patients with renal cell carcinoma have a varicocele, generally left-sided, caused by obstruction of the testicular vein. More common presentations for renal cell carcinoma are hematuria (50–60%), abdominal pain (40%), or a palpable flank mass (30–40%). However, the so-called classic triad in which all three of these symptoms are present occurs in less than 10% of patients who have renal cell carcinoma. The widespread current use of computed tomography and ultrasonography has led to increased detection of renal cell carcinoma in asymptomatic patients. In fact, these incidentally diagnosed tumors are more likely to be cured with surgery due to their smaller size at diagnosis. Approximately 5% of patients display paraneoplastic syndromes, including erythrocytosis, hypercalcemia, hepatic dysfunction (Stauffer's syndrome), and amyloidosis.

For Detailed Discussion: (1) Chapter 123, "Renal Cell Carcinoma." (2) Motzer RJ, et al. Medical progress: Renal-cell carcinoma. NEJM 1996;335:865. (3) Griffin E, Wilson JD. Disorders of the testes. In: Isselbacher KJ, et al, eds. Harrison's Principles of Internal Medicine.13th ed. New York:McGraw-Hill, 1994.

Answer 3.114.   **The answer is (d).**

One of the most important prognostic factors in determining the outcome for patients who have adenocarcinoma of the prostate is the Gleason grading system. This was developed by review of over 1000 prostate biopsy specimens from men entered in Veterans Administration cooperative studies. Although other prognostic systems based on pathologic findings have been proposed, the Gleason grade has retained its importance over time. Tumors are classified based on a score of 1 to 5 for the predominant differentiation, with a score of 5 indicating the least well-differentiated cells. A Gleason Type 5 pattern is characterized by the absence or paucity of glands and the presence of sheets of tumor cells. The degree of preservation of glandular architecture, rather than the number of mitoses, is the key feature in determining Gleason grade. Another number, also from 1 to 5, is assigned to the next most common pattern of histologic appearance in the biopsy specimen. Therefore, the possible Gleason scores range from 2 to 10. Although perhaps being the least helpful in the intermediate Gleason grades, the system predicts a 1% annual mortality rate for those who have Gleason scores of 2 or 3, and a 25% annual mortality rate for patients who have Gleason Grade 10 lesions.

For Detailed Discussion: (1) Chapter 126, "Neoplasms of the Prostate."

Answer 3.115.   **The answer is (c).**

Because prostate cancer does not cause symptoms until it is locally advanced or metastatic, there has been much interest in developing techniques that would detect early disease, potentially curable with local therapy alone. The standard approach for many years was an annual digital rectal examination in men over age 50 who had a life expectancy of at least 10 years. It is clear that both PSA and transrectal ultrasound examinations will add to the detectability of early cancers. However, many of the cancers detected by such techniques could be clinically unimportant, and current therapies may not have any effect on the natural history of the disease for these cancers. There is no question that the use of PSA and transrectal ultrasonography has caused a migration toward the detection of lower stage prostate cancer, with over 90% of cancer currently detected in screened populations being confined to the prostate itself. However, because transrectal ultrasound is expensive, subjective, and requires special training for its optimum performance, it is not currently recommended as a screening tool. Both the American Urological Association and the American Cancer Society recommend that healthy men over age 50 who have a life expectancy of at least 10 years have an annual digital rectal examination and PSA screening annually. African-Americans and those who have a family history of prostate cancer—groups at higher risk for the development of this disease—should have this screening strategy adopted by age 40. A PSA value of greater than 10 μg/mL has a positive predictive value of 53%, regardless of findings from digital rectal examinations. A PSA value of greater than 4 µg/mL in the presence of a negative digital rectal examination, carries only a 25% likelihood that the patient actually has adenocarcinoma of the prostate. Despite the recommendations by the American Cancer Society, no trials have conclusively shown a decrease in morbidity and mortality in the aggressively screened population compared with that of standard care without mandated screening. Such a randomized trial is under way, but the results are unavailable at this time.

For Detailed Discussion: (1) Chapter 126, "Neoplasms of the Prostate." (2) Mettlin C, et al. Defining and updating the American Cancer Society guidelines for the cancer-related check-up: prostate and endometrial cancers. CA 1993;44:42. (3) Catalona WJ, et al. Detection of organ-confined prostate cancer is increased through prostate-specific-antigen-based screening. JAMA 1993;270:948.

Answer 3.116.   The answer is (b).

During an extrafascial hysterectomy, the pubovesical fascia should not be separated from the cervix and should be excised with the specimen. The uterine vessels are skeletonized in order to lessen the need to slide the tip of the clamp off the cervix. The plane for the bladder separation from the cervix is created with sharp dissection because blunt dissection is more often associated with accidental entry into the bladder. Finally, the uterosacral ligaments are transected separately near the insertion into the cervix, freeing the uterus and cervix posteriorly.

For Detailed Discussion: (1) Chapter 130, "Neoplasms of the Cervix."

Answer 3.117.   The answer is (a).

Seventy percent of patients who have ovarian cancer are first seen at an advanced stage, with disease extending throughout the abdomen, frequently associated with ascites and omental metastases. It is precisely because of the vague and nonspecific nature of the symptoms produced by intra-abdominal carcinomatosis that patients are first seen in an advanced stage. In any patient with this history, the finding of a complex cyst on an ovary must be considered to be malignant. Although this is a typical presentation for advanced ovarian cancer, patients with breast, stomach, or colorectal cancer can have ascites and intra-abdominal carcinomatosis. However, in the absence of other historical or physical examination findings consistent with an alternative diagnosis, the patient should be considered to have ovarian cancer and should be referred for laparotomy, preferably by a gynecologic oncologist. The goal of surgery will be to establish a diagnosis and tumor stage, but it is important also to perform maximal surgical cytoreduction. One of the most important prognostic factors in ovarian cancer is whether or not a patient can be rendered maximally debulked (residual tumor mass not greater than 2 cm in diameter) after surgery. The treatment of choice after surgery is a platinum-based chemotherapy regimen.

For Detailed Discussion: (1) Chapter 133, "Ovarian Cancer."

Answer 3.118.   The answer is (d).

The surgical mainstay for renal cell carcinoma is radical nephrectomy: resection of the kidney, peritoneal fat, and ipsilateral adrenal gland. Based on a low likelihood of involvement in the ipsilateral adrenal gland, many experts now recommend that adrenalectomy be reserved for patients who have large upper pole lesions or abnormal-appearing adrenal glands as revealed by radiographic studies. Although lymph node metastases are clearly an adverse prognostic sign, the benefit of lymphadenectomy remains controversial. Nephron sparing surgery, employed if an absolute or relative contraindication to nephrectomy exists, is usually successful, with local recurrences occurring in less than 10% of patients. This more limited surgery may even be appropriate for the patient who has small localized tumor and a normal contralateral kidney. Involvement of the renal vein, including the inferior vena cava and even the right atrium, is common in patients who have renal cell carcinoma and is not a contraindication to surgery. Surgery in such cases is more complicated and has a higher operative mortality, but up to 50% of patients can be cured. Although nephrectomy could be justified in the rare patient with metastatic disease whose primary tumor is causing profound symptoms, there is a very low incidence of regression of metastatic deposits when the primary tumor is removed (less than 1%). The most common reason for failure after removal of the primary tumor is distant relapse, particularly in the lung.

For Detailed Discussion: (1) Chapter 134, "Gestational Trophoblastic Neoplasia." (2) Motzer RJ, et al. Medical progress: Renal cell carcinoma NEJM 1996;335:865.

Answer 3.119. **The answer is (d).**

This patient has clearly progressed from stable phase CML to the so-called blast crisis phase. Blast crisis is often heralded by an accelerated phase manifested by increasing constitutional symptoms and more marked splenomegaly. Blast crisis is defined as the presence of greater than 30% blasts in the peripheral blood and/or bone marrow. Given the pluripotent nature of the malignant cells in CML, the blast crisis may be erythroblastic, megakaryoblastic, lymphoblastic, or, as is the case in two thirds of the patients, myeloblastic. The lymphoid variety of blast crisis can be diagnosed by immunophenotypic studies that will document the presence of B-cell or possibly T-cell antigens. If a lymphoid origin for the blasts can be documented, then it is reasonable to use vincristine and prednisone (probably with the addition of anthracycline) as initial therapeutic management rather than the more myelosuppressive approach that would be required for treatment of the myeloid blast crisis (eg, 3 days of anthracycline plus 7 days of ara-C or high-dose ara-C). At least 50% of patients who have a lymphoid blast crisis will respond to vincristine-prednisone–based therapy. However, once a patient enters blast crisis, therapy must be considered palliative; in a younger patient who has a histocompatible sibling donor, allogeneic transplantation could be considered in the second stable phase, but the results in terms of long-term, disease-free survival are much inferior to those obtained when transplantation is performed earlier in the course of the disease.

For Detailed Discussion: (1) Chapter 143, "Chronic Myeloid Leukemia."

Answer 3.120. **The answer is (a).**

ALL in adults is a different disease biologically than ALL in children. This biologic difference is best exemplified by a 25 to 33% incidence of the Philadelphia chromosome [t(9;22)] in adults, yet less than a 5% incidence in children. The cytogenetic abnormality suggests that the leukemia has arisen from primitive hematopoietic elements, is associated with chemotherapy resistance, and presents an essential impossibility of cure without an allogeneic bone marrow transplantation. All balanced translocations are adverse prognostic signs in ALL. The incidence of L-3, or Burkitt's subtype, associated with the t(8;14) cytogenetic abnormality, is also higher in adults than in children. However, even in adults, this finding is relatively unusual, occurring in less than 5% of those who have ALL. Children have a higher likelihood of presenting at some point in their course with central nervous sytem involvement; however, the use of central nervous system prophylaxis, including cranial radiotherapy and/or intrathecal chemotherapy, has diminished the impact of this clinical problem. Although approximately 90% of adults under age 60 who have ALL will enter remission with newer, more intensive regimens, most of these patients are destined to relapse. Unfortunately, allogeneic bone marrow transplantation in adults with ALL in first remission has not been shown to be clearly superior to chemotherapy alone. Nonetheless, for those who are first seen with a balanced translocation, such as the Philadelphia chromosome, allogeneic transplantation must be considered as the treatment of choice, because it offers the only opportunity for cure.

For Detailed Discussion: (1) Chapter 145, "Acute Lymphocytic Leukemia in Adults."

Answer 3.121.   **The answer is (c).**

This patient is seen with a classic history and immunophenotypic results that are consistent with a diagnosis of chronic lymphocytic leukemia (CLL). This, the most common leukemia, is characterized by a proliferation of mature-appearing B lymphocytes that also express the nominal T-cell antigen CD5. The only other CD5–positive lymphoproliferative neoplasm is mantle cell lymphoma, which can be distinguished from CLL because of lack of CD23 expression. CLL is an indolent disease. Except for the relatively rare younger patient who has advanced disease and might be a candidate for high-dose myeloablative approach, treatment strategies in this disease must be considered palliative in nature. The purine analogue fludarabine may have supplanted the alkylating agent chlorambucil as the cytotoxic therapy of choice for patients with CLL who require systemic treatment, usually due to diffuse bulky adenopathy, or cytopenias related to bone marrow involvement. However, it is important to rule out an autoimmune hemolytic anemia, which can occur in up to 30% of patients, as the cause of an isolated anemia. Such Coombs'-positive hemolytic anemias must be actively sought for, because treating them requires corticosteroids alone, thereby sparing the patient unnecessary side effects of cytotoxic chemotherapy. Although the other staging studies listed are reasonable, it is important to exclude hemolysis by assessing reticulocytosis, evidence for red blood cell autoantibodies, and indirect hyperbilirubinemia.

For Detailed Discussion: (1) Chapter 147, "Chronic Lymphocytic Leukemia."

Answer 3.122.   **The answer is (e).**

This patient is seen with the new well-defined entity of Ki-1 anaplastic large-cell lymphoma. Typical features of this disease, in addition to the obligate Ki-1 (CD30) antigen expression, are skin involvement (including a relatively benign variant in which skin is the only site involved, obviously not the case here), and frequent finding of a t(2;5) translocation. Approximately 70% of the cases are of T-cell origin, with the rest being derived from null or B lymphocytes. Stage for stage, they behave in a similar fashion to their more typical B-cell–large-cell lymphoma (intermediate stage) counterparts. Because this patient has a systemic lymphoma, CHOP-based chemotherapy is warranted. Unlike the case for high-grade lymphomas such as lymphoblastic lymphoma and small noncleaved–cell lymphoma, central nervous system prophylaxis is not indicated.

For Detailed Discussion: (1) Chapter 150, "Non-Hodgkin's Lymphoma."

Answer 3.123. **The answer is (d).**

This patient has the classic presentation of lymphoblastic lymphoma. In contrast to most histologic subtypes of non-Hodgkin's lymphoma, lymphoblastic lymphoma is of T-cell origin in 80 to 90% of cases. Lymphoblastic lymphoma, clearly one of the high-grade non-Hodgkin's lymphomas, is typically seen in young adults and involves the anterior mediastinum. B type symptoms; bone marrow involvement, in which case the disease resembles T-cell acute lymphocytic leukemia; and central nervous system involvement are common. Unless emergency chest irradiation is required, routine chest radiotherapy is no longer necessary due to the efficacy of chemotherapy. Due to the likelihood of disease relapse at distant sites (even though this patient has localized disease), systemic chemotherapy with a CHOP–based regimen is warranted. Because of the likelihood of CNS involvement, most authorities recommend that prophylactic intrathecal methotrexate and cranial radiotherapy be administered after approximately two cycles of systemic chemotherapy. Several additional cycles of CHOP are then administered, with up to 1 year of "maintenance" therapy with oral methotrexate and 6-mercaptopurine to follow. Adverse prognostic factors for patients who have lymphoblastic lymphoma include elevated lactate dehydrogenase (LDH) levels, age greater than 40, and advanced stage of presentation (particularly an Ann-Arbor Stage IV). For patients who have localized disease, especially for those without elevations of serum LDH, cure rates in the 80% range have been reported.

For Detailed Discussion: (1) Chapter 150, "Non-Hodgkin's Lymphoma." (2) Picozzi VJ, et al. Lymphoblastic lymphoma. Semin Oncol 1990;17:96.

Answer 3.124. **The answer is (a).**

This patient is seen with an incidental finding of an M-spike (a monoclonal protein detected in the peripheral blood). The monoclonal immunoglobulin is of moderate level, and is not associated with lytic lesions, hypercalcemia, renal failure, plasma cell infiltration of the bone marrow, or any diagnostic criteria for multiple myeloma or other plasma cell neoplasm. Therefore, the diagnosis is monoclonal gammopathy of unknown significance (MGUS). Although some of these patients will eventually progress to frank multiple myeloma, early treatment for this incurable, indolent neoplasm is not indicated. Because the vast majority of patients (at least 80% of those with MGUS) will never have any problems secondary to a plasma cell neoplasm, observation is the most appropriate course. Gene rearrangement studies are not necessary, because by virtue of the monoclonal spike, it is already known that the patient has a neoplasm. Bone scanning is inappropriate for the work-up of known or suspected plasma cell neoplasm, because this technique is best for the detection of blastic metastasis, whereas myeloma produces bone lysis.

For Detailed Discussion: (1) Chapter 152, "Plasma Cell Tumors."

Answer 3.125.   The answer (a).

The mast cell diseases represent a spectrum of disorders from benign urticaria pigmentosa of childhood to mast cell leukemia, which has an aggressive and often fatal course. This child has typical urticaria pigmentosa that can be treated symptomatically, is not related to allergens, and will likely disappear by puberty. A more aggressive variant of the disease, systemic mastocytosis, is characterized by mast cell infiltration of reticulo-endothelial organs. Some patients who have systemic mastocytosis will eventually develop significant bone marrow involvement, with bizarre-appearing mast cells, and these patients will be diagnosed with mast cell leukemia.

For Detailed Discussion: (1) Chapter 153, "Mast Cell Leukemia."

Answer 3.126.   The answer is (e).

In contrast to adenomatous polyps, which have a high likelihood of malignant transformation, hyperplastic polyps are generally considered to be benign and not pre-malignant. Although such hyperplastic polyps may occur throughout the gastrointestinal tract because of their benign nature, colonoscopy is not warranted. Even in high-risk countries where the risk of gastric cancer associated with hyperplastic polyps may be as high as 4 to 8%, the polyp itself is not considered to be premalignant. Therefore, the finding of the polyp (or for that matter active gastritis) in and of itself is not a reason for either surgery or more aggressive screening approaches.

For Detailed Discussion: (1) Chapter 113, "Neoplasms of the Stomach."

Answer 3.127.   The answer is (a).

Because of the low prevalence of metastatic disease in patients who have low serum PSA levels (less than 8 ng/mL), low Gleason Grade tumors (less than Grade 8), or non–locally advanced tumors (less than stage T3), the value of bone scanning in these situations has been rightly questioned. In the presence of at least one such risk factor, false-positive bone scans are common. However, a patient with a higher level of PSA, an abnormal bone scan in the presence of a normal plain radiograph of that area (which therefore did not show benign bone abnormalities such as arthritis or benign enchondroma to explain the abnormal scan), the diagnosis of metastasis is highly likely. An MRI scan of the bone could be helpful in confirming the metastasis, but is probably not necessary in this case.

For Detailed Discussion: (1) Chapter 126, "Neoplasms of the Prostate."

Answer 3.128.   The answer is (c).

Although radical prostatectomy is associated with a high likelihood of disease-free survival when the tumor is pathologically confined to the gland, it is not uncommon that clinical Stage T2 lesions will be found to be pathologically Stage T3 (positive surgical margins or pathologic extension through the capsule). The rate of PSA nonprogression after radical surgery for patients in this category is 50 to 70%, which is similar to the long-term failure rate. Adjuvant radiotherapy given immediately post-operatively in patients who are determined to have pathologic Stage T3 lesions may increase the cure rate after surgery. Another viable approach, as was the case for this patient, is to wait until PSA progression occurs and offer radiotherapy. Approximately 50% of individuals treated in this fashion respond with a PSA level returning to undetectable; however, approximately half of such patients will eventually experience another PSA failure. A PSA failure is believed to represent a very high risk for eventual metastatic disease. It is possible that early hormonal therapy may be beneficial in patients who have positive margins or eventual PSA progression; however, the use of early hormonal therapy is currently being evaluated in randomized trials and cannot be recommended at this time.

For Detailed Discussion: (1) Chapter 126, "Neoplasms of the Prostate." (2) Mc-Carthy JF, et al. Effective radiation therapy for detectable serum PSA levels following radical prostatectomy; early versus delayed treatment. J Urol 1994;151:1575.

Answer 3.129. **The answer is (d).**

The optimal approach for patients who have clinically localized prostate cancer remains highly controversial. Although most patients are offered either external beam radiotherapy or radical prostatectomy, there is increased interest in formally studying a policy of watchful waiting. Watchful waiting is reasonable because many patients with localized prostate cancer, particularly those who have low Gleason Grades, will not die of their disease. Moreover, there is another subset of patients for whom local therapy could not possibly change the natural history of the disease, because micrometastases exist at the time of presentation. It seems quite likely that the modality associated with the greatest probability of cure is radical prostatectomy. Eighty percent of patients undergoing such surgery have a PSA level that is undetectable at 5 years compared with only approximately 50% of those undergoing definitive radiotherapy. However, radical prostatectomy requires that patients be in the hospital for approximately 5 days and lose between 4 to 8 weeks of work. The risk of incontinence is significant, with approximately 5% of those patients experiencing stress incontinence, and 1 to 2% having severe incontinence. Impotency is a major risk after radical prostatectomy; the so-called nerve-sparing approach may reduce the likelihood of impotency below the 70 to 100% rate quoted in earlier work. Incontinence is uncommon after radiotherapy in the absence of cancer recurrence. Impotency does occur in up to 50% of patients at 7 years. Approximately one third of patients undergoing definitive radiotherapy will develop proctitis with irritation and diarrhea, which is often quite treatable with steroid enemas. Therefore, treatment decisions are still difficult. It is important to note that the Veterans Administration cooperative clinical trials group, along with the NCI, has recently initiated a large prospective randomized trial of watchful waiting versus radical prostatectomy. This trial will require at least 10 years to complete. Comparisons of surgery and radiotherapy have never been evaluated in a prospective randomized clinical trial; one is therefore limited to comparing actuarial survival rates for similar prognostic groups treated with either modality.

For Detailed Discussion: (1) Chapter 126, "Neoplasms of the Prostate." (2) Fleming C, et al. A decision analysis of alternative treatment strategies for clinically localized prostate cancer. Prostate patients outcomes research team. JAMA 1993;269:2650.

Answer 3.130.   **The answer is (e).**

Because prostate cancer has an obligate dependence on androgens for growth, ablating such sex steroid production is the goal of treating symptomatic diffuse metastatic disease. Testicular androgens can be ablated by either orchiectomy or inhibiting pituitary gonadotropin release. Pituitary gonadotropin release may be inhibited by the synthetic estrogen DES; however, high doses (5 mg/d) of DES are associated with excess cardiovascular morbidity and mortality. A lower dose of DES (1 mg/d) is less risky in terms of vascular events, but suppresses testosterone to anorchidic levels in only 70% of patients. An intermediate dose of DES may have unwelcome side effects beyond those of hypercoagulability, such as gynecomastia, congestive heart failure, and impotence. Therefore, the current standard strategy to achieve medical castration is to use luteinizing hormone releasing hormone (LHRH) analogues, either leuprolide or goserelin. These super-agonists actually stimulate LH and FSH (and therefore testosterone) secretion for the first 7 days, but with continued therapy, down-regulation of pituitary LHRH receptors occurs, and testosterone levels fall within 14 to 21 days. Leuprolide appears to be considerably less toxic than DES and equally efficacious compared with orchiectomy. The response rate to such androgen suppression is high; 70 to 80% of men experience a decrease in the PSA level, with a similar likelihood of symptomatic response. Extratesticular androgens also appear to have a role in promoting prostate cancer growth. So-called total androgen deprivation may be obtained by the combination of the anti-androgen flutamide with an LHRH analogue. Flutamide competes with circulating antigens for the androgen receptor and inhibits testosterone 5-α-reductase. Flutamide also has the advantage of blocking the flare that can occur with leuprolide alone. A randomized trial of leuprolide alone versus leuprolide plus flutamide depicts a small but significant survival advantage for the combined therapy. Patients who progress on such hormonal therapy are very unlikely to respond to additional hormonal manipulations, although "flutamide withdrawal" responses have been described in up to 25% of such patients.

For Detailed Discussion: (1) Chapter 126, "Neoplasms of the Prostate."

Answer 3.131.   **The answer is (a).**

The prevalence of bladder cancer could be markedly reduced in this country if exposure to environmental carcinogens could be minimized. The most important such inciting agent is cigarette smoking, which accounts for approximately one half of the incidence of bladder cancer in this country. Aromatic amines have long been known to increase the risk of bladder cancer. Exposure to these agents occurs in leather workers, rubber workers, painters, truck drivers, and aluminum workers. Long-term cyclophosphamide use has been associated with an increased risk of bladder cancer, which may occur in the absence of hemorrhagic cystitis. Geographic areas in which infection with the parasite *Schistosoma haematobium* is endemic have higher rates of bladder cancer; histologies are both squamous cell as well as transitional cell. The lifetime risk of developing bladder cancer is highest among white men (approximately 3%) compared with an approximately 0.5 to 1% risk for black men, white women, and black women. The mortality rate is falling in all groups, possibly because of an increased rate of early detection.

For Detailed Discussion: (1) Chapter 125, "Bladder Cancer." (2) Hankey B. Trends in bladder cancer incidence and mortality 1973–1989. JNCI 1992;84:1689.

Answer 3.132. **The answer is (b).**

This patient is seen with Stage T1 transitional cell carcinoma of the bladder of an intermediate stage of differentiation. The lesion is T1 because it extends beyond the basement membrane of the mucosa into the lamina propria but not into the muscularis propria. This patient therefore has superficial bladder cancer, which includes lesions that range from Grade Ta (mucosa only) to a more histologically undifferentiated version of T1. The likelihood of progression to a form of bladder cancer with ominous overtones, such as a tumor that invades muscle and actually has metastatic potential, varies according to the stage and grade. Stage Ta tumors have a 2% likelihood of progression compared with a 48% likelihood for Stage T1 Grade 3 tumors. The patient in question has an approximately 20% likelihood of progression. Other factors that increase the risk of progression include multiple primary tumors, multiple recurrences, positive urine cytology after resection, and diffuse carcinoma in situ. The most appropriate approach for reducing the risk of eventual progression of such superficial tumors is the use of intravesical chemotherapy (thiotepa, doxorubicin, mitomycin-C) or immunotherapy with BCG. Mitomycin-C will reduce the risk of recurrence by approximately 15% based on randomized control study results. More aggressive forms of bladder cancer, such as T2 or T3 lesions that invade into muscle or fat, or T4 lesions that invade into adjacent structures, need to be treated more aggressively. The standard approach for such patients is radical cystectomy. The role of preoperative or postoperative radiotherapy is unclear. Partial cystectomy is being explored and may be appropriate for solitary cancers that are located in the region of the bladder that allows complete excision with a 2-cm, tumor-free margin. Remaining mucosa must have no evidence of atypia or carcinoma in situ. Whether or not perioperative chemoradiotherapy can increase the likelihood of successful bladder preservation remains unclear.

For Detailed Discussion: (1) Chapter 125, "Bladder Cancer."

Answer 3.133. **The answer is (e).**

Eighty percent of patients who have adenocarcinoma of the endometrium are postmenopausal, and most have bleeding as the presenting symptom. The staging system for endometrial cancer, once it is diagnosed, which is usually after dilation and curettage of the uterus, is based on pathologic results found at definitive surgery. Tumors confined to the endometrium are Stage I, and those with invasion into the cervix are Stage II. Local and/or regional spread (Stage III) may involve parametrial extension and/or cancer cells in ascitic washings (III A), vaginal involvement (III B), or metastasis to the pelvic and/or para-aortic lymph nodes. The likelihood of 5-year survival is strongly correlated with surgical stage, with survivals of greater than 80% for Stages I and II patients, but only 40% for patients who have Stage III disease. For those with Stages I or II disease, the likelihood of recurrence is influenced by histologic cell type (with the more unusual histologies, such as serous papillary, clear cell, and squamous cell cancers having a worse prognosis); grade (less well-differentiated tumors are worrisome); and the depth of myometrial invasion. Positive cytology appears to increase the risk of recurrence, but the magnitude of this effect is not clear. Based on the depth of invasion, this patient has FIGO (Federation Internationale de Gynecologie d'Obstetrique) Stage 1C disease and has a 5-year survival of approximately 75%. Benefits of adjuvant radiotherapy in this setting are unclear.

For Detailed Discussion: (1) Chapter 131, "Endometrial Cancer."

Answer 3.134.   **The answer is (e).**

The most important prognostic factors for patients who have AML are age and the presence of adverse cytogenetic abnormalities. Certain French-American-British (FAB) collaborating groups' classification subtypes correlate with well-defined (by cytogenetics) prognostic categories. The cytogenetic finding associated with the best prognosis is pericentric inversion of chromosome 16, which is associated with the so-called M4E subtype. Patients have myelomonoblasts (staining with both peroxidase and nonspecific esterase) associated with a population of dysplastic eosinophils that contain both eosinophilic and basophilic granules. Pure monocytic leukemia, characterized by nonspecific esterase cytochemical staining (sometimes associated with a translocation between chromosomes 9 and 11), is associated with extramedullary leukemia and a poor prognosis. Patients who have evolved from myelodysplastic syndrome and/or have had an antecedent hematologic abnormality (as might be inferred by the presence of dysplastic elements in association with the myeloblasts) also have a very poor prognosis. M0 AML, characterized by nondescript blasts that are cytochemically negative but immunophenotypically positive for myeloid antigens, also does not respond well to standard chemotherapy. FAB subtypes M6 and M7 are less likely to respond to therapy. The M6 subtype, acute erythroleukemia, is defined based on the presence of greater than 50% of the nucleated cells being erythroblasts in association with greater than 30% of the non-erythroid cells being myeloblasts.

For Detailed Discussion: (1) Chapter 142, "Acute Myeloid Leukemia in Adults."

Answer 3.135.   **The answer is (b).**

This patient is initially seen with Stage III diffuse large-cell lymphoma, a subtype of intermediate grade lymphoma. The patient has two adverse prognostic factors in the age-adjusted (for patients ≤60 years of age) international index of intermediate stage lymphomas, namely an elevated LDH level, and the presence of Stage III disease (as opposed to Stages I or II). The other adverse prognostic factor is poor performance status (ECOG [Eastern Cooperative Oncology Group] ≥2), and therefore this patient is in the high intermediate prognostic category, with a 5-year disease-free likelihood of approximately 50%. However, studies have not yet shown an advantage for the administration of intensified CHOP or more complicated regimens to treat patients with poor-risk lymphoma. Intrathecal prophylactic therapy is not required for patients with intermediate grade lymphoma, especially those patients without bone marrow involvement. The regimen of doxorubicin, vinblastine, dacarbazine, and bleomycin is more appropriate for patients with Hodgkin's disease (and not for those with non-Hodgkin's lymphomas). Although a combined chemoradiotherapy approach has been shown to be beneficial for Stages I and II disease, the standard approach for Stages III and IV disease is combination chemotherapy. Total nodal irradiation is not used in patients who have diffuse large-cell lymphoma. Whether or not patients like this one who has several adverse prognostic features will be better served by a more intensified chemotherapy approach with or without early transplantation remains a question for ongoing clinical research studies.

For Detailed Discussion: (1) Chapter 150, "Non-Hodgkin's Lymphoma." (2) Shipp MA, et al. A predictive model for aggressive NHL: The international non-Hodgkin's lymphoma prognostic factors project. NEJM 1983;329:987.

Answer 3.136.   **The answer is (d).**

The therapeutic strategy for children who have acute lymphoblastic leukemia has represented a paradigm for the treatment of patients of all ages who have various malignancies. Approximately 90% of patients who have standard risk ALL may be cured. Standard risk is defined according to the following criteria: the absence of true B cell (L3) morphology, the absence of significant leukocytosis (greater than 50,000/mm^3), ages 1 to10, and the absence of a balanced translocation. The application of somewhat more intensive therapy to patients in the high-risk category has led to apparent improvements in outcome. From a historical standpoint, an early advance was the recognition that the central nervous system was a sanctuary site for relapse; once patients began to receive prophylactic therapy, either with radiotherapy and/or with intrathecal chemotherapy, the cure rate for children with ALL improved markedly. The addition of daunorubicin, and probably L-asparaginase, to the backbone of vincristine and prednisone for induction has been a significant advance. Although the optimal duration of maintenance therapy is unclear, patients who cannot receive adequate long-term maintenance therapy (a surrogate marker is insufficiently high serum mercaptopurine levels) are more likely to relapse. The benefits of high-dose ara-C therapy have been restricted to patients who have AML.

For Detailed Discussion: (1) Chapter 164, "Acute Lymphoblastic Leukemia in Children."

Answer 3.137.   **The answer is (d).**

The majority of tumors arising in the newborn are benign, most of these being teratomas and other germ cell tumors. Only 32 malignant solid tumors in neonates were found in a 40-year review of the experience at the M D Anderson Cancer Center. Of the tumors listed, neuroblastoma is easily the most common lesion seen in the first 30 days of life. A greater proportion of these tumors arise in the thorax as opposed to the abdominal sites, which are the most common in older patients. Hepatoblastoma and Wilms' tumors are exceedingly rare in the neonate. Of note, the so-called "infantile" fibrosarcoma is seen about as frequently in this age group as neuroblastoma. However, according to some authors, the excellent outcome in patients who have these soft-tissue tumors calls into question their "true" malignant nature.

For Detailed Discussion: (1) Chapter 158, "Special Features of Surgery for Children with Cancer." (2) Parkes SE, et al. Neonatal tumours: A thirty-year population-based study. Med Pediatr Oncol 1994;22:309. (3) Xue H, et al. Malignant solid tumors in neonates: A 40-year review. J Pediatr Surg 1995;30:543.

Answer 3.138.   **The answer is (a).**

Many pediatric tumors exhibit a benign behavior, and the concept of spontaneous regression is well documented. Young patients who have neuroblastoma may survive even with minimal treatment. Children who have retinoblastoma do not require complete surgical excision, because other local tumor control methods and adjuvant systemic therapy are effective. The biology of "infantile" fibrosarcoma is poorly understood, but the vast majority of these patients survive in the long term without radical surgery. The addition or omission of chemotherapy and radiotherapy have not consistently affected outcome. The long-term survival in most pediatric patients who have lymphoma is related more to the effectiveness of systemic chemotherapy and does not depend on surgical excision. Pediatric patients with liver tumors remain the outstanding example of how successful complete tumor resection is critical. Many of the current chemotherapy strategies are planned so that tumor mass can be adequately reduced to allow the patient to become a surgical candidate.

For Detailed Discussion: (1) Chapter 158, "Special Features of Surgery for Children with Cancer." (2) Pierro A, et al. Preoperative chemotherapy in "unresectable" hepatoblastoma. Pediatr Surg 1989;24:24. (3) Reynolds J, et al. Chemotherapy can convert unresectable hepatoblastoma. J Pediatr Surg 1992;27:1080.

Answer 3.139. **The answer is (a).**

A patient who is at high risk for recurrence of colon carcinoma should be followed up with a routine blood work-up, including a CEA level; CT scans of the abdomen; and colonoscopy. However, the true sensitivity and specificity of CEA is controversial. A number of studies have examined the role of CEA in surveillance of patients with colon carcinoma. Although there are a number of reasons for this marker to be elevated, including benign peptic ulcer disease, jaundice, cirrhosis, or tobacco abuse, certainly a rise in the CEA level should be monitored for an upward trend. If indeed the CEA level continues to rise, then imaging studies should be performed in order to determine the presence of an intra-abdominal recurrence. Radio-immunoguided approaches have become more common, although their true utility has not been determined. In addition, whole body PET scan is valuable for determining the presence of recurrent disease, but its sensitivity and specificity have not yet been determined on a large-scale basis. If all staging studies are negative and there is no evidence of extra-abdominal disease, then a second-look laparotomy should be performed. Studies of large groups of patients have demonstrated that the use of CEA determination tends to demonstrate disease approximately 2 to 3 months sooner than symptoms alone.

For Detailed Discussion: (1) Chapter 121, "Adenocarcinoma of the Colon and Rectum." (2) Moertel CG, et al. An evaluation of the carcinoembryonic antigen (CEA) test for monitoring patients with resected colon cancer. JAMA 1993;270:943.

Answer 3.140. **The answer is (e).**

Villous adenomas, tubulovillous adenomas, and tubular adenomas are considered precancerous lesions. Although only 1% of tubular adenomas less than 1 cm in size will harbor occult metastases, this percentage increases tenfold for larger tubular adenomas and may be up to 30% for those lesions greater than 2 cm. Approximately 10% of neoplastic colon polyps are villous adenomas. As compared to the tubular adenomas, the villous adenomas are usually sessile, and their usual presentation is rectal bleeding, mucous discharge, or secretory diarrhea. Overall, approximately two thirds of villous adenomas contain cancer, and half of these are invasive. The risk of malignancy in a tubular villous adenoma is greater than in tubular adenomas but less than in villous adenomas. Hyperplastic polyps are not precancerous.

For Detailed Discussion: (1) Chapter 121, "Adenocarcinoma of the Colon and Rectum."

Answer 3.141. **The answer is (d).**

Although carcinoid tumors are most commonly found incidentally at the time of appendectomy and represent only 0.1% of all surgically removed appendices, occasionally patients will first be seen with a carcinoid syndrome characterized by flushing, diarrhea, and asthma-like symptoms. If the tumor is greater than 1 cm in size or if there is evidence of nodal metastases, a right hemicolectomy is recommended. Patients who have smaller tumors are usually adequately treated with appendectomy alone. Adjuvant therapy has not been of any value, and therapy is usually recommended only for those patients who develop recurrent disease and carcinoid syndrome symptoms. Single agents such as 5-FU and streptozocin have some activity in this disease. More recently, patients have been treated with the somatostatin analogue octreotide for control of carcinoid symptoms. Although these tumors are usually radioresponsive, there is usually little role for the use of this treatment in the palliation of carcinoid syndrome symptoms.

For Detailed Discussion: (1) Chapter 121, "Adenocarcinoma of the Colon and Rectum."

Answer 3.142. **The answer is (e).**

Patients who have rectal carcinoma have a 25 to 50% chance of local recurrence alone or in combination with distant metastases. The presence of nodal metastases and deep wall invasion are significant risk factors for locoregional failure. Several studies have demonstrated the importance of adjuvant radiotherapy. In addition, a combination of 5-FU and radiotherapy has been shown to be superior to radiotherapy alone, and the rate of locoregional recurrence is markedly reduced. However, the sequence of treatment employing pre- or postoperative irradiation is unknown, because the studies comparing these techniques are hindered by differences in disease staging at surgery caused by the treatment alone. However, it is clear that adjuvant 5-FU infusional therapy and radiotherapy of the pelvic region is most effective for local control of rectal cancer.

For Detailed Discussion: (1) Chapter 121, "Adenocarcinoma of the Colon and Rectum." (2) O'Connell MJ, et al. Improving adjuvant therapy for rectal cancer by combining protracted-infusion fluorouracil with radiation therapy after curative surgery. NEJM 1994;331:502.

Answer 3.143. **The answer is (d).**

In an elderly patient who appears to have metastatic colorectal carcinoma, local therapy alone is likely the best palliation of pain and perhaps bleeding. However, this patient is likely to develop an obstruction and would best be treated with a diverting colostomy. There is little role for the use of 5-FU therapy or preoperative radiotherapy combined with a more aggressive surgical approach. Intraoperative radiotherapy is under current investigation in the treatment of a locally advanced or recurrent rectal carcinomas, but this treatment has little role in the patient who has metastatic disease.

For Detailed Discussion: (1) Chapter 121, "Adenocarcinoma of the Colon and Rectum."

Answer 3.144. **The answer is (c).**

Although the cause of squamous cell carcinomas of the anus is unknown, there are several studies that demonstrate the association of papillomavirus, in particular condyloma acuminatum, in the development of this disease. More recently, there has been an increase in anal carcinomas in single and/or divorced men and women, which suggests that it may be caused by unusual sexual behavior—particularly anal intercourse. There is no increased incidence in anal carcinoma in those patients with excessive tobacco use, constant anal pruritus, or poor anal hygiene. Although *p53* mutations have been demonstrated in a large number of cancers, there are no data to suggest that these mutations are the causative agent in the development of anal squamous cell carcinoma. Although benzenes and fluorohydrocarbons are important carcinogens for hepatomas, it is unclear whether the aforementioned agents have any role in the development of these rare cancers.

For Detailed Discussion: (1) Chapter 122, "Neoplasms of the Anus."

Answer 3.145. **The answer is (d).**

The treatment for squamous cell carcinomas of the anus has undergone a revolution due to the advances outlined by Nigro and associates at Wayne State University. (Nigro ND, et al. An evaluation of combined therapy for squamous cell cancer of the anus. Dis Colon Rectum 1984;27:763). These researchers have demonstrated that rather moderate doses of preoperative irradiation (3000 Gy) and 5-FU infusion with mitomycin can dramatically reduce the need for extensive procedures such as abdominoperineal resection. A patient such as this one should receive neoadjuvant therapy, with resection of the residual disease, including the inguinal node metastases. Patients who have primary cancers greater than 5 cm in size or recurrent disease can often be salvaged with additional chemotherapy and radiotherapy and, if necessary, more aggressive surgical approaches. Although inguinal node metastases can be managed by external beam radiotherapy, inguinal node dissection is probably equally effective. Some investigators manage the inguinal nodes by external beam radiotherapy alone and then employ inguinal node dissection for those patients who develop recurrent disease at that site. Neither chemotherapy nor radiotherapy alone is as effective as the combination approach.

For Detailed Discussion: (1) Chapter 122, "Neoplasms of the Anus."

Answer 3.146. **The answer is (d).**

Anorectal melanoma is an unusual variant of cutaneous melanoma. The etiology of this disease is unknown, and it is unlikely due to sun exposure. Often these lesions are amelanotic and can be confused with a squamous cell carcinoma of this region. Often they are found in conjunction with hemorrhoids, which may delay the diagnosis. The tumors metastasize by both the venous and lymphatic routes, and although patients have traditionally been treated with abdominoperineal resection, there is no evidence to suggest that this more radical surgery decreases the rate of distant metastasis or improves long-term survival. There is no role for chemotherapy or radiotherapy in the treatment of early lesions. Although regional lymph node dissections have become an important aspect of the treatment of cutaneous melanoma, there is no role for prophylactic removal of the regional lymph nodes in anorectal melanoma.

For Detailed Discussion: (1) Chapter 122, "Neoplasms of the Anus."

Answer 3.147. **The answer is (d).**

Neoplasms of the glans penis are relatively rare. They constitute only 0.1% of cancer in the United States; this tumor is much more common in Asia, Africa, and Latin America, where penile cancer accounts for up to 12% of cancers in males. The etiology of this disease is unknown, although it is extremely rare in Israel, where circumcision is practiced at birth. Human papillomavirus types 16 and 18 have been associated with carcinoma of the penis and cervix. Men with psoriasis who have been treated with oral methoxsalen and ultraviolet A photo-chemotherapy have a higher incidence of penile cancer than the normal population. The treatment of this disease depends on the size of the primary lesion. Small lesions of 1 cm or less are usually treated with limited resection, although external beam radiotherapy appears to be equally effective for local control. Larger lesions may require more extensive resection that may be disabling. The size, thickness, and differentiation of the primary lesion are useful for estimating the risk of occult nodal metastases. In 1977, Cabañas (Cabañas RM. An approach for the treatment of penile carcinoma. Cancer 1977;39:456). described the sentinel node technique for determining the lymphatic drainage pattern from the primary lesion to the regional nodes and identifying the node most at risk for harboring metastases. Cutaneous lymphoscintigraphy is used to demonstrate the nodal basin in either unilateral or bilateral inguinal areas, and sentinel node biopsy can be performed to adequately stage the regional nodes. Inguinal lymph node dissection has been shown to be therapeutically beneficial in patients who have histologically positive regional node metastases. There is a limited role for chemotherapy, primarily in the setting of metastatic disease. Preoperative chemotherapy and radiotherapy have not been employed as in squamous cell carcinomas of the anus or esophagus.

For Detailed Discussion: (1) Chapter 127, "Neoplasms of the Penis."

Answer 3.148. **The answer is (c).**

Patients who have invasive carcinoma of the bladder are usually first seen with hematuria alone. The work-up includes evaluation of the urinary system, including cystoscopy and abdominal pelvic CT scan. Bone scan is typically reserved for those patients with symptoms or elevated alkaline phosphatase levels. Carcinoma in situ is generally well treated with intravesical therapy using mitomycin, doxorubicin, or BCG. However, those patients who have invasive carcinoma or high-grade lesions are best treated with a radical cystectomy. In addition, those patients who have diffuse carcinoma in situ are at high risk for recurrence, and they often have occult invasive disease. Similarly, those patients who fail intravesical therapy should undergo a radical cystectomy. Partial cystectomy is infrequently used unless there is a solitary lesion and random biopsies from remote areas of the bladder are negative. Although radiotherapy alone would represent insufficient therapy for those with invasive disease, urinary reconstruction is performed by intestinal conduits or continent cutaneous diversion, such as the Indiana or Koch pouch.

For Detailed Discussion: (1) Chapter 125, "Bladder Cancer."

Answer 3.149. **The answer is (b).**

Gastric lymphomas can be well controlled with external beam radiotherapy, although chemotherapy has been advocated as the most important modality. The use of chemotherapy in gastric lymphoma could obviate the need for either surgery and/or radiotherapy in some cases. There is no role for radiotherapy with leiomyosarcomas, premalignant lesions such as adenomatous polyps, or benign conditions of the stomach such as Ménétrier's disease or benign ulcers secondary to *H. pylori infection*. Recent data suggest that patients treated for *H. pylori* may be at increased risk for subsequent gastric carcinoma. Similarly, a number of studies have examined the use of external beam radiotherapy for patients who have locally advanced gastric carcinoma, although surgical resection remains the mainstay of therapy for this disease.

For Detailed Discussion: (1) Chapter 113, "Neoplasms of the Stomach."

Answer 3.150.   **The answer is (c).**

Gastrointestinal sarcomas are unusual and represent only a small fraction of all sarcomas. The most common histologic subtype is leiomyosarcoma. Most patients are first seen with symptoms that are indistinguishable from other benign or malignant gastric disease. The operative approach is based on the tumor's size and location, and the ability to obtain negative surgical margins. Patients should undergo limited resection in order to obtain free margins, because this is the most important prognostic factor for survival. Typically, small tumors of low grade have an improved prognosis, because they are technically easier to completely resect. There is no role for adjuvant or neo-adjuvant chemotherapy or radiotherapy in treating this disease. Although most patients will eventually develop an intra-abdominal recurrence to the liver, resection of the primary disease is performed for palliation and a small chance of cure. Patients who have isolated hepatic metastases can be salvaged by complete resection of the metastases.

For Detailed Discussion: (1) Chapter 113, "Neoplasms of the Stomach."

Answer 3.151.   **The answer is (b).**

There are a number of risk factors for gastric carcinoma, but they do not include previous gastric irradiation. *H. pylori* infection has recently been shown to be an independent risk factor for malignancy, although the etiology of this association is unclear. Chronic atrophic gastritis and previous gastric operation, typically for benign ulcer disease, have been associated with development of gastric carcinoma.

For Detailed Discussion: (1) Chapter 113, "Neoplasms of the Stomach."

Answer 3.152.   **The answer is (c).**

The standard approach for distal gastric carcinoma is subtotal gastrectomy, with resection of the proximal duodenum approximately 2 to 3 cm beyond the pylorus. There are limited data regarding the use of R1 and R2 nodal dissections. More extensive nodal dissections have not been shown to be of benefit. There is no role for esophagogastrectomy or total gastrectomy, because the complications of these procedures are much higher than those of a subtotal gastrectomy, and they are unlikely to confer a survival benefit to a patient who has a distal gastric lesion.

For Detailed Discussion: (1) Chapter 113, "Neoplasms of the Stomach."

Answer 3.153. **The answer is (b).**

Breast carcinoma in men accounts for 1% of all breast malignancies. However, this disease is rare and often is detected late because most cases of gynecomastia represent benign disease. Stage for stage, men may have a somewhat worse prognosis than women; however, treatment is typically the same for both sexes. Although the presence of BRCA-1 and BRCA-2 malignant gene mutations indicates a high risk for breast malignancies, neither of these tests is useful for screening a population.

For Detailed Discussion: (1) Chapter 136, "Neoplasms of the Breast."

Answer 3.154. **The answer is (d).**

Although cystosarcoma phylloides histologically resembles benign fibroadenomas, these tumors are typically larger than the average fibroadenoma. It is often difficult to differentiate the lesions by histology alone. However, both the large size and rapid growth rate are more indicative of a cystosarcoma phylloides. They are not multicentric, multifocal, or bilateral. Like most mesenchymal tumors, they tend to metastasize first by bloodborne pathways rather than the lymphatic system. In the absence of metastases, wide local excision and, if necessary, total mastectomy, are appropriate for management of these lesions.

For Detailed Discussion: (1) Chapter 136, "Neoplasms of the Breast."

Answer 3.155. **The answer is (e).**

Although DCIS was once a rare entity, it is becoming increasingly common due to early diagnosis of cancer with mammography. The treatment of DCIS continues to be controversial, because patients may have occult invasive disease at the time of presentation. This condition is typically not bilateral. Patients who have LCIS have up to a 70% chance of bilateral disease; LCIS should be considered a marker of subsequent risk for invasive carcinoma, rather than as a malignant or premalignant lesion.

For Detailed Discussion: (1) Chapter 136, "Neoplasms of the Breast."

Answer 3.156. **The answer is (d).**

The treatment for DCIS remains controversial. Patients with small tumors and low-grade histologies, including papillary, cribriform, and solid subtypes, can typically be managed with lumpectomy alone. Patients with comedo subtypes and larger primary lesions are at higher risk for multifocal disease and likely should have lumpectomy with postoperative radiotherapy, or as an alternative, total mastectomy. Patients with large tumors greater than 4.5 cm, comedo histology, high-grade tumors, and/or those that involve the surgical margins should not be considered for lumpectomy alone or in combination with postoperative radiotherapy. These patients and those who have suspicious microcalcification after segmentectomy should be treated with mastectomy. The presence of microinvasive disease is rare, and thus axillary lymph node dissection is typically not warranted in these patients.

For Detailed Discussion: (1) Chapter 136, "Neoplasms of the Breast."

Answer 3.157. **The answer is (e).**

Although typically the size; grade; architecture (either cribriform, papillary, or comedo); and degree of differentiation of the lesion have been useful in order to determine therapy, none of these factors have been demonstrated to be independently appropriate for determining the therapeutic approach for those who have DCIS. Newer techniques include determining the presence of *HER-2neu* oncogene overexpression, which is higher in comedo than noncomedo carcinomas. DNA flow cytometry has been used for invasive carcinomas, but recently has also been used in order to determine the S-phase fraction of non-invasive lesions. Newer techniques to determine the presence of sialyl-Tn expression have shown this marker to be associated with aneuploid and high nuclear grade tumors. Although the *p53* tumor suppressor gene has been associated with breast cancer and may indeed correlate with response to chemotherapy, *p53* overexpression has not been associated with DCIS.

For Detailed Discussion: (1) Chapter 136, "Neoplasms of the Breast."

Answer 3.158. **The answer is (c).**

A patient with a 2-cm breast carcinoma may have up to a 20% chance of harboring occult regional node metastases. Postmenopausal women with positive axillary nodes should be treated with tamoxifen, although there are data that suggest that CMF chemotherapy and tamoxifen may improve outcome over tamoxifen alone. There is no role for high-dose chemotherapy in this setting, and patients who have negative axillary nodes likely gain little benefit from tamoxifen. The problem with axillary lymph node sampling is that the incidence of inaccurate staging is unknown and may lead to understaging of the disease.

For Detailed Discussion: (1) Chapter 136, "Neoplasms of the Breast."

Answer 3.159. **The answer is (c).**

Patients who have locally advanced breast carcinoma ("inflammatory breast cancer") with involvement of the subdermal lymphatics have up to a 90% chance of having nodal metastases. Although most patients subsequently die of distant metastases, local disease control is imperative. Most regimens have combined preoperative combination chemotherapy followed by resection of the primary tumor and axillary lymph node dissection followed by postoperative radiotherapy and possibly additional chemotherapy. The combination approach allows for less aggressive surgical resection and ultimately may improve local disease control. Patients who are found to have locally aggressive disease may be candidates for high-dose chemotherapy and bone marrow or stem cell transplantation if they have had an initial response to cytotoxic therapy.

For Detailed Discussion: (1) Chapter 136, "Neoplasms of the Breast."

Answer 3.160. **The answer is (c).**

Patients with ipsilateral breast recurrence who have been treated by lumpectomy alone can be salvaged with total mastectomy. These patients are particularly at high risk for developing metastatic disease and should be considered for adjuvant therapy following surgical resection of the recurrence. Radiotherapy alone is not indicated, except following resection and perhaps if the recurrence is outside the irradiated field. There is no role for the use of tamoxifen alone in this setting, although it may be useful as an adjuvant therapy after mastectomy.

For Detailed Discussion: (1) Chapter 136, "Neoplasms of the Breast."

Answer 3.161. **The answer is (c).**

Retroperitoneal sarcomas constitute approximately 15% of all soft-tissue sarcomas. Most patients are first seen with an abdominal mass and nonspecific symptoms. These tumors are typically liposarcomas and less commonly leiomyosarcomas or fibrosarcomas. The differential diagnosis includes lymphomas or metastatic testicular carcinomas in men. Once the diagnosis is made, it is important to determine the potential for curative resection. Complete surgical resection is the primary treatment for retroperitoneal sarcomas; complete resection correlates with overall disease-free survival and long-term outcome. Although soft-tissue sarcomas of the extremities respond to chemotherapy and radiotherapy, the toxicity of treatment in the abdominal cavity is significant, and there are no data to support using this combination modality during initial treatment.

For Detailed Discussion: (1) Chapter 140, "Soft Tissue Sarcomas."

Answer 3.162. **The answer is (d).**

Patients who have retroperitoneal sarcomas should be followed up on a routine basis with CT scan of the abdomen. Some patients with locally recurrent disease will be salvaged with reresection. The benefit of repeat operation in patients with no symptoms is controversial. There is no role for chemotherapy or radiotherapy alone in this setting. Recent studies suggest there may benefit to intraoperative radiotherapy and postoperative external beam treatment, but the data are inconclusive.

For Detailed Discussion: (1) Chapter 140, "Soft Tissue Sarcomas."

Answer 3.163. **The answer is (c).**

Cystic neoplasms of the pancreas are a diverse group of lesions, including microcystic adenomas, mucinocystic neoplasms, intraductal mucin hypersecreting neoplasms, and solid and papillary retention cysts. Patients typically are first seen with abdominal fullness, and often CT scan findings are indistinguishable from a pancreatic pseudocyst. Biopsy is necessary to confirm the diagnosis of these lesions. Microcystic adenomas and mucinous neoplasms occur more commonly in women than in men, whereas solid and papillary epithelial neoplasms occur more commonly in young women. The cystic neuroendocrine tumors include gastrinomas, pancreatic polypeptide–producing tumors, glucagonomas, and insulinomas. All of these tumors are best treated by resection, because prognosis is typically much better than the more common adenocarcinoma of the pancreas. There are scant data to support the use of 5-fluorouracil chemotherapy and external beam radiotherapy in this setting. A patient who has advanced disease including hepatic metastases may be considered for chemotherapy and external beam radiotherapy as opposed to surgical resection.

For Detailed Discussion: (1) Chapter 119, "Neoplasms of the Exocrine Pancreas."

Answer 3.164.   The answer is (c).

Post-splenectomy sepsis is highest among patients who have their spleen removed for thalassemia or other reticuloendothelial system diseases such as Hodgkin's disease. The risk of overwhelming infection is lower in patients who have a splenectomy for trauma, ITP, or hereditary spherocytosis. Typically, infections caused by encapsulated bacteria such as *Streptococcus pneumoniae, Neisseria meningitidis,* or *Haemophilus influenzae* account for approximately 75% of cases. Patients who undergo splenectomy for staging should be vaccinated before splenectomy, in order to reduce the risk of overwhelming infection.

For Detailed Discussion: (1) Chapter 149, "Hodgkin's Disease."

Answer 3.165.   The answer is (c).

Age is an adverse factor with respect to cancer prognosis for many specific neoplasms. The incidence of cancer may be bimodal, as with ALL, where there are two distinct peaks, one at 4 to 7 years of age, and the other in persons over 50. The cure rate for pediatric patients with ALL is 60 to 80%. Although drug tolerance is somewhat better in younger patients, the most important reason for relatively poor results in older patients is tumor cell biologic differences. For example, hyperdiploidy, which correlates with a favorable prognosis, is more common in lymphoblasts obtained from children than adults. Conversely, balanced translocations, which are poor prognostic indicators, are more common in adults.

For Detailed Discussion: (1) Chapter 145, "Acute Lymphocytic Leukemia in Adults." (2) Chapter 164, "Acute Lymphocytic Leukemia in Children."

Answer 3.166.   The answer is (c).

Balanced chromosomal translocations that lead to novel proteins are frequently associated with neoplasia, particularly in patients who have hematologic neoplasms. In ALL, these translocations occur more commonly in adults and are associated with an adverse prognosis. *p53* mutations occur at a high frequency in patients with common adult epithelial tumors and in some AML patients. *p53* protects normal cells from damage by cycle arrest, which allows for repair of DNA damage and triggers chemotherapy-induced apoptosis in tumor cells. Thus, poorly responsive tumors commonly have *p53* deletion or inactivating mutations, whereas highly responsive tumors such as the pediatric cancers tend to have normal *p53*. Expression of the multidrug resistant gene is more common in patients who have secondary AML (after prior myelodysplasia or chemotherapy) and in untreated adults with AML. The marrow of an older patient with AML typically displays minor degrees of trilineage dysplasia, which implies derivation from a myelodysplastic syndrome and thus suggesting origin in a more resistant proximal hematopoietic cell.

For Detailed Discussion: (1) Chapter 142, "Acute Myeloid Leukemia in Adults." (2) Chapter 145, "Acute Lymphocytic Leukemia in Adults." (3) Chapter 164, "Acute Lymphocytic Leukemia in Children."

Answer 3.167. **The answer is (d).**

Non-Hodgkin's lymphoma, in contrast to Hodgkin's disease, is increasing in incidence, in part due to AIDS and transplantation-related immunosuppression. Patient age influences the pathology and stage of Hodgkin's disease. In persons over 40 or younger than 16, lymphocyte-predominant histology is more common. Hodgkin's disease has two age peaks that occur in the developed countries. In the developed countries, the younger age peak is predominant.

For Detailed Discussion: (1) Chapter 149, "Hodgkin's Disease."

Answer 3.168. **The answer is (e).**

Lymphocyte-predominant Hodgkin's disease is most commonly seen in males under 15 or over 40 years of age. This subtype is often localized to a single lymph node. Patients with mixed cellularity more often have systemic symptoms and more often have advanced stage disease. Nodular sclerosing Hodgkin's disease makes up 70% of patients in economically developed countries, but is less common in developed countries. The presence of granulomatous lesions in lymph nodes increases the likelihood of coexistent Hodgkin's disease, and may have favorable prognostic implications.

For Detailed Discussion: (1) Chapter 149, "Hodgkin's Disease."

Answer 3.169. **The answer is (c).**

EBV may play a causal role in the development of Hodgkin's disease. There is an excess incidence of Hodgkin's disease in individuals who have previously had infectious mononucleosis. Various techniques have been used to find EBV genome fragments in Reed-Sternberg cells of 30 to 50% of patients, especially those with mixed cellularity histology. The absence of an effective lymphocyte (polyclonal) response histologically may indicate a particularly immunosuppressed state and is predictive of a poor outcome. The lymphocyte-predominant variant with the distinctive lymphocytic and histiocyte Reed-Sternberg variants is negative for LEU-M1 (CD15), a marker that is typically expressed in the classic Reed-Sternberg cells of the mixed cellularity and nodular sclerosing subtypes. The Reed-Sternberg cell is clonal and may represent the true neoplastic cell. Patients who have the lymphocyte-depleted variant, which accounts for less than 5% of cases in developed countries, are usually seen with advanced disease.

For Detailed Discussion: (1) Chapter 149, "Hodgkin's Disease."

Answer 3.170. **The answer is (c).**

RS cells in patients with mixed cellularity or nodular sclerosing Hodgkin's disease express CD15 in contrast to RS cells from patients with the lymphocyte-predominant subtype. CD15 (My1) reacts with normal granulocytes as well. Ki-1, also known as

CD30, is commonly present on RS cells but is also expressed by activated B and T cells and large-cell anaplastic lymphoma. Other B-cell activation antigens such as the IL-2 receptor and HLA-DR may be expressed on RS cells. Antigen receptor gene rearrangement occurs, but rarely. The t(14;18) is characteristic of follicular, small cleaved cell B-cell lymphomas and is unusual in Hodgkin's disease. Transforming growth factor, produced by Reed-Sternberg cells, may stimulate the fibroblastic reaction seen in the nodular sclerosing subtype.

For Detailed Discussion: (1) Chapter 149, "Hodgkin's Disease."

Answer 3.171. **The answer is (e).**

The immune deficit in patients with Hodgkin's disease is present at the time of diagnosis and presumably precedes disease onset. Even in patients who achieve long-term remission with radiotherapy or chemotherapy, cellular immunologic deficits persist for years. Herpes zoster appears most commonly within the first year. Pneumococcal conjugated vaccines may be given following splenectomy, but ideally should be given preceding splenectomy to optimize response.

For Detailed Discussion: (1) Chapter 149, "Hodgkin's Disease."

Answer 3.172. **The answer is (e).**

The anatomic spread of Hodgkin's disease tends to involve central rather than peripheral lymph nodes. Hodgkin's disease in the early stages tends to spread by continuity to adjacent lymph nodes. In stage IV patients, however, there is evidence for hematogenous spread. Relapse at pretreatment sites of tumor after complete remission with chemotherapy is highly likely in Hodgkin's disease and substantially less likely in non-Hodgkin's lymphoma. With liver involvement, the spleen is almost always involved (but the reverse is not correct).

For Detailed Discussion: (1) Chapter 149, "Hodgkin's Disease."

Answer 3.173. **The answer is (d).**

Patients who relapse after combination chemotherapy, whether it be MOPP or ABVD, have a much lower response to treatment with the original combination. ABVD is superior to MOPP in that infertility and secondary tumors are much less common. The superiority of ABVD over MOPP is probably intrinsic, although in comparative studies downward dose modification with MOPP occurs more commonly than with ABVD. So-called hybrid regimens derived from the components of MOPP and ABVD, or MOPP–ABVD alternating regimens, are not superior to ABVD in terms of overall survival.

For Detailed Discussion: (1) Chapter 149, "Hodgkin's Disease." (2) Canellos G, et al. Chemotherapy of advanced Hodgkin's disease with MOPP, ABVD, or MOPP alternating with ABVD. NEJM 1992;327:1478.

Answer 3.174. **The answer is (e).**

Poutrier's abscesses consist of clusters of tumor cells in the epidermis. They occur relatively early in the disease and are not related to ulceration or infection. The most prominent area of infiltration of tumor cells is in the epidermis (not the dermis). Pruritis and erythematous lesions that wax and wane are early prominent manifestations of mycosis fungoides. The neoplastic cell in mycosis fungoides is the CD4 helper cell, which also loses antigens ordinarily expressed on T cells. Molecular biology studies, particularly those involving T-cell receptor rearrangements, are often relatively constant, which suggests clonality.

For Detailed Discussion: (1) Chapter 151, "Mycosis Fungoides and the Sézary Syndrome."

Answer 3.175. **The answer is (d).**

Topical corticosteroids are active against early lesions but tend to produce brief and incomplete responses. UVC (short wavelength UV) penetrates poorly. UVB alone is appropriate for most lesions, with UVA added (long wavelength, deep penetration) for deep-seated lesions. Electron beam therapy to the entire cutaneous surface is possible. This modality is highly effective in producing durable complete responses (50–90%, depending on the extent of the tumor). A randomized study of combination chemotherapy plus electron beam therapy produced higher and more durable complete remission rates than does standard therapy but no improvement in survival.

For Detailed Discussion: (1) Chapter 151, "Mycosis Fungoides and the Sézary Syndrome." (2) Kaye F, et al. A randomized trial comparing combination electron-beam radiotherapy in the initial treatment of mycosis fungoides. NEJM 1989;321:1784.

Answer 3.176. **The answer is (e).**

Topical nitrogen mustard applied repetitively to the skin is effective in mycosis fungoides, but its mechanism of effectiveness would appear to be mediated by immune mechanisms such as interaction with the epidermal Langerhans cell. Systemic absorption of nitrogen mustard apparently does not occur, and systemic toxicity, such as myelosuppression, is not observed. Interferon has substantial activity in mycosis fungoides, producing a 30% CR rate. Systemic 13 *cis*-retinoic acid is equally active. Circulating mycosis fungoides cells are responsible for the erythroderma of the Sézary syndrome. These cells have molecular and immunologic profiles similar to the tumor in the skin. The Sézary syndrome can be treated with extracorporeal photopheresis. The patient is given a photoactivating drug; the white blood cells are collected (leukapheresis), UVA-treated, and then returned to the patient. The therapy is well tolerated.

For Detailed Discussion: (1) Chapter 151, "Mycosis Fungoides and the Sézary Syndrome."

Answer 3.177. **The answer is (e).**

The patient has a squamous cell carcinoma of both vocal cords, which is not fixed. As such, it is a T1b lesion. The likelihood of a clinically positive lymph node is ≤2% at the time of presentation and 10% overall. The standard approach for a patient with this type of early-stage lesion is external beam radiotherapy. Chemotherapy is not required; excision is appropriate only for lesions limited to the midportion of the cord. With radiotherapy, voice quality is well preserved in more than 90% of patients. For

T1 lesions, approximately 6600 cGy will be delivered to a field extending from the thyroid notch to the bottom of the cricoid cartilage.

For Detailed Discussion: (1) Chapter 105, "Head and Neck Cancer."

Answer 3.178.   The answer is (c).

Smoking-related diseases exact an additional toll beyond their normal primary neoplasm from ex-smokers. Carcinoma of the lower airways is often more dangerous than the original primary lesion. Radiation-induced sarcomas are rare. Second aerodigestive malignancies occur at an annual rate of approximately 3%. Retinoids may be able to decrease this risk.

For Detailed Discussion: (1) Chapter 105, "Head and Neck Cancer."

Answer 3.179.   The answer is (d).

For completely excised low-grade parotid tumors, there is no known benefit to the addition of adjuvant radiotherapy and/or chemotherapy. MRI assessment of the parotids could provide useful baseline data, but is not considered part of standard management. Close clinical follow-up is called for.

For Detailed Discussion: (1) Chapter 105, "Head and Neck Cancer."

Answer 3.180.   The answer is (c).

Age is a risk factor for the development of prostate cancer, but this man is only 49, well under the mean age of onset. Diseases of the prostate such as benign prostatic hypertrophy, chronic prostatitis, or acute prostatitis due to sexually transmitted organisms are not predisposing factors. However, the incidence of prostate cancer is higher in African Americans compared with white men of similar age.

For Detailed Discussion: (1) Chapter 126, "Neoplasms of the Prostate."

Answer 3.181.   The answer is (e).

Most prostate cancers display a moderate degree of differentiation (Gleason grades 4–7). Poorly differentiated tumors (Gleason grades 8–10) are less common, but carry a poor prognosis. Cancers tend to occur in the peripheral zone, and are therefore not evenly distributed throughout the gland. Prostate cancer is rare, but not unheard of, before age 45. Intra-epithelial neoplasia is a precursor lesion.

For Detailed Discussion: (1) Chapter 126, "Neoplasms of the Prostate."

Answer 3.182.   The answer is (c).

If pelvic nodes are involved, radical prostatectomy is generally contraindicated. Noninvasive staging procedures are neither sensitive nor specific. Therefore, if the information is critical, laparoscopic-guided node biopsy is advisable (as opposed to the unnecessary aggressive laparotomy approach). A skeletal survey or bone marrow examination is not as sensitive as a bone scan for the detection of metastatic disease. A bone scan could be done preoperatively, but is likely to be negative given the low PSA level (unless the Gleason grade is high).

For Detailed Discussion: (1) Chapter 126, "Neoplasms of the Prostate."

Answer 3.183. **The answer is (e).**

Growth hormone secreting pituitary adenomas typically produce the acromegaly syndrome characterized by progressive enlargement of the hands, feet, and face. Metabolic effects of excess growth hormone production include hyperglycemia. Growth hormone releasing tumors tend to occur in middle-aged men. When the presentation is classic, as in this case, the diagnosis is straightforward. Those patients with serum growth hormone levels greater than 10 ng/mL usually have active disease. Magnetic resonance imaging is useful to find the location of the tumor. Transsphenoidal surgery is the treatment of choice, with the restoration of normal growth hormone levels occurring in approximately 80% of patients. Complications include anterior pituitary hypofunction, cerebrospinal fluid leak, and meningitis (each below 5% in likelihood). Medical therapy with long-acting somatostatin analogues such as octreotide may reduce symptoms and decrease growth hormone levels, but would not be appropriate for primary therapy. Radiotherapy may be beneficial and is an alternative to surgery, but is associated with a significant failure rate.

For Detailed Discussion: (1) Chapter 99, "Pituitary Neoplasms."

Answer 3.184. **The answer is (a).**

The rare patient with ovarian cancer who is first seen with a low-grade lesion limited to one ovary is highly likely (>90%) to be cured by surgery alone. There may be a role for combination chemotherapy in certain limited-stage patients who are at higher risk for recurrence. There has been no documented benefit for adjuvant radiotherapy approaches.

For Detailed Discussion: (1) Chapter 133, "Ovarian Cancer."

Answer 3.185. **The answer is (d).**

Computed tomography, although helpful, is not a definitive staging procedure for ovarian cancer. Marrow harvest to obtain a "rescue" for high-dose chemotherapy is relevant only for those refractory or relapsed patients who are enrolled in a relevant investigational trial. Paracentesis may be helpful diagnostically and for palliation, but is not an appropriate antineoplastic approach. Chemotherapy without laparoscopy is relevant only for stage IV patients.

For Detailed Discussion: (1) Chapter 133, "Ovarian Cancer."

Answer 3.186. **The answer is (d).**

Screening strategies such as measurements of CA-125 or detection of ovarian masses by TVUS are not known to (and probably would not be effective in) detecting and/or preventing ovarian cancer. There are no data to support a low-fat diet or exercise as preventative strategies. Combined estrogen-progestagen contraceptive pills have decreased the frequency of ovarian cancer, presumably by suppression of ovulation.

For Detailed Discussion: (1) Chapter 133, "Ovarian Cancer."

Answer 3.187. **The answer is (b).**

If the polyps were known to be benign, the patient would be unlikely to have a colonic neoplasm within 17 months. On the other hand, if the polyps were malignant or premalignant, the current symptoms could be secondary to a frank carcinoma, which is best ruled out by a colonoscopy. The history of travel to the tropics may not be relevant in a patient with known pre-existent colon pathology. A barium enema would be less discriminating than colonoscopy for detecting inflammatory mucosal lesions. Even the presence of ova or parasites would not exclude the possibility that the original polypoid lesion had been a carcinoma, now regrown. Inflammatory bowel disease or amebic ulcers could be recognized at colonoscopy, as could neoplastic lesions. There are scant data to recommend gastroscopy in the absence of upper gastrointestinal symptoms.

For Detailed Discussion: (1) Chapter 121, "Adenocarcinoma of the Colon and Rectum."

Answer 3.188.   The answer is (c).

The metastatic cascade follows an orderly sequence of at least five steps to establish a metastatic site. The metastatic phenotype must proliferate at the primary site, gain access to the circulatory system, bind to the proposed distant organ microvasculature, traverse the extracellular matrix, and proliferate as a metastatic parenchymal focus. Only a minority of dispersed malignant cells are able to complete all of these steps.

For Detailed Discussion Chapter: Chapter 111, "Metastatic Tumors in the Thorax."

Answer 3.189.   The answer is (a).

Long (>40 days) tumor doubling times are associated with a 63% rate of 5-year survival following resection and reflect a long disease-free interval. Patients with uncontrolled primary tumors or disseminated disease obtain no survival benefit from pulmonary resection. Fewer than four metastatic nodules are associated with a higher 5-year survival than four or more lesions, although the absolute number of metastases is not necessarily a contraindication if these metastatic foci have a long doubling time.

For Detailed Discussion: (1) Chapter 111, "Metastatic Tumors in the Thorax."

Answer 3.190.   The answer is (d).

The choice of surgical approach to pulmonary resection depends on the surgeon's discretion. Full thoracic exploration is performed before resection to include all pleural surfaces and the mediastinum. Extension of disease to the chest wall or major vascular or bronchial structures is not a contraindication to more extensive resection, with a 25% 5-year survival rate reported by Putnam in 1993.

For Detailed Discussion: (1) Chapter 111, "Metastatic Tumors in the Thorax." (2) Putnam JB Jr, et al. Extended resection of pulmonary metastases: is the risk justified? Ann Thorac Surg 1993; 55:1440.

Answer 3.191.   The answer is (b).

Regardless of the apparent stability of a large extremity mass, adequate histologic study of a biopsy specimen is indicated. Generally, frozen section examination is required to confirm that the specimen is representative of the lesion and adequate for diagnosis. Excisional biopsy is not indicated for this large lesion, but could be used for small tumors less than 3 cm in size. Longitudinal biopsy incision is preferred for extremity lesions due to easy incorporation into subsequent definitive surgical incisions. Fine-needle aspiration is useful in the hands of an experienced pathologist for diagnosis of malignant tumors and sarcomas.

For Detailed Discussion: (1) Chapter 140, "Soft Tissue Sarcoma."

Answer 3.192. The answer is (c).

There is no ideal or universally accepted classification system for soft-tissue sarcomas. Problems that arise in distinguishing cell origin include changes induced by metaplasia, several different cell types within the same tumor, and the degree of dedifferentiation. These problems can make histogenetic identification extremely difficult. The current AICC clinicopathologic staging system depends on the tumor size, lymph node status, evidence of distant metastasis, and histopathologic grade (TNMG). The most important prognostic factors for the majority of sarcomas are histopathologic grade and tumor size.

For Detailed Discussion: (1) Chapter 140, "Soft Tissue Sarcoma."

Answer 3.193. The answer is (b).

Brachytherapy is directed radiotherapy after surgery via deposition of radioactive materials through catheters placed at the time of surgery. This modality's use is particularly beneficial for high-grade sarcomas, improving local control from 65 to 90%. However, brachytherapy has no significant impact on low-grade tumors. Adjuvant chemotherapy has an important role in treating bone sarcomas, but has not been of conclusive benefit for soft-tissue sarcomas. In recent years, the use of limb sparing surgery has become accepted practice. Even for larger lesions (>5 cm), preoperative external beam radiotherapy can make a more limited surgical approach feasible.

For Detailed Discussion: (1) Chapter 140, "Soft Tissue Sarcomas."

Answer 3.194. The answer is (b).

Desmoid tumor or musculoaponeurotic fibromatosis is notorious for local recurrence. The principal treatment for this tumor is wide excision. Brachytherapy is generally not indicated because this is a low-grade malignant neoplasm. Like other soft-tissue sarcomas, MFH carries a prognosis that is dependent on size and grade of the primary lesion. Although rhabdomyosarcoma is chemoresponsive, complete tumor eradication can rarely be achieved. Even in the typical elderly (non–HIV-infected) patient with classic Kaposi's sarcoma, secondary malignancies do occur with higher-than-expected frequency.

For Detailed Discussion: (1) Chapter 140, "Soft Tissue Sarcomas."

Answer 3.195. The answer is (a).

Above the age of 1 and below the age of 10, prognosis in acute lymphoblatic leukemia is considered favorable. Ploidy, initial white blood cell count, and karyotypic changes can all add additional prognostic features. The prolonged period of symptoms without abnormalities in this patient's blood count cannot be considered a compromise of standards of good care. Concurrent testicular disease is not the only reason that males do slightly less well than females. In the absence of a complex translocation, which has an extremely poor prognosis, allogeneic transplantation in the first remission of ALL is not recommended. Intrathecal methotrexate is not given daily as prophylaxis; rather, weekly administration of intrathecal methotrexate is the norm.

For Detailed Discussion: (1) Chapter 164, "Acute Lymphocytic Leukemia in Children."

Answer 3.196. **The answer is (c).**

This boy has several features that imply a short survival: a Philadelphia chromosome, hyperleukocytosis, and age 11. Although the latter two prognostic features would not be enough, the Philadelphia chromosome, taken together with the hyperleukocytosis and age, predict extremely low curability with conventional therapy. Prophylactic testicular irradiation is no longer appropriate, because high-dose methotrexate with leucovorin rescue can prevent testicular disease. Five-year treatment is too long, even if chemotherapy was the proper choice for this boy.

For Detailed Discussion: (1) Chapter 164, "Acute Lymphocytic Leukemia in Children."

Answer 3.197. **The answer is (c).**

Recent data from the Cancer and Leukemia Group B (CALGB) demonstrate that, for patients who are younger than 60, high-dose cytarabine given after induction can double the likelihood of disease-free status compared with standard intensification. Immunotherapy has no established place in treating acute myeloid leukemia, nor does maintenance therapy. The best arm of the CALGB study employed four cycles of high-dose cytarabine ($3.0 \ g/m^2/3$ h on Days 1, 3, and 5).

For Detailed Discussion: (1) Chapter 142, "Acute Myeloid Leukemia in Adults." (2) Mayer RJ, et al. Intensive post-remission chemotherapy in adults with acute myeloid leukemia. N Engl J Med 1994;331:896.

Answer 3.198. **The answer is (c).**

Certain karyotypes have more favorable prognoses with improved, long-term, disease-free survival—genetic alterations such as translocations t(8;21), t(15;17), and an abnormal 16q22. In contrast, all other karyotypic abnormalities impart adverse prognoses. For those individuals with AML who appear to have a normal diploid karyotype, the prognoses lie somewhere in between. Although there is rough correlation of the karyotypic abnormality with morphology, it is not absolute. Karyotype outweighs age in defining leukemic prognosis. Bone marrow transplantation is not persuasively superior in first remission, and the results are significantly influenced by karyotype.

For Detailed Discussion: (1) Chapter 142, "Acute Myeloid Leukemia in Adults."

Answer 3.199. **The answer is (a).**

An isolated low-grade papillary lesion confined to the epithelium is considered to be carcinoma in situ. Urine cytology is frequently positive. Although papillary lesions are frequently widespread, because this lesion is singular, completely resectable, and low grade, no additional treatment is required. Repeat urinalysis for cytologic examination and annual cystoscopy for 5 years are prudent.

For Detailed Discussion: (1) Chapter 125, "Bladder Cancer."

Answer 3.200. **The answer is (c).**

When a patient with muscle invasive high-grade carcinoma has failed several local treatments, cystectomy is required. There are no data that convincingly demonstrate equivalence of radiotherapy for this situation; neoadjuvant chemotherapy is an attractive option based on certain, but not all, randomized studies. Cystectomy is the established choice.

For Detailed Discussion: (1) Chapter 125, "Bladder Cancer."

Answer 3.201. **The answer is (b).**

Tobacco smoking is a risk factor for bladder carcinoma, and may well have been present in this patient. A 2-cm pulmonary lesion might well be a lung cancer curable with surgery, as well as a single metastatic bladder lesion. This man should be treated like any other patient who has a solitary coin-shaped lesion in the lung, which at 2 cm requires resection for diagnosis and therapy.

For Detailed Discussion: (1) Chapter 125, "Bladder Cancer."

Answer 3.202. **The answer is (c).**

In an ultimately fatal disease, it is imperative that the diagnosis be unambiguous. Three kinds of Ph-negative chronic myeloid leukemias exist: specious negatives, in which a triple complex chromosomal rearrangement has occurred that involves chromosome 9, another chromosome, and chromosome 22, such that 22 does not appear smaller than normal; Ph-negative morphology, where nonetheless the bcr-abl rearrangement has occurred; and the rare true Ph-negative disease that by definition is not typical chronic myeloid leukemia. Awaiting determination of the BCR-ABL rearrangement will be of importance in prognosis and choice of therapy.

For Detailed Discussion: (1) Chapter 143, "Chronic Myeloid Leukemia."

Answer 3.203. **The answer is (e).**

Marrow fibrosis with islands of granulocytic and megakaryocytic hyperplasia are not inconsistent with any of the diagnoses offered. The modest number of promyelocytes and myeloblasts do not qualify for blastic transformation of CML. Splenomegaly is uncommon in the myelodysplastic syndrome. The neutrophilic granulocytosis and preserved platelet count would be unusual for myelodysplastic syndrome as is the absence of monocytes seen in chronic monocytic leukemia. Metastatic carcinoma to the bone marrow would also need consideration. Myelodysplastic syndrome is the least likely of the choices, although it would be unusual for essential thrombocytosis to exhibit splenomegaly and a left-shifted differential. Fibrosis should be absent in essential thrombocytosis.

For Detailed Discussion: (1) Chapter 143, "Chronic Myeloid Leukemia."

Answer 3.204. **The answer is (e).**

Gestational trophoblastic tumor is extremely vascular and cannot be locally excised or eradicated by curettage. Occult pulmonary metastases are present in a substantial number of patients. Combination chemotherapy may produce menopause, as may cisplatin. There are no long-term data for Taxol. Single-agent methotrexate or actinomycin D produce remission in 93% of patients, with salvage of all remaining patients by hysterectomy or combination chemotherapy.

For Detailed Discussion: (1) Chapter 134, "Gestational Trophoblastic Neoplasia."

Answer 3.205. **The answer is (b).**

Although there is a higher risk of subsequent molar pregnancy (1:150 compared with 0.6–1.1:1000 pregnancies), there is no increase in spontaneous abortions, tubal pregnancies, or congenital anomalies. A patient cured of gestational trophoblastic tumor may anticipate a normal pregnancy.

For Detailed Discussion: (1) Chapter 134, "Gestational Trophoblastic Neoplasia."

Answer 3.206. **The answer is (b).**

Ameloblastoma is an epithelial odontogenic tumor that partially recapitulates the early enamel organ. It is a slow-growing, radiolucent lesion noted in young adults. This tumor is locally invasive and has a great tendency to recur if incompletely removed. The resection margin should be 2 cm, if possible. Radiotherapy has no role, curettage is inadequate, and chemotherapy is untested. The tumor is nonmetastasizing, but in the absence of effective surgery, might recur.

For Detailed Discussion: (1) Chapter 106, "Odontogenic Tumors."

Answer 3.207. **The answer is (b).**

In a minority of patients flutamide can serve as a growth stimulant, presumably because of a mutated androgen receptor that is present in the regrown population. Short remissions occur with removal of flutamide. There is no basis for castration after a response to leuprolide.

For Detailed Discussion: (1) Chapter 126, "Neoplasms of the Prostate."

Answer 3.208. **The answer is (e).**

Although small-cell carcinoma can evolve out of adenocarcinoma of the prostate, prostatic biopsy should not be undertaken until small-cell carcinoma of the lung is excluded. The presence of increased bronchovascular markings on a chest radiograph might well have been due to pulmonary edema and congestive heart failure, but might preclude easy recognition of a neoplasm that has small-cell pathology. If positive results from a CT scan of the lung were noted, bronchoscopic biopsy would be relevant. In the presence of negative results from a CT scan, prostatic biopsy would be appropriate, even if the prostate were not appreciably enlarged. Other sites of origin of small-cell carcinoma must also be considered. Elevation of the prostate specific antigen level could be not be relied on to indicate prostatic origin of the small-cell carcinoma. PSA staining of the node would be useful if the results were positive, but would not exclude prostatic origin if the results were negative. For Detailed Discussion: (1) Chapter 126, "Neoplasms of the Prostate."

Answer 3.209. **The answer is (d).**

There is no established role for high-dose chemotherapy in treating metastatic prostate cancer. Although IV morphine may be necessary in his final weeks, the patient can potentially have months to years of comfortable life after ^{89}Sr radioisotope therapy. His pain is too widespread to anticipate response from external beam radiotherapy. Pamidronate has not been described as benefitting osteoblastic metastasis.

For Detailed Discussion: (1) Chapter 126, "Neoplasms of the Prostate." (2) Porter AT, et al. Results of a randomized phase III trial to evaluate the efficacy of strontium 89 and external beam irradiation in the management of endocrine resistant metastatic prostate cancer. In J Radiat Oncol Biol Phys 1993;25:805.

Answer 3.210. **The answer is (c).**

Radical prostatectomy is popular and produces long-term, disease-free status for T1 and T2 tumors. In contrast to radiotherapy, surgery is most frequently used for younger men, although rigorous comparative data are not available. A policy of watchful waiting may be appropriate and is being evualated in randomized trials. Testosterone administration would not be safe in the presence of possible micrometastases.

For Detailed Discussion: (1) Chapter 126, "Neoplasms of the Prostate."

Answer 3.211. **The answer is (c).**

The description best fits serous adenocarcinoma of the peritoneal surface, which closely resembles ovarian carcinoma in its pathogenesis and management. The absence of a pancreatic mass on CT scan, a CEA level of 6, and a CA-125 level of 350 lend no credence to the need for ERCP. Maximal cytoreduction before chemotherapy improves the outcome of chemotherapy for ovarian cancer. Although paclitaxel and cisplatin are the chemotherapy regimen of choice, they are best applied after cytoreduction. A reassessment of the ovaries in the pathology laboratory is also in order, no matter how long before the ovaries were removed.

For Detailed Discussion: (1) Chapter 156, "Neoplasms of Unknown Primary Site." (2) Strand CM, et al. Peritoneal Carcinothetosis of Unknown Primary Site in Women. Ann Intern Med 1989;111:213.

Answer 3.212. **The answer is (b).**

The presentation is that of a midline germ cell tumor. After meticulous palpation of his testes excluded a primary site there, the risks of therapy without a histologic diagnosis versus the hazards of surgery come into question. An intercostal incision parasternally, (Chamberlain procedure) should be able to retrieve a tumor specimen without causing pneumothorax or hemorrhage, although tracheal intubation is a minor concern. A needle biopsy may not give a representative sample, and might lacerate a distended vein. Immediate treatment after diagnosis with cisplatin, etoposide, and bleomycin should elicit maximal benefit. CHOP is not the chemotherapy of choice, and radiotherapy is not equal to BEP.

For Detailed Discussion: (1) Chapter 110, "Primary Germ Cell Tumors of the Thorax."

Answer 3.213.   **The answer is (c).**

The "anaplastic neoplasm" and nodal enlargement pattern are suggestive of lymphoma, although metastatic carcinoma or metastatic melanoma are the classic differential diagnoses, and a negative cytokeratin result is a strong point against the carcinoma; also, a negative S-100 protein result is a strong point against melanoma. The positive leukocyte common antigen indicates a hematopoietic cell. Expression of epithelial membrane antigen, although characteristic of carcinomas, can also occur in lymphomas. Vimentin, too, can sometimes be a positive finding in lymphomas. Chromogranin, which is a positive finding in neuroendocrine carcinomas, was negative in this patient. Electron microscopy of the axillary node will not be necessary. The chemotherapy of choice for lymphoma is the CHOP regimen.

For Detailed Discussion: (1) Chapter 156, "Neoplasms of Unknown Primary Site."

Answer 3.214.   **The answer is (c).**

Although the patient will need preoperative assessment of risk factors and malnutritional status, most surgeons would obtain further information concerning resectability before preceding with this case. Repeat upper endoscopy with attempt at biopsy should also be considered. Radiotherapy is rarely of use in the preoperative treatment of small bowel tumors. A Whipple procedure may not be indicated in this situation, especially if the tumor is benign.

For Detailed Discussion: (1) Chapter 120, "Neoplasms of the Small Intestine, Vermiform Appendix, and Peritoneum."

Answer 3.215.   **The answer is (b).**

Most small bowel obstructions are benign, and even if they are malignant, the operation (which should include resection of mesentery and lymph nodes) would be the same. Reducing the intussusception would only prolong the procedure, because a bowel resection would certainly follow. Leaving an obstructing lesion and potentially compromised bowel is not an option.

For Detailed Discussion: (1) Chapter 120, "Neoplasms of the Small Intestine, Vermiform Appendix, and Peritoneum."

Answer 3.216.   **The answer is (c).**

Appendiceal carinoids of greater than a centimeter in diameter should be treated with right hemicolectomy. Metastatic disease should be searched for and resected, if possible. The treatment of carcinoid, even if metastatic, is surgical, so debulking should be attempted

For Detailed Discussion: (1) Chapter 120, "Neoplasms of the Small Intestine, Vermiform Appendix, and Peritoneum."

Answer 3.217. **The answer is (e).**

No one treatment for metastatic carcinoid is uniformly successful. Multimodality therapy offers the best chance of palliation. Both chemotherapy and surgical ligation or intra-arterial hepatic chemotherapy are effective treatments, but intraperitoneal chemotherapy has not been shown to be effective.

For Detailed Discussion: (1) Chapter 120, "Neoplasms of the Small Intestine, Vermiform Appendix, and Peritoneum."

Answer 3.218. **The answer is (a).**

In the face of asymptomatic low-grade non-Hodgkin's lymphoma, with no other evidence of rapid progression, bulky symptomatic masses, cytopenias, or B-cell symptoms, close monitoring of the path of this patient's disease is the best option. There is no evidence to support CHOP or fludarabine as initial therapy over single alkylating agents. At the present time, high-dose therapy should be reserved for protocol investigations.

For Detailed Discussion: (1) Chapter 150, "Non-Hodgkin's Lymphomas."

Answer 3.219. **The answer is (e).**

The most appropriate choice is high-dose therapy if the disease remains sensitive to re-induction therapy. The use of CHOP alone or radiotherapy is only palliative. A subset of patients (<20%) who respond to re-induction therapy, which is administered for a total of six cycles, may be long-term survivors without autologous transplantation.

For Detailed Discussion: (1) Chapter 150, "Non-Hodgkin's Lymphomas." (2) Freedman AS, et al. Autologous bone marrow transplantation in B-cell non-Hodgkin's lymphoma; very low treatment-related mortality in 100 patients in sensitive relapse. J Clin Oncol 1990;8:1.

Answer 3.220. **The answer is (b).**

Splenomegaly, leukocytosis, leukocyte alkaline phosphatase, and increased red blood cell masses are common to both polycythemia vera and secondary polycythemia. It is true that splenomegaly would be relatively unusual in secondary erythrocytosis. Erythropoietin levels are not elevated in polycythemia vera, which represents an autonomous proliferation of the red blood cells, whereas secondary polyoythemia occurs in renal or hepatic diseases that cause erythrocytosis.

For Detailed Discussion: (1) Chapter 154, "Polycythemia Vera and Essential Thrombocythemia."

Answer 3.221. **The answer is (b).**

Repeated phlebotomy leads to a significant excess of thrombotic episodes in the elderly, which are not controlled by aspirin and dipyridamole. Hydroxyurea may safely decrease the risk. Chlorambucil and ^{32}P are clearly leukemogenic in patients with polycythemia vera who also have a higher-than-background rate of conversion to AML.

For Detailed Discussion: (1) Chapter 154, "Polycythemia Vera and Essential Thrombocythemia."

Answer 3.222. The answer is (e).

Expensive work-ups based on a high marker level should not be undertaken unless the laboratory value is confirmed. The Day-20 level may still represent disappearance of a high preoperative level. If the level returned to normal, no further search would be necessary, although baseline status of liver and lungs is useful information. There is no clear role for chemotherapy in the postoperative setting other than for treating Dukes B or C colon cancer; in this instance, the patient had metastatic disease.

For Detailed Discussion: (1) Chapter 121, "Adenocarcinoma of the Colon and Rectum." (2) Moertel CG, et al. An evaluation of the carcinoembryonic antigen (CEA) test for monitoring patients with resected colon cancer. JAMA 1993;270:943.

Answer 3.223. The answer is (a).

Delay in diagnosis in order to undertake a therapeutic trial is unacceptable when other means are available that could lead to definitive diagnosis and therapy. Response to antituberculosis medicine could be quite slow. A change in anti–HIV medications may be helpful in any event and may result in an improvement in the pulmonary disease, especially if it is caused by Kaposi's sarcoma.

For Detailed Discussion: (1) Chapter 155, "Neoplasms in Acquired Immunodeficiency Syndrome."

Answer 3.224. The answer is (b).

Kaposi's sarcoma has a distinctive epidemiology within the group of all HIV–infected patients. This neoplasm is rare in IV drug users, women, or those acquiring the infection through blood products. There may well be an independent virus responsible for Kaposi's transmission. Kaposi's has occurred in several homosexual men who were HIV–negative.

For Detailed Discussion: (1) Chapter 155, "Neoplasms in Acquired Immunodeficiency Syndrome."

NS-3 - 4106.

(Box in)

Box5- 25+

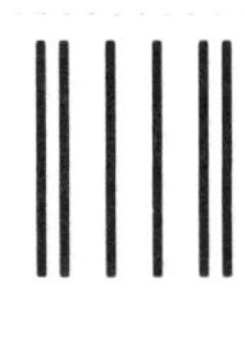

| |||| |

BUSINESS REPLY MAIL

FIRST CLASS   PERMIT NO. 724   BALTIMORE, MD

POSTAGE WILL BE PAID BY ADDRESSEE

Williams & Wilkins
P.O. Box 1496
Baltimore, Maryland 21298-9656